ALSO BY IRA RUTKOW

Seeking the Cure: A History of Medicine in America

James A. Garfield

Bleeding Blue and Gray: Civil War Surgery and the Evolution of American Medicine

Surgery: An Illustrated History

American Surgery: An Illustrated History

The History of Surgery in the United States 1775–1900: Volume II, Periodicals & Pamphlets

The History of Surgery in the United States, 1775–1900: Volume I, Textbooks, Monographs & Treatises

EMPIRE
OF THE
SCALPEL

THE HISTORY OF SURGERY

Ira Rutkow

SCRIBNER

New York   London   Toronto   Sydney   New Delhi

Scribner
An Imprint of Simon & Schuster, Inc.
1230 Avenue of the Americas
New York, NY 10020

First Scribner hardcover edition March 2022

SCRIBNER and design are registered trademarks of The Gale Group, Inc., used under license by Simon & Schuster, Inc., the publisher of this work.

For information about special discounts for bulk purchases, please contact Simon & Schuster Special Sales at 1-866-506-1949 or business@simonandschuster.com.

The Simon & Schuster Speakers Bureau can bring authors to your live event. For more information or to book an event, contact the Simon & Schuster Speakers Bureau at 1-866-248-3049 or visit our website at www.simonspeakers.com.

Interior design by Wendy Blum

Manufactured in the United States of America

1   3   5   7   9   10   8   6   4   2

Library of Congress Cataloging-in-Publication Data

Names: Rutkow, Ira M., author.
Title: Empire of the scalpel : the history of surgery / Ira Rutkow.
Description: First edition. | New York : Scribner, 2022. | Includes
bibliographical references and index.
Identifiers: LCCN 2021048634 (print) | LCCN 2021048635 (ebook) |
ISBN 9781501163746 (hardcover) | ISBN 9781501163760 (ebook)
Subjects: LCSH: Surgery—History.
Classification: LCC RD19 .L33 2022 (print) | LCC RD19 (ebook) |
DDC 617—dc23/eng/20211104
LC record available at https://lccn.loc.gov/2021048634
LC ebook record available at https://lccn.loc.gov/2021048635

ISBN 978-1-5011-6374-6
ISBN 978-1-5011-6376-0 (ebook)

For Alex and Benjamin, two A²G²s.
May your futures be filled with happiness, health, love, and success

CONTENTS

CONTENTS

AUTHOR'S NOTE

Why is the amphitheater crowded to the roof, by adepts as well as students, on the occasion of some great operation, while the silent working of some well-directed drug excites comparatively little comment? Mark the hushed breath, the fearful intensity of silence, when the blade pierces the tissues, and the blood of the unhappy sufferer wells up to the surface. Animal sense is always fascinated by the presence of animal suffering.

Henry J. Bigelow, *An Introductory Lecture*, delivered at the
Massachusetts Medical College, 1849

Surgeons must be very careful
When they take the knife!
Underneath their fine incisions
Stirs the Culprit, — Life!

Emily Dickinson, *Poems*, 2nd series, 1891

This book is about the history of surgery and examines the relationship between my profession and society. The clearest indication of modern surgery's impact on our lives is the reasonable certainty that virtually no one in the industrialized world will escape having an illness for which effective treatment requires a surgical operation. This extraordinary fact is supported by a recent World Health Organization report that estimates the global number of surgical procedures at hundreds of millions per year; in America alone, tens of millions are performed annually.[1] Indeed, a case can be made that many aspects of modern surgery, such as breast augmentations, cataract removals, gender reassignment operations, heart transplants, hip and knee replacements, and procedures for obesity, have become mainstream cultural benchmarks. That few of us pause to think about the magnitude of these statistics, that we have such inherent faith in this mystifying branch of the medical world, is nothing short of remarkable.

There is no denying that the rise of surgery and confidence in its practitioners is among the most profound of changes that separate current existence from past eras. Yet, despite the debates, the headlines, and the table talk that surround surgical operations, most of us have no idea how surgeons arrived where they are or of the ins and outs of what they do. None of this is surprising, because surgery's inner sanctum is closely guarded. After all, surgery began as a quasi-religious, supernatural craft, as intriguingly admired as it was singularly feared (it still is in many cultures); there are not many events in life that are as simultaneously life frightening and lifesaving as a surgical procedure.

Few would disagree that surgery is concealed from the world by its jargon and rituals. For instance, to simply enter an operating room necessitates an act of supplication to the surgical gods. Surgeons must first put on a cap and mask to separate themselves from the outside world. If the patient is to be closely approached, then an anointing wash of antiseptic soap and cleansing water followed by the sliding on of sterile rubber gloves and the donning of a germ-free gown (the surgeon's priestly robe?) are required to further isolate and purify the encounter. Nonphysicians seeking entry into this mysterious realm and its secrecies are usually met by locked doors.

Empire of the Scalpel addresses this glaring silence and tells surgery's story; from its subjective Stone Age origins to its objective roots in the classical world of Europe and finally its rise to scientific and social supremacy in the United States. No other approach captures the growth of surgery in all its dramatic and gory complexity. I devote attention to European surgery because its evolution, from Greek and Roman Antiquity to the rise of barber-surgeons in the Middle Ages, followed by the emergence of centers of surgical excellence in England and France during the seventeenth and eighteenth centuries, and concluding with Germany's predominance at the end of the nineteenth and beginning of the twentieth centuries, developed in ways that served as the wellspring of modern surgery.

European surgery's dominance arose from the technical expertise of its practitioners, the credibility of their professional organizations, and the perception that surgical therapies worked well. Its status as the international leader in surgery ended with the First World War. The conflict destroyed much of the Continent—if not its physical features, then a large measure of its finances and passion for scholarly and scientific pursuits. The result was a global vacuum in surgical education, research, training, and therapeutics. It was only natural for surgeons from the United States, the industrialized nation least affected physically and psychologically by the war, to fill the void.

Over the last century, the rise of surgery is intimately bound up with the United States' development as an international leader in cultural, political, socioeconomic, and scientific affairs. I have little doubt that the world would not have surgery as it presently exists, with its triumphs, tragedies, and contradictions, without modern America and, quite possibly, vice versa. Moreover, given that I was born and live and work in the United States, it only seems natural that my history of surgery reflects an American tilt. None of this is to suggest that each nation in the world does not have its own fascinating, unique, and worthy surgical story to tell. The reality is that what began as the surgery of Europe and became the surgery of America was transformed into the surgery of the globe.

I focus on "Western" Medicine because its relationship to surgical illnesses evolved in ways that made it successful and worldwide in appeal. "Eastern" Medicine, exemplified by Indian practices, enjoyed numerous surgical achievements, especially plastic and reconstructive procedures, including development of a renowned method to reconstruct the noses of individuals who suffered a traumatic injury. However, these successes did not markedly sway the overall organizational, scientific, and technologic developments of Western surgery that became the global norm. Surgery in China did not flourish due to Confucian tenets that concerned the sacredness of the human body along with restrictions against human anatomical studies. As late as the nineteenth century, human anatomy was still being taught by means of diagrams and artificial models rather than cadaver dissection. Japanese aversion toward the performance of surgical operations surpassed that of the Chinese. Once the religious stigmas attached to caring for the bleeding, the wounded, and the dying were overcome, Japanese surgeons were able to develop their craft. However, as in China, this progress occurred much later than in Western civilization.

Condensing surgery's story into a single, accessible volume is a challenge. Surgeons are detail oriented. You want your surgeon to be somewhat obsessive-compulsive. Orderliness and perfectionism are necessary because a steadfast attention to specifics can spell the difference between surgical success and surgical failure. Similarly, *Empire of the Scalpel* must pay close attention to a myriad of facts and, at the same time, be reasonably concise. In no way is this book the complete story of surgery; it is not a tell-all account of every well-known knife bearer of the past. A balancing act is called for.

On one hand, the history of surgery is a series of awe-inspiring discrete triumphs. These include the unanticipated discovery of anesthesia in 1846 and, a century later, the Nobel Prize–winning, seemingly impossible feat of transplanting a kidney. Many of the singular breakthroughs are worthy of their own books, tales of men and women standing on an intellectual and technologic precipice as they conquer the surgical unknown. On the other hand, surgical advances often move in slow, almost imperceptible steps. The rise of the profession as a recognized specialty and the growth of organized surgery with its accompanying societal concerns of credentialing, education, and licensing took centuries to achieve. Neither of the accounts—the distinct or the gradual, the scientific or the socioeconomic—is complete without the other. They must be grafted together to convey the complexity, genius, and vibrancy of surgery's development.

Similarly, two overarching and linked themes, both reflective of basic human nature, are also central to surgery's story. The first is antipathy toward a contemporary and/or rival, noted by the conflicts between the public and physicians, physicians and surgeons, and surgeons and surgeons (these types of disagreements date back to Antiquity and continue through the present). The second theme is an inclination to dismiss scientific or technical advances that contradict deeply held, often-erroneous views. Whether caused by economic concerns, ego gratification, social disparities, or other competing interests, these disputes and jealousies impacted the evolution of surgery in ways that cannot be disregarded.

An additional admonition concerns the fact that the history of surgery has been largely dominated by white men. There is no disputing that, as far back as the Middle Ages, there were women who had a role in providing surgical services for their households or the poor. However, with the growth of the male-dominated Catholic Church in the sixteenth century and their care of the sick, females were forced aside and discouraged from performing any form of surgical therapy. Even with the beginnings of modern surgical training at the start of the twentieth century, the road for female surgeons remained difficult. Nevertheless, the opening of the Woman's Medical College of Pennsylvania and the London School of Medicine for Women provided fresh opportunities in surgery. Yet, despite the increasing presence of female surgeons, few held positions of authority or leadership or exerted any semblance of control over the governance of surgery until the mid-1970s.

Empire of the Scalpel is meant to be a comprehensive and revelatory history, one that is educational and entertaining and showcases the development of the profession within the rich tapestry of human life in which it evolved. As a popular narration, it is intended for a wide audience, laypersons and physicians alike—since surgical terminology can act as a barrier to the uninformed, this book is as free of the surgeon's tongue as possible. Its words inform readers as to what scalpel wielders have accomplished, individually and collectively, the impact of their thoughts and actions, and why my profession should be regarded as a scientific marvel and societal juggernaut.

Plainly stated, *Empire of the Scalpel* aims to change the way people think about surgery by helping them understand its character while exposing its conduct. I say this with the firm conviction that surgery has played a major and, certainly in the Western world, expanding role in human society, one that will, figuratively and literally, shape future generations. For this reason, the many interfaces between surgery and other spheres of human endeavor need to be examined to reveal how cultural and socioeconomic conditions have influenced surgery and vice versa; events in literature and theater, music and the visual arts, sports and recreation, and philosophy and religion are important adjuncts to this narrative. The interweaving of such nonsurgical historical facts with the main body of information imparts a greater sense of timeliness to the writing.

To the extent that my own experiences and perspectives shape the narrative, I offer the following. I have devoted my adult life to Medicine,* as both a surgeon and a historian. I believe that my understanding of the subject (the combination of a surgeon's skills and a historian's scholarship) has given me unique insights to tell surgery's story. When trained historians deal with this material, albeit skillfully, their perspective is necessarily limited by their "outsider status" and not having toiled in surgery's vineyards. Conversely, I remain in awe of the expertise of scholars who have studied the many epochs and subjects covered in this book. Their historical insights and writings aided me in synthesizing surgery's tale since I freely admit to not having in-depth knowledge of more than a few eras and themes.

---

* Throughout *Empire of the Scalpel*, I use "Medicine" to signify the totality of the profession and "medicine" to indicate internal medicine as differentiated from neurology, obstetrics, pediatrics, radiology, surgery, et cetera.

Lastly, I confess to being an inveterate storyteller; more precisely, a "surgical raconteur." History provides an explanation for past behaviors and my approach is to let those who have died speak for themselves—the living will not be found in these pages. I am neither a critic, moralist, philosopher, nor soothsayer. Similar to one of my boyhood heroes, Sergeant Joe Friday on the 1950s and 1960s TV series *Dragnet* and his signature businesslike catchphrase, I am interested in "just the facts." I am a sleuth, a surgical private eye. I enjoy relating anecdotes about my profession and the individuals who have populated it, their whys and wherefores, their sense of self, and, most important, their decencies and deficiencies.

Empire of the Scalpel is the result of five decades of learning and listening and attempts to show how every surgeon, knowingly or unknowingly, reflects a testimony to their profession's past. In addition, I hope this book is meaningful and relevant to the lay reader, even more so to those about to confront a surgeon and his or her scalpel. Most importantly, my research and writing has furthered my optimism about the future of surgery and the enduring bond between surgeons and patients. The essential quality of this relationship is an abiding interest in mankind, and all that it entails in caring for another human being.

PRELUDE

As no man can say who it was that first invented the use of clothes and houses against the inclemency of the weather, so also can no investigator point out the origin of Medicine—mysterious as the sources of the Nile.

Thomas Sydenham, *Medical Observations*, 1676

If there were no past, science would be a myth; the human mind a desert. Evil would preponderate over good, and darkness would overspread the face of the moral and scientific world.

Samuel D. Gross, *Louisville Review*, 1856

On the evening of July 4, 1975, John Quigley, a forty-three-year-old salesman from Southie, a working-class Irish community in Boston, was out on the town with his wife, Maureen. They were celebrating John's recent promotion and had driven toward the city's Esplanade, where they joined the crowd of 170,000 who watched Arthur Fiedler conduct the Boston Pops on America's "birthday." It was a balmy fun-filled evening of fireworks, Frisbees, music, picnics, and swaying bodies. Afterwards, the Quigleys were driving home when their car was hit by a drunk driver. Although their injuries seemed minor, the Quigleys were taken by ambulance to nearby Boston City Hospital.

An urban emergency room on a Friday night, especially at the beginning of a holiday weekend, can be a gritty and hectic place. Doctors and nurses scramble about while the flashing lights, the bloodstained bandages, the stretchers askew, and the half-eaten pizzas lay bare the chaotic atmosphere. Life and death hang in the balance as the staff determine which individuals might die if care is not immediately given versus those who can wait with less threatening situations. For the Quigleys, this meant an hour or so of passing the time before they would be fully evaluated. In a bare, curtain-enclosed side cubicle, John quietly lay on a stretcher. Maureen sat beside him. Together, they listened to the sounds of Medicine at work.

Around midnight, a doctor poked his head in and told the Quigleys he was there to examine them. "I'm fine," Maureen said. "I feel okay." Physicians are taught to observe, to listen, and to pay attention to words and actions. In Maureen's case, the doctor agreed with his patient. Other than her being upset by the ordeal, Maureen's examination was unremarkable.

John's situation was different. The ambulance driver mentioned that when John was first seen he was out of sorts—"groggy" was the description—and may have suffered a brief loss of consciousness. John's version of the events was not the same. "It wasn't much of an accident," he related, "just us getting bounced around. Nothing bad. Maureen was okay, but I hit my head and cut my scalp. Before I knew it, an ambulance was there." On the ride to the hospital the attendant said that John regained his senses and joined in the conversation.

John's vital signs, his blood pressure, breathing, pulse, and temperature, were all normal. The doctor examined his ears, eyes, and neck, listened to his heart and lungs, felt his abdomen, and flexed his extremities. John's hearing, seeing, smelling, tasting, and touching were unremarkable. The same was true of the neurological evaluation that tested his brain, the spinal cord, and the nerves that arose from these areas. The doctor assessed John's mental status and found that he spoke clearly and knew where he was as well as the date and time. John's balance was fine; he easily stood up and walked up and down the corridor without assistance. Nothing was out of the ordinary. "Other than a little headache, I'll be okay," John said.

Everything about John appeared normal except for a nasty-looking 2.5-inch gash on the right side of his scalp. Dried blood matted John's hair and the tissue surrounding the laceration was swollen and tender. The doctor parted the wound to see whether he could feel an underlying skull fracture. The bony surface was smooth with no evidence of breaks, roughness, or splintering. To complete the evaluation, the ER physician ordered routine blood tests, an electrocardiogram, a urinalysis, and X-rays of John's chest and head—computerized axial tomography (CAT) or magnetic resonance imaging (MRI) scans were not yet available. As a matter of precaution, John was admitted to the hospital's neurology service for an overnight observational stay. While he waited to be transferred to a room, the neurosurgical service was asked to send someone to repair his scalp.

*   *   *

I was twenty-six years old, eight weeks out of medical school, on my third night of call duty on Harvard's fabled neurosurgical service, and about to meet the Quigleys. BCH, as Boston City Hospital was commonly referred to (it is presently part of the Boston Medical Center), is one of the most storied institutions in America's medical past, a valued national resource that counts among its own a who's who of American Medicine. From Nobel Prize winners to medical and public health school deans to celebrities who sought treatment, BCH's impact on health care has been outsized. I felt privileged when I matched for a general surgical residency there. It was my first choice and Beth, my wife of three years, and I were excited about the move from St. Louis, where I had attended medical school, to Boston with its business, cultural, and educational opportunities. There was one overriding flaw in our naïve enthusiasm: the surgical resident's on-call schedule. I was about to become an intern (in present-day jargon I was a "PGY-1," in my first postgraduate year from medical school or a first-year surgical resident) and did not appreciate the mental and physical rigors of a general surgical training program.*

Some context is necessary to understand these difficulties.

Surgical training is strenuous. My on-call schedule was an unrelenting every other night, a grind that would continue for five years. What did that entail? When I reported to the hospital on Monday morning, there was a full day of patient and operating room obligations ahead of me. That night, I was on call and responsible

---

* The first two years of a general surgical residency are focused on the development of basic skills in general surgery and other surgical specialties, including cardiothoracic surgery, ear, nose, and throat surgery, emergency and trauma surgery, neurosurgery, orthopedic surgery, pediatric surgery, plastic surgery, and urologic surgery. During the final three years of a general surgical training program, further experience is obtained in general, colorectal, critical care, endocrine, oncologic, transplant, and trauma surgery. Upon completion of a general surgical training program, individuals are eligible to take a series of examinations given by the American Board of Surgery and become board-certified in surgery. Once certification is achieved, they are then eligible for additional certification offered by the American Board of Surgery in the subspecialties of: Hand Surgery; Hospice and Palliative Medicine; Surgical Critical Care; Pediatric Surgery; Surgical Oncology; and Vascular Surgery.

for admitting new patients and responding to emergencies. Whether I slept was a matter of serendipity. Tuesday was another twelve to fourteen hours of tedious work on the wards, clinics, and assisting at operations. That evening, no longer on call, I was home but usually not before 7:00 pm. Back in our apartment, my fatigue was all-consuming and my sleep was deep. Wednesday and Thursday were a repeat of Monday and Tuesday. Friday was a full workday but not an on-call night. The weekend was daunting. It began with early morning rounds on Saturday, typically at 6:30, and continued through Monday evening. By Monday night, I had been in the hospital, with little guarantee of sleep, for over sixty hours. The coming week I had full workdays Monday through Friday and was on call Tuesday night, Thursday and Friday nights, and off on Saturday and Sunday.

The hallowed tradition of every other night surgical training stretched back to the nineteenth century. Over the years, the more prestigious the surgical residency, the stronger the belief in an all-consuming approach to training. At BCH, the two-week cycle of every other night call with its 135-hour workweek was considered essential for the continuity of care afforded patients and the quality of education provided to residents. Indeed, the mantra voiced by many surgeons-to-be lamented that the singular problem with an every other night surgical training program was they missed half the cases. The sad reality was that such an on-call schedule was unsafe: unsafe for the patient and unsafe for the resident.

Starting in the late 1990s, due to an increasing number of reports of clinical errors believed to have arisen from overworked and sleep-deprived house staff, regulations were put in place to limit the number of hours any individual in a graduate medical training program in the United States (i.e., internships, residencies, and fellowships) could be in a hospital. Among the new national standards, the workweek was capped at eighty hours and overnight call of no more than once every three nights and less than twenty-four hours consecutively. The ogre that was every other night surgical training programs had mercifully ended.

* * *

At around one thirty in the morning, the *beep-beep-beep* of my pager went off. I was on one of BCH's large multi-bed surgical wards talking to the charge nurse. For an intern, the nursing staff (at the time it was mostly female) was a source of professional knowledge and motherly advice. They had practical experience in caring for patients. It mattered little whether the discussion concerned clinical questions or personal affairs; nurses helped untested surgical house officers get through their days and nights. I told Nancy (she wasn't much older than me) that I was needed downstairs in the ER to tend to someone with a head injury. She pointedly said, "Make sure he doesn't have a blown pupil." I had been on the neurosurgical service for only four days and had a limited understanding of what a "blown pupil" meant. However, as I walked down a back stairway, I paused on a landing to look over my pocket-sized book on neurosurgical emergencies.

When I finally met the Quigleys, shortly before 2:00 am, John had just returned from the X-ray suite. His studies were normal with no suggestion of a skull fracture. I introduced myself and explained that I would stitch his head wound. There was the usual grilling that interns face. "You look so young!" "Do you know what you're doing?" "How many of these have you done?" Even though these were my first days as a surgical house officer, I had received a fair amount of experience with scalp lacerations as a medical student. John appeared anxious and Maureen noted that he didn't seem totally back to his normal self.

In my reading about blown pupils, one fact stood out: *the lucid interval*. The chapter stressed that with bleeding on the brain from a blow to the head, despite being initially knocked unconscious, some patients go on to have a temporary improvement lasting several hours, a so-called lucid interval (the time it takes for a collection of blood to increase in size before it causes symptoms), after which their condition rapidly deteriorates. The lucid interval is a time bomb that can easily fool the unsuspecting. I made sure to closely examine John's pupils. Everything appeared normal, so I went about gathering the material I needed to sew his scalp laceration.

John's wound was jagged and not simple to repair. I shaved the hair surrounding the wound, injected his scalp with an anesthetic, and placed green sterile cloths over his head. I couldn't see John's face, but I could talk to him. I had been working for a half hour and thought all was well when John mentioned that his headache was getting worse. "Give me a few more minutes," I said. "Let me finish the last two stitches and we'll be done." "Okay," was his reply.

Several minutes later the drapes came off and I was staring at a patient who was going downhill rapidly. John's speech was garbled and he seemed drowsy. I snatched my flashlight and shined it in his eyes. I couldn't believe what I saw. John's right pupil was lifeless. It was blown. I was terrified, not only because John was near death's doorstep, but I feared that I had missed the earlier signs. What about his increasing headache? What about Maureen saying her husband didn't seem right? What about the time that I kept John under the drapes, away from direct vision? I panicked and needed help.

I ran to the front desk and told the ER's attending doctor what I found. He dropped everything, followed me back to the cubicle, and confirmed what I already knew. "We need to get him to the operating room, immediately," shouted the physician. "Call your chief resident and get him in here."

I explained what was going on to Maureen. She was scared. I was more scared.

*   *   *

John's brain had suffered an insult and the injury would try to kill him. Like all humans, John's brain was cushioned in a soothing pool of cerebrospinal fluid and enveloped by the dura mater, a thick fibrous membrane that lies, lightly attached, to the inside surface of the skull. These multiple layers of protection are necessary because the brain is soft and fragile—only slightly more substantial than tofu in consistency—and susceptible to damage, especially from blows to the head. When John was jostled during the accident, he not only cut his scalp; his brain was shaken and twisted inside its liquid bed also. The split-second back-and-forth motion pushed it against the unyielding barrier of John's skull. Like a rubber ball when it is squeezed and let go, his brain had been momentarily deformed and then returned to its normal shape, then distorted and bounced back again until the rebounding stopped.

In everyday language, John had experienced a concussion. As his brain compressed, recoiled, and rotated, various pathological and physiological events took place. Clusters of John's neurons—the brain consists of roughly 100 billion of these cells—were torn asunder. Waves of electrical brain impulses, representing his conscious state, were abruptly discharged. The torrent of electric activity overwhelmed anything John was experiencing. Anxiety, bewilderment, pain, and pleasure were erased by the massive outpouring of electrical activity. Like a boxer on the receiving end of a stunning punch, John was knocked unconscious. His brain stem, the part of the brain that is structurally continuous with the spinal cord, continued to maintain its life-regulating control of blood pressure, breathing, and heart rate. It would take several minutes for John's brain and its overburdened neurons to reboot and his grogginess to abate before he regained his wits and could engage in meaningful activity and conversation.

But it was not just John's brain's electrical activity that went awry; there was also the issue of torn blood vessels. The human brain is heavily traversed by these vascular conduits, which carry the nourishment necessary for its intense activity. They receive almost 15 percent of the heart's entire output. Among the more important vessels is the middle meningeal artery, which nourishes the dura mater. The artery runs in a groove on the inside of the skull, near the temple. The bone of the cranium is relatively thin in this spot and a vicious blow to the head can shear the vessel off its attachments. Arteries are under higher blood pressure than veins, and bleeding from a torn middle meningeal artery will be sizeable. This is where Nancy's warning about a blown pupil turned relevant.

When the middle meningeal artery bleeds, an expanding collection of blood, called a hematoma, accumulates in the space between the brain and the skull. Such a hematoma is a nasty foe, one that silently and slowly morphs into a fiendish killer— Robert Atkins, the diet doctor, Gary Coleman, the actor, and Natasha Richardson, the actress, died from such an untreated surgical emergency. As the accumulation of blood enlarges it causes the brain and the brain stem to shift position. They are pushed downward, their structures are squeezed, and life hangs in the balance.

Once the brain stem is tightly jammed, the heartbeat becomes irregular, breathing slows down, and speech becomes slurred. The patient complains of dizziness, double vision, headache, and coma looms. For a physician, the most telling and ominous sign of brain stem injury is dilation of the pupil on the side of the head injury. The nerve that controls pupillary response runs along the brain stem. When the brain stem is squeezed, this oculomotor nerve is rendered nonfunctional and the pupil no longer responds to light. The powerless pupil is large and round or, in medical parlance, fixed and dilated. The pupil is considered "blown" and, suddenly, the most urgent of all surgical emergencies confronts the doctor. Their patient will die unless the skull is immediately opened, the blood clot removed, and the bleeding stopped.

* * *

In the operating room, everything was underway. The anesthesiologists were monitoring John's vital signs. Fortunately, his heart rate and breathing were holding steady. The nurses had the instrument trays and gowns and gloves laid out. The chief neurosurgical resident arrived. Minutes later, the attending neurosurgeon walked through the door. He was an august, nationally known Harvard professor, tall, thin, gray haired, and scholarly. There was little chitchat between them while they scrubbed. I was shunted off to the side until the attending asked who I was. Once the chief resident explained the situation and my involvement, I was told to join them at the operating table.

The action went into high gear. Betadine, an orange-brown antiseptic solution, was applied. The stitches that I had earnestly placed just minutes before were unceremoniously removed. Scalpel in hand, the surgeons extended John's laceration. This larger opening was to ease their entry into his skull. A trephination or circular drill was called for. I watched in awe as the chief resident bore down on John's head to create a nickel-size opening, a "burr hole." The tool produced a powerful whirring noise. Barely visible plumes of pulverized skull escaped, accompanied by the smell of burnt bone and blood. Few words or glances were exchanged: "retract . . . drill . . . suction . . . retract . . . drill . . . suction." The circular drill bit penetrated as deep as the bone, stopping short of the dura. Everything happened fast and methodically. "We're there," said the professor.

The bulging dura came into view. The chief resident took a scalpel and split its membranous fibers. Immediately a gelatinous maroon-colored blood clot oozed out of its confines. With a bit more suctioning, we were looking at the surface of John's brain. Inspection showed no more active bleeding. Through it all, John's vital signs remained steady, harbingers of a good outcome. Calmness settled over the operating room as the attending surgeon stood back from the table and told the chief resident to finish up. In John's case, the small button of removed skull was not replaced. Instead, a small plastic tube was inserted through the hole to help drain any residual hematoma. His scalp was closed around the tube to support it. Over time, the bony edges of John's burr hole would regenerate new growth, thus decreasing the size of his defect. In other types of operations on the skull involving a larger piece of removed bone, the segment is often placed back and secured with metal mesh, wire, or screws. Once repositioned, the bone will heal naturally, although the screws and wire can sometimes be felt under the scalp but are not painful.

When the professor took off his gown and gloves, he asked to speak with me, privately. Terrified by what I viewed as my errors in judgment, I was certain I was about to be severely admonished, if not dismissed outright from the program. The professor ushered me into a side lounge. "I know you're tired," he said. "Probably even a little scared. Internship, staying up all night, and dealing with an intracranial bleed are not fun." I was too anxious to respond. He looked at me, shook his head, and smiled. "You saved John's life. If it wasn't for what you did, the guy might not be alive."

I felt relieved, and more than relieved, I was reassured. The professor asked if I understood the historical significance of what I had just seen. I was uncertain what he meant. Obviously, a life had been saved and I'd gained invaluable clinical experience. But I remained puzzled by the question. He told me that he was a student of surgical history and thought it important for surgeons to understand their profession's past. The Harvard don then explained that a trephination was the earliest operation known to mankind and how, thousands of years ago, cavemen chiseled holes into the skulls of other cavemen for spiritual reasons, probably to release evil forces. By this time, it was almost four in the morning. As the professor left, he turned to me. "Keep in mind," he said, "your experiences are tied to the experiences of all the surgeons that have gone before." The elegance and simplicity of his observation would define and guide my career.

* * *

Boston City Hospital, with its numerous multistory redbrick buildings, many constructed during the closing years of the nineteenth century, is a testament to the grandeur of American Medicine's past. Each structure had a well-earned name; there were twenty-six in all, including the Sears Pavilion, the Peabody Pavilion, the Marie Curley Pavilion for Children, the Thorndike Memorial Laboratory, the Dr. John J. Dowling Surgical Building, and the Mallory Laboratory. Whether I wandered through the rabbit warren–like maze of underground tunnels that connected one building with the next or took an aboveground stroll from Harrison Avenue and the white-domed administration building built in 1864 to Albany Street and the smoke-stacked power-generating plant that was overhauled in 1955, BCH was one of the nation's largest living medical museums.

Everywhere I turned, I met surgical history head on. I read about the earliest use of surgical antisepsis in America in 1867 at BCH. I was regaled by a surgeon with firsthand knowledge of a young Cassius Clay who, three days before the defense of his world heavyweight boxing crown against Sonny Liston in November 1964, was admitted to BCH for an emergency hernia repair. The bout was delayed six months. A big thrill came in April 1977 (I was preparing to leave Boston and transfer to the famed Johns Hopkins Hospital in Baltimore) when John J. Byrne, one of BCH's retired chiefs of surgery, presented me with an inscribed copy of a book he had authored on the history of the institution. "To Ira Rutkow," he wrote, "A gift to a budding career in studying medical history." Surgery's past proved a powerful voice and I wanted to hear and learn more.

Almost forty-five years later, I still can't say exactly why my curiosity was so piqued. Was it triggered by the Harvard professor's comments? Probably, at least in part. At the same time, my growing interest in surgical history served as a valued respite from the daily grind of surgical training itself. For as long as I could remember, I wanted to be a physician, largely coaxed by my mother's persistent refrain, "Look, the hands of a doctor." As far as surgery, there was the series of grandfatherly talks from my mom's father, a kosher butcher in Newark, who told me he was a "surgeon of animals," but I would be a "surgeon of people." Family opinions aside, by my junior year in medical school I was certain I wanted to be a surgeon, an individual who saved lives and made definitive and precise decisions. Yes, I sought the ego gratification and social prominence that being a surgeon afforded, along with the triumphal feeling that accompanied a successful surgical operation. But, as I would learn, I needed something to complement the purely clinical side of surgery, beyond the "guts and gore." I began to study the sources and evolution of my craft.

I had never previously demonstrated any formal interest in studying the past. I did not take history courses in college, never completed a systematic reading of history texts, and had little knowledge of how to conduct historical research or assess historical evidence. Slowly, however, I began to probe into surgery's yesteryears. Although beleaguered by the day-to-day bustle and stress of surgical training, I began to understand how my experiences were indeed part of that continuum that stretched back centuries. I recognized a fabric made up of innumerable strands, each one a captivating story filled in itself with complex personalities and celebrated accomplishments.

Bit by bit, I developed a framework, a skeleton so to speak, that allowed me to situate my story and others within surgery's long evolution. For instance, the New York Doctors Riot of 1788, when crowds, sparked by anger over human dissections, called for the hanging of surgeons (Alexander Hamilton and John Jay attempted to quell the disturbance), harked back to the sixteenth-century saga of Andreas Vesalius and his crusade to accurately describe human anatomy while trying to appease the conservative clergy who clamored to have him burned at the stake for studying corpses. My learning how to administer local anesthesia brought to mind the life of

William Halsted, the meticulous and taciturn Johns Hopkins surgeon, who, in the late nineteenth century, discovered the technique by repeatedly injecting his skin with cocaine and observing how it numbed the area. Sadly, Halsted ended up a lifelong drug addict.

As my historical studies progressed, I became acquainted with a body of literature that was surprisingly original, yet crudely eloquent in style. Reading the words of my predecessors became a research laboratory; they helped explain how individuals and their societies behave in relation to health, sickness, and surgical intervention. I came to the realization that an appreciation of history allows one to better understand the chain of influences that define his or her professional development. Linkages between the past and present do exist. They needed to be mined, brought to the surface, and exposed. A surgical lifetime later, this book relates what that journey taught me.

* * *

I was off for the holiday weekend and did not see John again until early Monday morning. When I arrived, he was sitting up in bed; a large bandage swathed the top of his head, through which peeked the drainage tube. John looked at me with a smile on his face and a ready thank-you. He said he didn't remember much but that Maureen had filled in the gaps. We spoke and discussed the entire chain of events. "I'm so glad you did what you did," he said. "And I'm so glad you're okay," I responded. BCH was awakening for the start of another workweek and I told John I had a full day and night call in front of me. "I'll see you later," I promised as I pulled the curtain back around his bed. "Leave it open," John requested. "I like the view."

PART I

BEGINNINGS

1.

GENESIS

Those about to study medicine and the younger physicians should light their torches at the fires of the ancients.

Karl von Rokitansky,
Handbuch der Pathologischen Anatomie, AD 1846

Then give place to the physician, for the Lord hath created him: let him not go from thee, for thou hast need of him. There is a time when in their hands there is good success.

Ecclesiasticus 38:12

The history of surgery begins not with Mesopotamian cuneiform script or Egyptian hieroglyphic writing, nor with Greek and Latin words, but with holes, holes in ancient human skulls that tell extraordinary tales of pain and suffering and healing and recovery. The skulls are found throughout the globe, many dating back ten thousand years, to a time when Stone Age humans roamed the earth. The startling thing is that these holes were man-made. Of the numerous achievements that make up surgery's story, perhaps none is more astonishing than the realization that cavemen practiced neurosurgery, successfully.

In 1865, a physician with an interest in medical archeology was exploring a megalithic tomb in the Massif Central region of southern France, when he made a fascinating discovery. There, in the mountainous countryside, lying half-exposed, alongside one of the grave's vertical stone supports, was a human skull that was missing a large section of its cranium. Finding ancient bones among the ruins was not unusual, but something about this noggin seemed off. Despite the hole in his head, there was no evidence that this individual had sustained a violent death-wielding blow—no jagged splinters of bone protruding from a viciously punched-out hole were anywhere to be seen. Instead, deep and precise grooves, and other curvilinear indentations, suggested that the missing piece had been somehow purposely detached, as if removed by hand. The mystery deepened when the doctor noticed that a segment of the hole's edge was smoothed over with a polished sheen. He had never come across anything like this and speculated that the skull was used as a drinking cup, perhaps in religious or spiritual ceremonies. Over time, suggested the physician, the bone edges had been worn smooth by the lips and teeth of the multitude who drank from it.

The doctor showed the skull to several of his colleagues who had more expertise in bone pathology. One pointed out that the shiny area was actually new bone growth, the result of an effort by the skull to heal and seal itself. More importantly, explained the specialist, bones that make up the skull develop slowly and cease growing once an individual dies. This was no Neolithic chalice meant to soothe those who imbibed an ancient elixir. Instead, whoever this Stone Age human was, he had survived for several years following the intentional removal of a large portion of his skull.

The finding was met with amazement and doubt. At a time when surgeons were first beginning to understand the complexities and dangers of modern neurosurgery, it did not seem possible that a Stone Age caveman could have undergone a successful neurosurgical operation. Yet a growing number of similar prehistoric trephined skulls, found in other parts of the world, soon corroborated this theory.

The medical communities were abuzz with the news. The most renowned physicians and surgeons of the day voiced their opinions as to what the skull revealed. How did Stone Age humans, thousands of years prior to the discovery of anesthesia and antisepsis, successfully perform such complicated surgery? A number of methods were suggested, all of which, undoubtedly, required the most stoic of patients and the most brazen of "surgeons." First, the patient had to have his or her hair and skin scraped away before the Stone Age equivalent of a modern knife bearer started to bore into the skull. The simplest and crudest technique would have been to scratch a hole in the cranium, using a sharpened rock or shell. Or perhaps the surgeon had furrowed or scored the skull in a tic-tac-toe intersecting pattern with a sharpened flint stone, thus freeing the segment of center bone. If these practices were not harrowing and painful enough, a crude hammer and chisel could have been used to fashion a series of small holes that were then connected by grooves, allowing the loosened middle section to be lifted out.

One thing is certain: despite the crudeness of the procedure and lack of pain relief and cleanliness, having part of one's skull cut away, thousands of years ago, did not necessarily condemn an individual to death. The critical question is why: Why would a prehistoric man have a hole created in his head and what motives guided the hand of a Neolithic surgeon? Was there a therapeutic basis or religious and spiritual reasons? Was the operation meant to benefit the patient in this life or the one that followed? And who was responsible for performing such surgical procedures? What was his or her psychological makeup?

Much that is written about the ancient skulls is pure conjecture. There are no eyewitness accounts of a prehistoric trephination. Despite all the suppositions, one thing is fairly certain: religion and spirituality went hand in hand with actual therapy in prehistoric times. After all, the idea that evil life forces can exist in one's head is an ancient superstition. In primitive times, a hole created in the skull could have been perceived as an escape route for magical and sinister spirits. The weak and infirm might have submitted to trephination as a way to relieve disabilities thought to reside in the head; in present-day terms, treatment for convulsions, epileptic fits, mental illness, migraines, or other neurological maladies.

Trephination for solely magical or spiritual reasons is certainly antiscientific. However, it appears that, distinct from those whose craniums were opened for mystical purposes, some seriously injured individuals were truly aided by the Stone Age surgeon's use of trephination. Numerous ancient skulls show evidence of burr holes created as treatment for traumatic head injuries. Coma, the major consequence of an acutely fractured skull, could have been reversed by removal of pushed-in bone fragments and wounded brain tissue. For the Neolithic surgeon, to bring the near dead back to life would have been a commanding show of competence and power.

Everything has a beginning, a birth from which its story emerges. For surgery, prehistoric surgeons and their trephinations represent the naissance, the Big Bang of its evolutionary tree. And, much like our ancestors' DNA determines who we are as human beings, vestiges of the caveman's surgical essence—his authority, his derring-do, his psyche, and his skills—course through every modern surgeon's body.

* * *

In room 3 of the Richelieu wing, on the ground floor of the Louvre Museum in Paris, stands one of the most revered objects in all of surgery: a seven-and-a-half-foot-tall black basalt stele, shaped like a huge index finger, on which are engraved 282 laws promulgated by the legendary Hammurabi, ruler of the Amorite dynasty of ancient Babylon. With its inscribed and sculptured surface, this stone slab, dating back thirty-eight hundred years, is not only a work of art and history but also the most complete legal compendium of Antiquity, and has been called "one of the most important artifacts in the history of humans."[1] To put its age in perspective, the pillar was carved hundreds of years before Moses and the laws of the Bible, twelve centuries before the birth of Buddha and Confucius, and two and a half millennia prior to when Muhammad founded Islam.

Hammurabi was a fearsome warrior king who united the many small kingdoms that made up the Fertile Crescent of Mesopotamia, the lush region in the Middle East bounded by the Tigris and Euphrates rivers. Hammurabi's code formalized laws that regulated individuals and their society and recognized the concept of obligations and privileges such that the strong should not oppress the weak and wrongs must be made right. The decrees also included a code of behavior that regulated the practice of Medicine—mankind's oldest written guidelines for any profession.

In 1901, during an archeological dig at the site of ancient Susa in present-day Iran's Khuzestan Province, this relic was found, broken in several pieces. Cleaned and reassembled, the stone was soon displayed in the Louvre. This final welcoming journey was far different from the column's troubled past. After Hammurabi had his legal code inscribed in Akkadian cuneiform—Akkadian was the daily language of Babylon—the structure was placed in the center of one of the city's public squares. Like an incessant wagging digit, the stele's admonishments were not easily overlooked or dismissed. For over five hundred years the pillar survived in Babylon, but in the twelfth century BC it was plundered and taken to Susa, where it was defaced and flaunted as a trophy of war. Thirty-one centuries later the stone relic was unearthed and brought to Paris.

Like their Neolithic ancestors, Babylonian medical treatments were "unscientific," based on demons, gods, omens, and sorcery. This belief system presented the surgeon, or at least those individuals who wanted to practice the craft of surgery, with a major dilemma. The priestly class, which included physicians, appealed to various gods to cure the ill through the casting of magical rites and supernatural spells. The opposite was true of the surgeon who looked mostly to his crude instruments to heal. Once they relied on man-made probes, saws, and scalpels, the surgeon was considered to have lessened his dependence on soothsaying and the gods.

In the eyes of Babylonian society, the surgeon was tainted as a healer, not fit to be included in the priestly caste, and relegated to a much lower social standing. One result of this downgrading was the notion of *caveat chirurgicus*, "let the surgeon beware." As written in Hammurabi's code—of the stele's 282 decrees, numbers 215–223 relate to surgery—to risk failure meant the knife bearer would suffer physical and financial consequences:

> 218. If a surgeon has treated a gentleman for a severe wound with a bronze lancet and has caused the gentleman to die, or has opened an abscess of the eye for a gentleman with the bronze lancet and has caused the loss of the gentleman's eye, one shall cut off his hands.
> 219. If a surgeon has treated a severe wound of a slave or a poor man with a bronze lancet and has caused his death, he shall render slave for slave.[2]

Notwithstanding Hammurabi's regulations, little is known of Babylonian surgical techniques. What constituted a "severe wound" or an "abscess of the eye" is open to wide speculation. Whether other types of surgical operations were performed also remains a matter of guesswork. Surgeons in Babylon might not have been considered the equals of priest/physicians, but these knife bearers and their procedures were not easily dispensed with. Then again, the severity of punishment meted out for an unsuccessful surgical case must have made the individuals who practiced surgery circumspect in their choice of operations.

Priest/physicians regarded surgery as strictly a manual trade, rather than a learned profession; a less cultured task and something unbecoming. The lesser respect that Babylonians accorded surgeons, the notion that they were baser individuals who worked with their hands, in contrast to pious and thoughtful physicians, left an indelible mark on Medicine for millennia to come. Why is easily explained, and the consequences far-reaching. It was a prejudicial attitude that pitted the brash surgeon against the discreet physician, the doer versus the thinker, the uneducated versus the educated, and would underscore surgery's story for the next four thousand years.

* * *

In 1858, Edwin Smith, an American expatriate and antiquities dealer, settled in Luxor, site of the ancient Egyptian city of Thebes. He was an interesting blend of Egyptologist and entrepreneur who combed the stalls of the area's antiques sellers looking for the next great find. Four years later, he bought a tattered fifteen-foot-long papyrus covered in black and red ink with hieratic, a form of cursive Egyptian hieroglyphs. Smith was told that the roll had been lying in a noble's tomb for over three thousand years and was newly discovered. More likely, it had been plundered by local thieves who made their livelihood ransacking pharaoh-era grave sites. Smith knew enough hieratic to recognize the papyrus as a medical treatise, but despite his attempts to translate the text, nothing came of it.

A half century later, following Smith's death, his family presented the document to the New York Historical Society, where it would lay forgotten. That is, until 1930, when James Breasted, the widely respected director of the Oriental Institute of the University of Chicago, published a translation of the entire papyrus (in 1948, the scroll was donated to the New York Academy of Medicine, where it remains today). He found the crumbled manuscript to be more than just a simple treatise on health care. In fact, Breasted proclaimed the now-named Edwin Smith Papyrus to be the world's "earliest known scientific [surgical] document," one that illustrated how, for the first time, "the human mind peered into the mysteries of the human body, and recognized conditions and processes due to intelligible physical causes."[3]

When Breasted translated the Smith text he found that the scroll, although written by a scribe around 1600 BC, appeared to be a copy of a manuscript authored several centuries earlier. The most fascinating aspect of the Smith Papyrus is what it does not contain. There are no farfetched charms and jumbles of prayers. Instead, the facts are presented in a forthright and practical manner. Just as intriguing as the want of the supernatural was Breasted's "conjecture"[4] that a surgical treatise of such obvious importance may have been composed by or directly reflected the views of the renowned Imhotep.*

---

* Towering over everyone in the world of Egyptian Medicine was Imhotep, a man for all seasons who lived around 2625 BC. He was chief vizier to Pharaoh Djoser, architect of the Step Pyramid of Sakkara, high priest at Heliopolis, a dabbler in astrology, astronomy, and engineering, and a revered philosopher and poet. But, above all, Imhotep is considered mankind's earliest recognized physician/surgeon. His eminence was such that, within several hundred years of his death, Imhotep was elevated to the status of a god and worshiped as the principal Egyptian deity of healing.

And it is through the clarity of an ancient surgeon's thinking that modern surgery's story takes shape.

In a world reliant on the occult, Imhotep, or whoever the author was, wrote about the brain and skull, ears and face, neck and throat, arms and shoulders, and ribs and spine in an impassive and impersonal voice. What makes the Smith Papyrus truly unique is that it reads like a modern textbook, an all-in-one surgical encyclopedia of dos and don'ts. Babylonia and Hammurabi provided rules that governed surgical engagement, but Egypt and the pharaohs supplied surgeons with day-to-day working instructions.

The primitive anatomical observations in the Smith Papyrus are apt and colorful. For the first time, the word "brain" appears. The undulating grooves on the surface of the brain (known as the sulci) are likened to "those ripples that happen in copper through smelting." In a fractured skull, the pulsations of the exposed brain are said to "throb and flutter under your fingers like the weak spot of the crown of a boy before it becomes whole for him"[5]—thus demonstrating a clear understanding of the fontanelles, the gaps in a child's skull that close by adulthood. But it is not only the anatomical observations that are remarkable for their surgical wisdom. Explanations of physiological conditions are revealed with surprising clarity. The strength of the pulse and its rate were used as an indicator of a patient's well-being. Strokes are detailed along with an awareness of the relation between the location of a brain injury and the side of the body involved. A fracture of the neck with damage to the spinal cord is linked with paralysis, involuntary urination, as well as priapism, the persistent erection of the penis.

What the Smith Papyrus makes obvious is that surgery and magic did not share common ground. The individuals in ancient Egypt who treated surgical problems saw what needed to be fixed (e.g., superficial abscesses, broken bones, bulging tumors, grievous injuries, necrotic fingers and toes, rotten teeth, et cetera) and treated them in as objective a manner as the times permitted. This contrasted with those who practiced medicine, a field still mired in prescientific subjectivity. It is impossible to treat illnesses such as cancer, heart failure, gastrointestinal conditions, and respiratory disorders when there is no insight as to what causes them.

For thousands of years, the healing arts in Egypt were unaffected by foreign influence. The rational and the supernatural held sway, but around 500 BC Greek physicians came to Egypt. Under their influence, Egyptian Medicine was replaced by different ways of thinking, including the beginnings of evidence-based therapies as well as speculative mumbo jumbo. Before long, little was left of the ancient medical ways other than a dismal sort of alchemy and sorcery. The tenets of Egyptian surgery, its independence from the mystical and its rationality of action, fell silent. But the Greek emphasis on fair-minded inspection and unbiased observation in gathering medical knowledge, along with objectivity and practicality in the practice of surgery, would provide the light that continued to move the craft forward.

2.

EXODUS

No good physician quavers incantations
When the malady he's treating needs the knife

Sophocles, *Ajax*, fifth century BC

The good physician [surgeon] is he who knows how to employ the right
remedies at the proper time; the poor one, he who, in the presence of a
serious illness, loses his courage, becomes flustered, and is unable to devise
any helpful method of treatment

Aeschylus, sixth/fifth century BC

Around 1100 BC, various peoples, later collectively identified as "Greeks," emerged in the lands encircling the Aegean. Over centuries, and through a series of conquests, these communities coalesced and were themselves subjugated in the fourth century BC by a neighboring king, Alexander the Great. He is one of Antiquity's most successful military leaders and, at the height of his victories, Alexander's realm stretched from the Adriatic Sea in the west to the Indus River in the east, including the lands of Egypt to the south. During his adolescence, Alexander was tutored by the Greek philosopher Aristotle. Not unexpectedly, the future sovereign became a great admirer of Hellenic traditions and his later resettlement of Greek colonists throughout his empire created a cultural diffusion that profoundly affected world history.

In 331 BC, at the mouth of the Nile Delta, Alexander established his new capital, the city of Alexandria with its harbor guarded by a celebrated lighthouse, one of the Seven Wonders of the Ancient World. Eight years later, at age thirty-two, Alexander died under mysterious circumstances. His successor declared himself King Ptolemy, the first in a long line of family claimants to the throne of the pharaohs. The Ptolemaic reign lasted until 30 BC and the death of Cleopatra, the last ruler of an independent Egypt. Subsequently, her family's kingdom became a province of the newly established Roman Empire.

Ptolemy was a classicist and humanist. Among his favored projects was the construction of a library, part of an effort to gather, in one place, all the knowledge of the ancients. This building, the renowned Alexandrian library, was an architectural marvel with its lecture halls, observatory, research rooms, and zoological gardens. Well-paid scholars translated manuscripts from past civilizations as adroit scribes endlessly copied one document after another. It is said that seven hundred thousand handwritten papyrus scrolls were eventually housed on the library's shelves with Aristotle's private collection as the nucleus. In 48 BC, this celebrated storehouse of wisdom burned down during a period of political unrest sparked by the appearance of Julius Caesar and his Roman legions.

Ptolemy's intellectual curiosity encompassed the healing arts. He decreed that all writings on medicine, dating back to the Hippocratic teachings of the fifth century BC, be gathered under a single title. The king's interest in Medicine arose from Greek philosophic speculations about health and sickness that were a key component in their discourses regarding life and nature. The collection of over seventy works became known as the *Corpus Hippocraticum* and marks the beginnings of mankind's enduring medical and surgical literature; the compilation would exert a profound influence on Western thought. It's unknown whether a single person authored the *Corpus* or, as is more likely, it was derived from a circle of doctors associated with the individual named Hippocrates.*

---

* Hippocrates was considered the personification of all that a physician should be. He was forthright, kindhearted, prolific, and, above all, a man of the people. His earliest biographers tell of Hippocrates's birth on the island of Cos, located in the southeastern Aegean Sea, and that through his mother, Phaenareta, he was descended from the Greek god Hercules. Hippocrates's father, Heraclides, a renowned doctor, was his first teacher. It is believed that Hippocrates's education continued under the guidance of Democritus, the formulator of the atomic theory, Gorgias, a philosopher, and Herodicus, the father of sports medicine. At the end of Hippocrates's formal schooling, he traveled widely, paying attention to illnesses and their relation to the environment and nature. Posterity claims Hippocrates as the "Father of Medicine," the one individual who defined and epitomized the story of health care in ancient Greece. The

What is significant is the Hippocratic-based conviction that health and illness can be explained through an understanding of nature, apart from the shackles of religion and speculation. Pre-Hippocratic Greek healers regarded disease as being of supernatural origin, caused by angry gods or demonic possession. The underlying concepts in the *Corpus* opposed these beliefs. There is not a single mention of evil spirits in the entirety of the writings. Instead, what the *Corpus* offered was a biologic-based approach to disease.

The followers of Hippocratic-style medicine believed that ill health was not a punishment brought by angry gods but the consequence of lifestyle choices, environmental issues, and other mitigating factors including mind-set and social class. They called for an analytic approach to healing, one independent of dogmatism and hearsay and, instead, based on inspection and observation. In the view of medical historian Fielding Garrison, the Hippocratic healer was "the exemplar of that flexible, critical, well-poised attitude of mind, ever on the lookout for sources of error, which is the very essence of the scientific spirit."[1]

Despite this appeal for objectivity, Greek medical practices remained far removed from the science of modern Medicine. For example, the fundamental concept in the *Corpus* is that to be healthy, an individual must exist in a steady state with nature. The shortcoming in Greek thinking was not the message; the quest for balance and oneness with the universe remains pervasive even in today's world. The miscue was in the explanation of how the equilibrium was maintained.

The Greeks believed that equilibrium with the natural world depended upon the proper balance of four fluids or humors—black bile, blood, phlegm, and yellow bile—that silently flowed through the body. Illness arose from an imbalance in these humors. Winter colds were due to an abundance of phlegm while summer diarrhea was caused by an overflow of yellow bile. Depression occurred when there was a profusion of black bile. On the one hand, too much blood resulted in inflammation. On the other hand, the routine loss of blood was associated with a renewal of life, observed in menstruation and childbearing. Bleeding was seen as beneficial and led to the practice of bloodletting, formulated by the Greeks, systematized by the Romans,

---

reality is that a confusion of facts surrounds his very being. Historians agree that around 460 BC, on an island off the coast of present-day Turkey, a person with the name Hippocrates was born. However, barely two hundred years after this man's death no biographer could tease out the truths versus the myths. Virtually every statement concerning the life of Hippocrates is unsubstantiated.

performed by men who titled themselves surgeons, and used well into the closing decades of the nineteenth century AD. Above all, the humoral theory appealed to Greek physicians and their need for rationality. Unlike diseases that involved invisible workings inside the body, the four fluids were visible, leaving no question as to their existence. It was a case of "seeing is believing."

*   *   *

Objectivity and pragmatism were also evident in the craft of surgery. Over time, Greek surgeons learned that wounds should be kept dry, except for an occasional application of wine on the dressing. Fractures were reduced, a term used to describe how a bone is fixed or set after an injury and the ends of splintered bones removed when they punctured the skin. Fractured pieces of bone must be put in close proximity to one another so that proper healing can occur and permanent functional loss or deformity is avoided. Bladders were catheterized to remove bladder stones. The consequences of pressure on the brain from a fractured skull were understood; trephination was employed as a cure.

Once the *Corpus* was available as a manuscript, Greek knife bearers had a written how-to guide for surgical operations, as well as the first technical descriptions of an operating room and its appurtenances. From lighting ("there are two kinds, the common and the artificial") and positioning of the patient ("avoid shrinking down, shrinking from, turning away, and maintain the figure and position of the part operated upon") to instrumentation ("they may not impede the work, and there may be no difficulty in taking hold of them") and posture ("when sitting, his feet should be raised to a direct line with his knees, and nearly in contact with one another"), meticulousness was the message. This fastidiousness extended to the surgeon's personal grooming ("the nails should be neither longer nor shorter than the points of the fingers") and his manual dexterity ("the surgeon should practice with the extremities of the fingers . . . all sorts of work . . . endeavoring to do them well, elegantly, quickly, without trouble, neatly, and promptly").[2]

While there is much in the surgical writings of the *Corpus* that is faulty and remote from modern surgical practices, the advice was cautious and practical. The work became the most widely quoted surgical literature for the next five centuries. Despite the *Corpus*'s shortcomings—for instance, the presence of pus was mistakenly considered a vital element of wound healing—Hippocratic-influenced surgery established the lasting model of the altruistic and virtuous surgeon. Professionalism was spelled out in the most well-known of the *Corpus*'s writings, the Oath of Hippocrates.

* * *

One of the most awe-inspiring days of my life was May 9, 1975, when I stood in Kiel Auditorium for my graduation from the Saint Louis University School of Medicine and recited with my classmates the Hippocratic Oath. Accompanied by Beth, my parents, my in-laws, and my grandmother-in-law, I was admitted to the profession of medicine by echoing many of the same words that doctors had spoken for twenty-five hundred years:*

> I will respect and show gratitude to my deserving teachers . . . ,
> I will carry out that regime which . . . shall be for the benefit of my patients;
> I will keep them from harm and wrong . . .
> My own life and my professional practice I will keep guiltless and right . . . ,
> I will not permit considerations of race, religion, nationality, party politics, social standing, or financial circumstances to interfere with my attending my patient.
> I will maintain the honor and noble traditions of the medical profession . . . ,
> My colleagues shall be as my brothers.

The Oath was a pledge of trust to my patients and peers, a vow to serve others and to share my craft's knowledge with succeeding generations. These two obligations are my direct link to the Hippocratic thinking that separated religion from science and dogmatism from open-mindedness.

The original Oath set Medicine's moral high ground. At the same time, it

---

* The origins of the Hippocratic Oath are obscure and modern scholars do not attribute it to Hippocrates but believe it was written a century or two after his death. Over the millennia, the Oath has been modified and even superseded as a declaration of professional ethics by more politically correct versions. I took an adaptation adopted by the Saint Louis University School of Medicine in 1954.

sowed confusion, as its prohibitions against performing an abortion and assisting a suicide conflicted with the fact that some Hippocratics engaged in those activities. This ambivalence broadened when it came to the practice of surgery. The original Oath specifically forbade cutting: "I will not use the knife; not even on sufferers from stone, but will withdraw in favor of such men as are engaged in this work."[3]

The proscription established an unmistakable division between Hippocratic-influenced physicians and the class of individuals who performed surgical operations. Like that of their Babylonian predecessors, who consigned surgery to a lesser standing within Medicine, the Greeks left the craft and its work of the hand to itinerant craftsmen and roustabouts. This clear-cut separation is reflected in the etymological derivation of the words "surgery" and "medicine." "Surgery" originated from the ancient Greek *cheiros* (hand) and *ergon* (work) and was then modified into the Latin *chirurgia*, which led to the French *chirurgien* and finally the English "surgerie." In contrast, "medicine" is derived from the Latin *medicus*, meaning "a learned physician."

As Greek medical and surgical thinking spread throughout the Mediterranean, it found a new base in Rome. Over the course of a millennium, the consolidation of Greek and Roman medicine, centered on the precepts of the *Hippocratic Corpus*, created a new type of learned doctor who cared directly for the patient rather than relying on the beneficence of demons and gods. This unification of practice and theory was primarily seen through the written works of several prominent physicians who recorded their discoveries during the Roman Empire.

3.

PROLIFIC PENS

The medical profession is the only one in which anybody professing to be a physician is at once trusted, although nowhere else is an untruth more dangerous.

Pliny the Elder, *Natural History*, AD 77

Only a poor physician gives up.

Seneca the Younger, *De Clementia*, AD 55

Following the fall of Egypt to Caesar in the closing decades of the first century BC, the Roman Empire came to dominate the Mediterranean world as well as much of Europe and wide swaths of the Middle East. This sizeable kingdom absorbed many Greek traditions and became the progenitor of Western civilization. Despite the Romans' intellectual and technical vigor, exemplified by their achievements in public health—including the construction of multi-level aqueducts, paved streets, public sewers, and well-ventilated dwellings—when it came to personal health, they showed little respect for physicians and their training. In general, middle- and upper-class Roman citizens had an aversion to manual labor; it was unthinkable for them to engage in anything as physically and socially unbecoming as "doctoring."

The antipathy toward physicians changed over time, as itinerant Greek healers settled in Roman territory and became leaders of the growing medical community. The influx of Hellenic doctors led to the spread of Hippocratic beliefs throughout the Roman Empire. As the need for physicians outpaced the supply of immigrant healers, servants and slaves assumed more health care–related responsibilities. It was not uncommon for members of the lower classes to be taught medical and surgical therapies by Greek mentors, so that Roman families would always have a "doctor" in the house.* The use of slaves and other social outcasts to perform surgical operations reinforced the long established and demeaning attitude toward healers who worked with their hands.

* * *

Even if Romans considered themselves divorced from the physical practice of Medicine, they did not shun writing about it. Two authors wielded the most influential and prolific of surgical pens: Aulus Cornelius Celsus, a vendor of Medicine's past, and Galen of Pergamon (located near the modern Turkish city of Bergama), who repositioned Hippocratic thinking in ways that brought it both backward and forward.

Celsus was the first of the Encyclopedists, a group of men who over the centuries attempted to summarize the existing knowledge in "all fields." With equal competence, Celsus wrote on agriculture, jurisprudence, military science, medicine, philosophy, rhetoric, and surgery. He lived in Gallia Narbonensis, a Roman province located in what is now southern France, during the reign of the emperors Tiberius and Caligula, in the first century AD. Celsus was not a physician but a wealthy landowner who wrote in Latin for his fellow patricians. His encyclopedic compilations, partially based on Greek sources, totaled at least twenty-one books, of which only the eight on Medicine survive.

This octuplet, known as *De Medicina*, is the oldest recognized medical treatise following the *Corpus Hippocraticum* and provides a wealth of information on surgical affairs from their mythical beginnings to the dawn of the Christian era. Celsus

---

* A notable example is seen in the life of Luke the Evangelist. He lived, probably as a slave, in the Greek city of Antioch in ancient Syria, where he labored as a physician. In Luke's middle age, he was brought into the household of Paul the Apostle, a Roman citizen. Luke became one of Paul's main disciples and accompanied him on numerous missionary journeys throughout the empire. Luke cared for Paul while he evangelized and during his final stay and martyrdom in Rome in AD 67. Two decades later, Luke died, possibly also as a martyr, near Thebes, Greece. The Catholic Church venerates Luke as one of the patron saints of surgeons—among the feast days set aside for his remembrance is October 13, coincidentally my birthday!

starts with a history of the craft and deftly moves to a listing of surgical conditions. He describes operative techniques for each body region, from the head to the toes, including those for abscesses, cataracts, fractures, hernias, and varicose veins. Celsus's account of urologic surgery included a section on the restoration of penile foreskin! Apparently, there were Jews in the Roman Empire who curried political titles and social acceptance by cloaking their religious affiliation. But what particularly set Celsus apart from his contemporaries was his belief that surgery was an integral branch of Medicine and should not stand alone:

> [P]art of the art of Medicine is that which cures by the hand . . . the effects of this treatment are more obvious than any other kind; inasmuch as in diseases since luck helps much, and the same things are often salutary, often of no use at all, it may be doubted whether recovery has been due to medicine or a sound body or good luck. . . . But in that part of medicine which cures by hand, it is obvious that all improvement comes chiefly from this. . . . This branch, although very ancient . . . was unwisely separated from the rest of medicine, and began to have its own professors.[1]

As the first major medical author writing in Latin, Celsus translated hundreds of Greek medical terms into the language of ancient Rome. Many of these words remain in modern professional usage. I recall, fifty years ago as a freshman medical student, memorizing the four cardinal signs of inflammation enunciated by Celsus, ones that he urged every surgeon to be on the lookout for: "calor, dolor, rubor, tumor; calor, dolor, rubor, tumor." This assonant phrase, with its English rendition—"heat, pain, redness, swelling"—is tattooed onto every surgeon's psyche. Even today, these four rhyming words jingle in my brain and represent my personal connection to Celsus and his two-thousand-year-old pen.

*   *   *

The modest surgical developments during Antiquity conclude with the voluminous writings of Galen, one of the most accomplished and outlandish personalities of the Greco-Roman era. In his day, Galen was Medicine's superstar: an over-the-top mixture of egotism, erudition, intuition, and narcissism. He was the most talented of all medical investigators of Antiquity. His work influenced the development of anatomy, medicine, pathology, pharmacology, physiology, and surgery for the next fifteen centuries.

Galen's medical and surgical interests knew no bounds; neither did his temperament. Galen's name was derived from the Greek adjective *galernos*, meaning "calm"; he was anything but. Galen was self-absorbed and self-righteous, while his writings reveal his contentious behavior (they contain much in the way of autobiographical information). Galen was boastful and demeaning. He ridiculed his rivals, called them asses and buffoons, and claimed that they knew nothing and he understood everything:

> I have done as much to medicine as Trajan did to the Roman Empire, in making bridges and roads throughout Italy. It is I alone that have pointed out the true method of treating diseases: it must be confessed that Hippocrates had already chalked out the same road . . . as the first discoverer . . . he opened the road, but I have rendered it passable.[2]

Galen was born in AD 129 to a learned and wealthy architect ("My great fortune was to have as my father a most good tempered, just, efficient, and benevolent man."); and a woman with anger management problems ("My mother, on the other hand, was so irascible that she would sometimes bite her serving-maids, and was constantly shouting at my father and quarrelling with him.").[3] He received a broad-based medical education that included several years of study in Alexandria augmented with travels throughout the lands that bordered the Mediterranean Sea. By the time the twenty-eight-year-old Galen returned to his hometown of Pergamon, he was the celebrated author of manuscripts on anatomy and physiology and a highly regarded doctor. Galen's skills with fractures and dislocations, head injuries, lacerations, and draining blood and other fluids from wounds of the chest and abdomen served him well; he was shortly appointed surgeon to the city's stable of gladiators.

For five years, Galen enjoyed a unique window into the workings of the human body. Since Roman law forbade human dissection, the horrific wounds suffered by the battlers provided a living anatomy laboratory that was impossible to replicate. The spilled brains, the throbbing heart, the undulating intestines, and the shattered bones offered a young surgeon trying to understand the inside mysteries of man a remarkable but still limited learning experience.

Because Galen did not appreciate the detailed specifics of human anatomy (he never performed or witnessed a full human dissection), his backyard contained a menagerie of apes, calves, goats, monkeys, pigs, and sheep, all of which fell victim to his curiosity and dissecting prowess. Compelled to apply animal findings to humans, Galen described, for example, a jumbled network of nerves and vessels found at the base of calf brains and, erroneously, said this same complex existed in humans. He claimed, again incorrectly, that the human liver had fingerlike extensions that clasped the stomach, similar to what he saw in pigs, and that these lobes assisted the two organs in changing food into blood. As Galen's writings increased and his reputation grew, the inaccuracies caused by his extrapolating human anatomical data from animals also spread. If his methods were criticized, the egotistical Galen was unmoved:

> Now let me once and for all make this general statement to apply to my whole [anatomical] treatise so as not to be forced to say the same thing repeatedly: I am now explaining the structures actually to be seen in dissection, and no one before me has done this with any accuracy. Hence, if anyone wishes to observe the works of Nature, he should . . . either come to me, or consult one of my associates.[4]

Despite Galen's status as the hometown son who had made good, he considered Pergamon one of life's provincial way stations. Seeking a more fitting city in which to demonstrate his skills, he moved to Rome. Galen arrived with an impressive show-and-tell of live experiments. His flair for self-promotion was apparent when, before an enthusiastic audience, Galen took a pig and methodically severed the nerves in its neck. As each fiber was cut, the struggling animal continued to squeal until Galen came to the recurrent laryngeal nerve. He had previously shown how this structure allowed the vocal cords to open and close. With one nimble slice, Galen severed the nerve and the pig's squealing ceased, dazzling the astounded Romans.

Flaunting the virtues of his medical education and backed by his grounding in the arts and humanities, Galen became a favorite of the elite. They showered him with encomiums. Galen basked in the limelight while reminding the public that his patients came from the highest levels of Roman society, including Emperor Marcus

Aurelius and his son Commodus. "As you well know," Galen told his followers, "[the emperor] was continually speaking of me as the first among physicians and unique among philosophers."[5] Under the protection of these benefactors, Galen, a lifelong bachelor with few outside interests, pursued his scientific investigations with vigor and continued to practice and write until his death at age seventy.

The breadth and volume of Galen's works are staggering. They form almost half of all extant ancient Greco-Roman medical writings and, if the *Corpus Hippocraticum* and *De Medicina* are removed from that list, Galen's contributions approach 85 percent. He was among the few physicians who wrote about surgical procedures. However, in contrast to Celsus, Galen believed that surgery should be separated from and viewed as a lesser mode of treatment within the whole of Medicine. By implication, Galen maintained the ancient Greek conviction that the craft of surgery was a minor element of the art of healing—not worthy of study by reputable physicians—and could be mostly left to the uneducated and the unskilled.

More than anything, Galen was a systematizer, an individual who brought order to things. This characteristic reflected his personality: definitive, independent, and precise. Galen's zeal for organization led to his crowning scientific achievement: the classification of every illness as excesses of Hippocrates's four bodily fluids. For example, Galen considered cancers the result of superfluous black bile, colds an accumulation of phlegm, fevers a surfeit of blood, and liver diseases an abundance of yellow bile. To reduce these imbalances and restore humoral equilibrium, Galen championed bloodletting and fluid evacuation. Whatever the disease, the patient's age, the time of the year, or even the weather, Galen provided a simple therapeutic approach: bleed by opening a vein and supplement with an enema to produce diarrhea and/or an emetic to bring about nausea. Like his straightforward remedies, Galen's clinical end point was also clear-cut: the bled patient was to be made woozy or lapse into a faint.

Bleeding was a messy affair and most Greco-Roman physicians were loath to perform it. Instead, it was slaves and men from the lower classes who became prized for their surgical skills at incising veins. In turn, their successors carried on what became a family avocation. Over the centuries, faith in bloodletting intensified as Galen came to be regarded as the leading authority on all matters medical and surgical.

Two hundred years after Galen's death, the Western Roman Empire fell and the Middle Ages engulfed Europe. During Antiquity, Galen's light transformed Medicine; over the next fifteen centuries it glowed even brighter. However, replete with anatomical and physiological errors, its glare suppressed fresh ways of thinking. With Galen established as Medicine's leading authority so, too, were his erroneous beliefs, exemplified by his obstinacy that monkeys and pigs had the same anatomy as humans and the lungs were not involved in oxygenating the blood. Galen was a speculator. What he could not see or understand he concocted. And, at a time when medical and surgical conjecture ran rampant and dissections and vivisections on humans were strictly prohibited, those looking for answers were content to believe in Galen's imaginations.

4.
DARKNESS, THEN DAYLIGHT

The greatest good is to be wise, the greatest evil is to suffer physical pain.

Saint Augustine of Hippo, *The Soliloquies*, c. AD 410

The surgeon should have a perceptive eye, ideas that are always lucid, of the nature that will enable him always to act with promptness and assurance.

Jehan Yperman, *La Chirurgie*, c. AD 1310

W hen the Western Roman Empire began to fragment in the fourth century AD, the Catholic Church became a major unifying force as it went about crushing all opposition to its doctrines. The Church's spiritual appeal, the presence of an efficient hierarchical organization, and its embrace of feudal life led to its total domination of medieval society.* Secular schools of learning withered and a

---

* The Middle Ages or medieval period lasted from the fall of the Western Roman Empire in the fourth century AD to the beginning of the Renaissance in the fifteenth century AD. The early Middle Ages, from the late fourth century AD through the beginning of the ninth century AD, are referred to as the Dark Ages, a time of pervasive bigotry, cruelty, and ignorance underscored by a lack of social progress. Danger and death were ever present and the best chance of some form of safety for the common people was to have their land and possessions conveyed, voluntarily or coerced, to the most powerful nobleman in the region and place themselves under his safeguard. As this practice grew, feudalism developed and western Europe disintegrated into small fiefdoms, each under the hegemony of a strong-arm leader.

dogmatic form of thinking, centered around Church canon, became the standard. Intellectual development suffered along with Medicine's progress. Rationality and science took a backseat to the conviction that illness was divinely inflicted, only to be lifted through endless prayer and godly intervention.

As the Church flourished, the physical landscape of western Europe became dotted with abbeys, cathedrals, and castles. Monasticism thrived and monasteries, with their facilities for care of the sick and weak, became natural places of congregation. Monks, who rejected the Hippocratic belief that diseases could be explained through an understanding of biology and nature, assumed the role of "medical practitioners" and resorted to the miraculous healing power of Jesus Christ, the saints, and holy relics.

*   *   *

Because Church authorities had little regard for Greco-Roman attitudes toward illness, the study of Hippocratic and Galenic texts waned. But, in the Byzantine Empire, the tradition of Hippocratic-Galenic medical practice continued. This kingdom, also known as the Eastern Roman Empire, was a carryover from the fallen Western Roman Empire, though situated in the Greek-speaking, eastern part of Europe and the Mediterranean. The political makeover was set in motion in AD 330, when Emperor Constantine the Great transferred the capital of what remained of the Western Roman Empire from Rome to Byzantium (later renamed Constantinople). The Byzantine Empire was distinguished by two key features: a focus on Greek rather than Latin culture, and the practice of a form of Orthodox Christianity (later termed "Greek Orthodox").

During its lengthy history, the borders of the Byzantine Empire underwent numerous shifts that proved important to the subsequent interplay between cultures. In the sixth century AD, under Justinian I, an aggressive military campaign resulted in the recapture of much of the territory of the Western Roman Empire, including North Africa and Italy. One hundred years later, a new enemy of the Byzantines, the Muslims, won a series of victories against them and established an Islamic caliphate that extended across the lands of Egypt, Palestine, and Syria. When Muslim fighters crossed the Mediterranean's Strait of Gibraltar, their kingdom reached into Spain and southern France. During the ninth and tenth centuries, Byzantine armies drove the Muslims back, but Islam's influence had already impacted Western society.

Efforts were made to contain this spread, particularly by Christian soldiers, known as Crusaders, who, under papal authority, began a series of holy wars to recover the Holy Land and other areas under Muslim rule. The conflicts were fought between AD 1096 and 1271, but despite repeated attempts, the recapture of these territories was less than successful.

* * *

The integration of communities along the borders of the Byzantine and Islamic empires had refocused attention on Greco-Roman medicine. This interest was guided by Byzantine physician/scholars and fostered by the zeal of their Muslim counterparts eager to study past authorities. Indeed, the medical and surgical knowledge from Antiquity might have vanished had not the center of learning shifted to the Arab world. It was the flowering of Islam in the Middle East and North Africa and on the Iberian Peninsula that produced hotbeds of scholarly activity where intellectuals preserved the writings from the Greco-Roman eras through translations into Arabic, Persian, and Syrian.

The Byzantine and Muslim academicians concentrated their efforts on Galen, revered as Antiquity's foremost philosopher-physician and the prophet who elevated Hippocrates to godlike status. Galen was considered a clinical pragmatist and his interpretation of natural and religious phenomena appealed to theologians who found in his writings a rational basis for their own studies on faith and healing. Moreover, at a time when independence of thought was not encouraged, Galen's authoritarian manner attracted followers who preferred dogmatic, steadfast leadership. For these supporters of the vast scope of his writings, disagreement with Galen's beliefs and methods was considered medical and surgical heresy. The blind acceptance of Galenism led to a lack of progress in Medicine and was among the reasons why physicians and their clinical activities were separated from surgeons and their performance of operations.

Early in the Middle Ages, erudite Byzantine Greek writers, led by Paul of Aegina, a physician/surgeon who studied and practiced in Alexandria during the seventh century AD, considered it their task to spread Galen's influence. They combined elements from Galen's and other scholars' works into massive compendia of Greek and Roman medicine. Paul's manuscript, *Epitome Medicae Libri Septem* (Seven books of medicine), attempted to summarize all surgical knowledge and shaped the "Galenism" that dominated later centuries. Paul claimed that the surgical patriarchs had basically said all there was on the subject and he was only a respectful admirer ("I have compiled this collection from the works of the ancients and have set down little of my own."[1]). In short order, Paul's work was translated from Greek to Arabic and incorporated into the texts of the principal Islamic physicians.

Of the numerous manuscripts written in Arabic, the *Kitab al-Tasrif* (The method of medicine), composed in the eleventh century AD by Abul Qasim (known as Albucasis), had the longest-lasting effect on surgery during the Middle Ages. He was born in Muslim Spain, in a small village outside of Cordova; little other biographical information is available. Albucasis's straightforward advice and personal observations reveal a cautious and conscientious surgeon. Like other surgical texts of the period, Albucasis borrowed freely from Paul's *Epitome* but without mention of any attribution. What most set Albucasis apart from his contemporaries was an honesty about the state of surgery, a frankness that revealed the pitiful status of the craft:

> The skilled practitioner of operative surgery is totally lacking in our land and time; so that the knowledge of it is on the point of being blotted out and its remains lost; and there is nothing left of it except a few traces in the books of the Ancients; where, however, it has been so corrupted by the hands of scribes, and subjected to errors and confusion, that its meaning has become obscured and its value diminished.[2]

Albucasis was correct in his assessment. Much like the children's game "telephone," in which one person whispers a phrase into the ear of the next person through a line of people until the last player announces what he or she was told, the later versions of Hippocrates and Galen had undergone numerous renditions. In telephone, inaccuracies accumulate in the retellings, so the statement announced by the last person usually differs significantly from that of the first. The same problem of cumulative errors can be found in the back-and-forth copying, editing, and translating of Hippocrates's and Galen's texts. These handwritten manuscripts were never the same relative to their original intent, not that their earlier versions were more scientifically accurate than later copies.

Moreover, the newer translations emphasized surgical principles that were regressive in nature and would stagnate the development of surgery throughout the

Middle Ages. Some of the misguided concepts, including the perception that pus (i.e., a thick, whitish-yellow fluid that results from the accumulation of white blood cells, liquefied tissue, and cellular detritus and is commonly a sign of infection) was an essential factor in wound healing, or the unrelenting use of bloodletting, dated back to the time of Hippocrates. Other obstacles resulted from Galen's errors, such as his belief that blood, in its movement through the body, passed from the right to the left side of the heart via invisible pores, instead of coursing through the lungs before returning to the heart. This particular miscue prevented physicians from understanding the human circulatory system until the middle of the seventeenth century AD. Muslim commentators had their own flawed ideas and proscriptions. Among them was obedience to a religious-based notion that it was unclean or unholy to touch a corpse. Thus, human dissection was banned and, as Albucasis pointed out, surgical activity limited in the Muslim world.

*   *   *

Over time, the practice of monastic-based medicine in the West became more restrictive, especially after the Gregorian reforms of the eleventh century forced those in holy orders to live in greater conformity with the Church's doctrines. In AD 1130, at the Council of Clermont, monks were told they could no longer practice both general medicine and civil law. Thirty-three years later, at the Council of Tours, an infamous phrase, *Ecclesia abhorret a sanguine* ("the Church abhors the shedding of blood"), was stated publicly. At the Fourth Lateran Council in AD 1215, Pope Innocent III reinforced this admonition when he proclaimed, "No cleric is to be put in command of cavalry, archers, or others of the same kind who shed blood, nor are subdeacons, deacons, or priests to exercise that part of surgery involving cauterization and incision."[3] An additional canon law stated that anyone who caused the unintended death of a person—including the fatal outcome of a surgical operation—was forever barred from the priesthood.

These declarations were not intended as overt attacks on surgery. But, by adhering to Galen's assertion that surgery was a lesser form of medical care, while maintaining that the shedding of blood and causing a death secondary to a surgical procedure were incompatible with ecclesiastical status, the Church restricted the educated class from performing any type of operation. In effect, the Church disposed the world of surgery to the less learned members of medieval society and treated the individuals who performed surgical operations as servile practitioners. A contemporary observer of the medical scene noted:

> O God, why in our day is there so great a difference between the physician and the surgeon! The physicians have abandoned operations to laymen, since they disdain, as some of them say, to work with their hands.[4]

The surgeon's role fell mostly to uneducated barbers who had been frequenting monasteries since the late eleventh century AD, when beards were banned. Initially, barbers, with their indispensable razors, shaved the monks, cut their hair in the styles of specific religious orders, performed periodic bloodletting, and assisted clerics in the care of medical and surgical patients in the monastery. Over time, the barbers were also asked to trim bunions, corns, and nails, lance boils, as well as pull rotten teeth, dress wounds, and amputate mangled fingers and toes.

By the fourteenth century AD, surgical techniques had matured at the hands of these individuals who were now known as "barber-surgeons." Without a formal educational system, the illiterate barber-surgeons learned the craft of surgery as apprentices and handed their invaluable knowledge down through families. Eventually, due to necessity or preference, the barber-surgeons no longer confined their activities to monasteries but traveled through the towns and villages of Europe as purveyors of the craft of surgery. Some of the barber-surgeons even went so far as to narrow the scope of their clinical activities; one operated on hernias, another on tumors, others treated cataracts, and some grew skilled at bloodletting. Despite the political and socioeconomic slights that came with being an uneducated knife bearer, it was the legion of obscure barber-surgeons who, through their devotion to the craft, ensured surgery's ultimate survival.

* * *

The first stirrings of revival of Greco-Roman-based Medicine in western Europe occurred in Salerno, a seaside settlement on the west coast of Italy, thirty miles south of Naples. The region was a cultural crossroads and legend holds that the medical school in Salerno was founded in the ninth century AD by an Arab, a Greek, a Jew, and a Latinist. This tale contains some metaphoric truth that likely symbolizes the social fusion that factored into the institution's origins. The reality was that from the late tenth century AD onward, Arabic translations of the Greco-Roman masters, particularly Hippocrates and Galen, began to appear in western Europe and were soon retranslated back into Latin; Salerno was their first and most important site of entry.

What set the Salerno medical school apart from its contemporaries was the presence of a lay administration. In AD 1140, Roger II of Sicily, known for his intellectual curiosity and religious skepticism, assured Medicine's freedom from total clerical domination when he decreed that anyone who practiced medicine and surgery in his realm was required to pass a battery of tests to be administered by secular-based physicians. Decades later, Roger's grandson Frederick II of Hohenstaufen was even more explicit when he bestowed on Salerno's faculty the sole authority to approve all physicians and surgeons for practice within his kingdom.

Frederick II's edict was important because it raised the standards of European medical education and brought both physicians and surgeons under control of formal learning. What's more, Frederick II endorsed human anatomical dissection as an essential component of medical and surgical training. Despite the requirement of proper schooling, the course of study for surgeons was markedly shorter and less comprehensive than for physicians, perpetuating the surgeons' inferior educational and social standing. Some Salernitan knife bearers responded by pursuing the physician's broader training prior to obtaining their instruction in surgery.

It was not long before surgeons associated with the School of Salerno authored their own texts on surgical topics. *Practica Chirurgiae*, by Roggerio dei Frugardi (known as Roger of Salerno), was the era's preeminent manuscript and earliest original surgical work in the West. Roger's sources were primarily from Byzantine compilations of Greek and Roman writings but supplemented with observations from his personal experience (minus the magic spells and incantations used by the monks). As Roger's reputation spread, his *Practica Chirurgiae* and its systematic approach to surgery provided a broad foundation for future surgical texts. Thus, the School of Salerno and its progressive views can be considered the birthplace of modern Western surgery and Roger its midwife.

The intent of Frederick II's law widened when similar ordinances were introduced in Spain in AD 1283 and, a half century later, in Germany. Paralleling these developments, disciples of Roger disseminated his teachings throughout Europe, eventually making their way as far north as Scandinavia. Of the physicians who passed on the Salernitan traditions, Theodoric Borgognoni was the most influential. He studied medicine at the University of Bologna while also becoming a Dominican friar. Later in Theodoric's career, he served as personal physician to Pope Innocent IV and was eventually named by Clement IV as Bishop of Cervia, a small town within the province of Ravenna. In AD 1267, Theodoric completed his major work, the *Chirurgia*, a lengthy treatise that covered all aspects of surgery. The manuscript broke with many time-honored surgical practices handed down from the ancient Greeks and their Arabic translators. Among these, Theodoric insisted that the practice of encouraging the development of pus in wounds was incorrect and should be replaced by a "dry" treatment plan:

> It is not necessary . . . as Roger and [other surgeons from the School of Salerno] have written, as many of their disciples teach, and as all modern surgeons profess, that pus should be generated in wounds. No error can be greater than this. Such a practice is, indeed, to hinder Nature, to prolong the disease, and to prevent the conglutination and consolidation of the wound.[5]

* * *

By the beginning of the fourteenth century AD, the civil wars and political instability that engulfed the region's city-states caused Italian leadership in surgery to wane. Paris assumed Salerno's role as the gathering place for up-and-coming surgical talent. France's standing as surgery's lodestar was initially guided by an Italian refugee, Guido Lanfranchi, known as Lanfranc of Milan. He was a defrocked cleric—Lanfranc paid scant attention to his vows of celibacy and had several children—who had received a university degree in medicine and devoted his professional life to the practice and teaching of surgery.

Due to the civil unrest in his homeland, Lanfranc fled Italy for Lyon, but ambition drove him to Paris, a city that had become the educational and intellectual center of western Europe. There, in AD 1295, he showcased the full capabilities of Italian surgery by inviting French surgeons to witness a series of surgical operations, an event unprecedented for his time. The following year, Lanfranc completed his *Chirurgia Magna* (Grand surgery), which he expediently dedicated to Philip IV of

France. Covering general principles of surgery, the work served as one of the foundations of medieval French surgical teaching.

Lanfranc, the first renowned surgeon in France, sought to establish his craft as a scholarly endeavor, equal in stature with the practice of medicine. He was a bitter critic of uneducated barber-surgeons and other unqualified knife bearers and took a determined stand against them and the continuing divide between surgery and medicine. "Good God!" he exclaimed in the *Chirurgia*:

> Why this abandoning of operations by physicians to lay persons, disdaining surgery, as I perceive, because they do not know how to operate . . . an abuse which has reached such a point that the vulgar begin to think the same man cannot know medicine and surgery . . . however, no man can be a good physician who has no knowledge of operative surgery; a knowledge of both branches is essential.[6]

Despite Lanfranc's reputation and his currying favor with the royals, he never obtained a position on the medical faculty of the University of Paris because of his lack of celibacy—the school was supervised by the French kings and the Church. Instead, he affiliated with the recently established Collège de Saint Côme (College of Saints Cosmas and Damian),* a loosely organized association of "educated" surgeons, which was destined to play an important role in the history of surgery.

Following Lanfranc's death, his teachings were carried on by Henri de Mondeville, the first renowned native-born French surgeon. De Mondeville was raised in Normandy, studied in Montpellier and Paris, and served as a surgeon to Philip IV and his successor Louis X. Much like Lanfranc, de Mondeville was a bold but practical surgeon who crusaded for the respectability of surgery as an honorable craft. He constantly chided the Church and its hierarchy to explain how, if priest/physicians were expected to take care of all manner of illness, could these men not practice both medicine and surgery?

---

* According to popular lore, Cosmas and his twin, Damian, were the youngest of five brothers who belonged to a Christian family of some distinction in the Roman province of Syria in the fourth century AD. The twins were traveling physicians who gave their services freely to those in need. During the persecution of the Christians that occurred in the reign of Emperor Diocletian, Cosmas and Damian were tortured and beheaded. They soon received sainthood for what were regarded as miraculous medical and surgical cures and have since been considered the major patron saints of physicians and surgeons.

De Mondeville was particularly blunt in his contempt for his contemporaries and the way they treated wounds. Like Theodoric, he fiercely opposed the Hippocratic-Galenic conviction that the presence of pus was an essential element in the process of wound healing. De Mondeville insisted that pus was not only unnecessary but also dangerous to a patient's recovery. His advice was simple: wash a wound clean and control bleeding by styptics or compression of the blood vessels. The clamor that followed his modest suggestion is a striking example of two related and recurrent themes in the history of surgery, gratuitous hostility toward a contemporary/rival and the dismissal of surgical advances that contradict deeply held, often-erroneous views. As de Mondeville explained:

> It is rather dangerous for a surgeon to operate differently than is the custom of the other surgeons. I have experienced this in the treatment of wounds. . . . I have suffered the disdain and shameful words on the parts of laymen and of our colleagues, the surgeons; and even threats and dangers . . . at each change of dressing. I have endured disputes and words so violent that half-vanquished and fatigued with all the opposition, I would have been close to renouncing this treatment and abandoning it entirely, had it not been for the support of other personages who have seen wounds cared for in the camps by my method.[7]

A far cry from the colorful personality of de Mondeville but, nonetheless, his successor in advancing French surgery was Guy de Chauliac, an erudite and sober cleric who studied medicine and surgery in Toulouse, Montpellier, and Paris. He eventually settled in Avignon, where he served as personal physician/surgeon to Popes Clement VI, Innocent VI, and Urban V. Avignon, with its imposing edifice the Palace of the Popes, contained a superb papal library. De Chauliac had ready access to all the great medical works of past civilizations. The availability of this literary treasure led him, during the mid-fourteenth century, to write his own *Chirurgia Magna*, a masterpiece of surgical erudition, with over thirty-three hundred references to more than one hundred authors, almost nine hundred quotations from Galen, and a thorough review of the history of surgery. De Chauliac was considered a skilled technician and, like de Mondeville, called for surgery to be taken out of the hands of the uneducated and itinerant. Unlike his other predecessor Lanfranc, de Chauliac's standing in the Church provided authority to his surgical teachings. De Chauliac's views concerning the responsibilities of the surgeon and the needs of his patients, along with his teachings in *Chirurgia Magna*, dominated French surgery and Western Medicine for the next three centuries.

* * *

At the start of the thirteenth century, the practice of surgery in Paris was in the hands of two classes of individuals who were at constant odds with each other, the large group of illiterate barber-surgeons and a smaller faction of "educated" surgeons. As time passed and the number of men (or women) who performed surgical procedures and their technical abilities rose, each side recognized a growing necessity to protect their economic and social interests. Around AD 1270, these concerns were partially addressed when Louis IX granted his approval for the "educated" surgeons of Paris to meet as a loose confederation and affiliate themselves with the newly constructed parish church of Saints Cosmas and Damian, located in the city's academic enclave, home to the University of Paris. The move to the educational district was an attempt by these knife bearers to gain quasi-scholastic status by appearing to be members of the medical faculty at the university. They were not.

In AD 1311 aware of the increasingly chaotic state of affairs between the "educated" surgeons and the "uneducated" barber-surgeons, Philip IV decreed that only individuals who underwent an examination administered from a royally authorized source would be allowed to practice surgery in Paris. Without discussing the situation with their rivals, members of the College of Saints Cosmas and Damian usurped the royal order and began testing for clinical proficiency. As heightened jealousies and strife continued to mark the city's surgical scene, an informal association of barber-surgeons arose to safeguard their rights. Paralleling the "educated" surgeons' goals to attain or at least maintain the semblance of university recognition, the barber-surgeons had their own notions on how to enter the ranks of recognized scalpel wielders. In AD 1372, they obtained, from Charles V (through the intermediary of his personal barber-surgeon), their own charter. This royal edict sanctioned their professional ambitions and granted them official recognition as a Guild of Barber-Surgeons. Most important, the surgeons of the College of Saints Cosmas and Damian were warned not to hinder the development of the Guild of Barber-Surgeons.

Not unexpectedly, the surgeons of the College and the barber-surgeons of the Guild clashed. These arguments intensified as the growing number of barber-surgeons supplanted the smaller faction of surgeons in performing surgical operations, particularly bloodletting. Suspicions abounded, egos were bruised, as the ever-changing discords and liaisons between these two groups reflected the growing number of individuals who performed surgical procedures. Still, surgery remained a bloody and meddlesome affair, but sensible men among the two surgical societies no doubt understood that the infighting and jealousies could lead to nothing but regrets and troubles. The growing efforts to strive for some form of unity presaged the Renaissance and the eventual maturation of modern surgical thought.

PART II

FOUNDATIONS

5.

THE HUMAN
ROAD MAP

A chirurgien should have three diverse properties in his person. That is to say, a heart as the heart of a lion, his eyes like the eyes of a hawk, and his hands as the hands of a woman.

John Halle, *Historiall Expostulation*, 1565

Can honor set to a leg? No. Or an arm? No.
Or take away the grief of a wound? No.
Honor hath no skill in surgery then? No.

William Shakespeare, *Henry IV*, c. 1597

By the fifteenth century, surgery was being freed from the shackles brought on by the mistranslations of Galen and Hippocrates as well as the stifling influence of the Church and its bans on human dissection and surgical operations. Despite surgery's reawakening, in the absence of a working knowledge of anatomy and an inability to control the triumvirate of bleeding, infection, and pain, the scope of a knife bearer's work was limited. Surgery was inevitably a last resort, performed only for matters of life and death. Moreover, those few patients who underwent a surgical operation suffered through a truly frightening ordeal. In the direst of medical straits, they were fully conscious and restrained with blood-encrusted leather straps or by the hands of assistants as their flesh was opened with a dull and rusty scalpel. It made no difference whether the procedure was performed in the grimy room of a barber's shop or a grand chamber in a king's castle; spasms of pain racked the patients while the walls echoed their unworldly screams.

When the individuals who called themselves surgeons performed an operation it was strictly for the cure of an ailment that was located externally, on, or just beneath the skin: to enter the abdomen was a foolhardy venture, while opening the chest, joints, and skull was even more reckless. Conversely, medical treatment dealt mostly with "internal" problems. Hence, the present-day terms "internal medicine" and "internist."

Regardless of the limited and terrifying nature of surgical intervention, operative surgery in the prescientific era was considered a valued therapy. Despite their narrow technical and therapeutic appeal in performing procedures largely limited to the body's surface (e.g., amputations, superficial tumor removal, setting fractures, teeth extraction, et cetera), surgeons were guided by objective findings. Knife bearers could physically perceive the problem they addressed. Individuals who practiced medicine rendered care in a more subjective manner, generally for illnesses whose causes were neither seen nor understood (e.g., anemia, emphysema, hepatitis, syphilis, et cetera). Not until the nineteenth century would advances in pathology and physiology provide "internists" with objective evidence more closely approximating that of surgeons. They were no longer surrounded by a dense diagnostic and therapeutic fog.

Fifteenth- and sixteenth-century surgeons did not await the diagnostic and pathological/physiological revolution needed by physicians. Despite surgery's imperfect knowledge and hard-nosed amputation/extirpation approach to disease, much like a broken clock that shows the correct time twice a day, surgeons occasionally cured, always with brutal self-confidence. What surgery needed for its further advancement was the elucidation of four basic but crucial clinical fundamentals: 1) an understanding of human anatomy; 2) the ability to control bleeding; 3) minimizing the risk of infection; and 4) reducing pain. Taken together, these four issues were more critical than advancing the mechanics involved in a surgical operation. Without these foundational elements, mere technical improvements in surgical technique were doomed to failure. And, like Alexandre Dumas's musketeers' creed, "All for one and one for all, united we stand, divided we fall," the four fundamentals had to work in concert for an operation to succeed. None could stand alone.

The first two, a knowledge of human anatomy and a way to contain hemorrhage, began to be resolved in the mid-sixteenth century. Without an anatomical road map to serve as a guide, scalpel wielders were stymied in making technical decisions. But even with such detailed information, surgeons need to see where they are headed. Bleeding floods and obscures the structural roadway and makes forward progress difficult, if not impossible. The craft of surgery advanced no further until the advent of modern anesthesia in the late 1840s. The accessibility of pain-free procedures meant that haste in the operating room was no longer a surgeon's prime concern. Though the burden of discomfort was relieved, the growth of surgery remained stalled for several more decades until the grave problem of postoperative infection was resolved with the discovery of germs followed by an understanding of the principles of antisepsis. Not until the four foundational elements were in place could surgery blossom as a modern science and bring about the clinical triumphs and socioeconomic initiatives that promoted professionalization and specialization.

* * *

The Renaissance—the magnificent parade of the arts, humanities, natural sciences, and social sciences that occurred from the fourteenth to the seventeenth century in western Europe—marked the transition from the Middle Ages to modern civilization. It was spurred by a revival of scholasticism that looked to improve the secular world through the rebirth of ancient concepts integrated with novel approaches to everyday dilemmas. From the invention of the pivot compass that allowed mariners such as Columbus, Hudson, Magellan, and Verrazzano to navigate their ships without reference to the stars, or the shift toward realism in the arts, as noted in the paintings of Botticelli, El Greco, Raphael, and Titian, and the written works of Cervantes, Donne, Marlowe, and Rabelais, humanism and intellectualism guided the Renaissance.

These new attitudes were particularly apparent in the sciences, where long-standing shibboleths were brought to an end. Copernicus reconnoitered our place in the universe by placing the sun, rather than the Earth, at the center of the solar system; Mercator drew his map of the world with its location of the continents. An eagerness to question and seek new knowledge had a vast impact on the development of surgery, fueled by the invention of the printing press and widespread use of gunpowder.

Few substances had a greater effect on civilization than gunpowder, an explosive mixture of charcoal, potassium nitrate (saltpeter), and sulphur. It altered the art of warfare and affected the whole fabric of society. Gunpowder was introduced into Europe in the mid-thirteenth century and warfare turned deadlier and injuries more dreadful, conspicuous for their staggering amount of blood and tissue loss. Because of surgeons' lack of knowledge about anatomy and their inability to control bleeding (let alone infection and pain), they were less than effective as they treated awful wounds.

It was not until the mid-sixteenth century that a detailed understanding of the structure of the human body came about largely due to the repudiation of Galenism by Philippus Aureolus Theophrastus Bombastus von Hohenheim (aka Paracelsus) followed by the anatomical studies of Andreas Vesalius and their dissemination owing to the invention of the moveable-type printing press. There is no certainty as to the date of the creation, or the name of the discoverer, of moveable components used to print books and documents. However, Johannes Gutenberg, a goldsmith from Mainz, Germany, is regarded as the strongest claimant to the honor. Around 1440, Gutenberg devised a brass hand mold that allowed individual letters and punctuation marks to be cast out of metal. Gutenberg combined his moveable type with two other important innovations of his own, a hand-mechanized printing press and a viscous oil-based ink that made it possible to print on paper and parchment. Within a half century of Gutenberg's breakthrough, printing businesses could be found throughout Europe. Printed books and documents were less costly to produce than handwritten manuscripts and allowed texts to be easily copied, with fewer errors. The demand for printed volumes was immense and led to a use of vernacular dialects (i.e., French, German, Italian, Spanish, et cetera) in books and a decline in Latin's status.*

---

* A key aspect of early book printing was the codex, a book-style layout consisting of bound sheets of paper, papyrus, or parchment with handwritten contents. By the start of the Middle Ages, the codex had replaced the handwritten scroll—the leading book form in the ancient world—and it is considered the most important development in the history of the book prior to printing itself. This is understandable because codices held a number of practical advantages over scrolls: compactness, convenience of reading by turning pages, and less cost since both sides of a leaf could be written on. The earliest printed books appeared in the mid-fifteenth century; works on Medicine were not published until several decades later. This meant that the written efforts discussed in earlier chapters (e.g., Hippocrates's *Corpus Hippocraticum*, Paul of Aegina's *Epitome Medicae Libri Septem*, or Roger of Salerno's *Practica Chirurgiae*, et cetera) were not available in printed form, if ever, until centuries after the deaths of their authors. For example, in 1478 Celsus's *De Medicina* first became available in printed book format, fifteen centuries after the manuscript was initially composed, while de Chauliac's *Chirurgia Magna* was written in 1363 but not published until 1490.

* * *

Books on Medicine largely ignored religious dogmas and specious ideologies and promoted new relations between society and the healing arts as they focused on solving ordinary medical and surgical problems. This was particularly evident in the activities and writings of Paracelsus (it was said he chose his nom de plume to indicate intellectual superiority over the ancient Roman Encyclopedist Celsus), a controversial figure but among the most original medical thinkers of his century. Paracelsus had an unconventional education far removed from that era's mainstream university curriculum, including time spent in the mines and metallurgical laboratories in the Tyrolean countryside. Whether Paracelsus ever obtained "formal" medical education and training is an open question. His detractors questioned his right to title himself Doctor of Medicine, but none could gainsay his vast knowledge of medicine, surgery, and health-related folklore. He was also familiar with alchemy, astrology, and other occult sciences. Paracelsus was assertive, clever, insolent, and more than willing to denounce long-standing traditions as he emerged as the medical establishment's most prominent faultfinder:

> When I saw that nothing resulted from medical practice but pain, killing and laming, I decided to abandon this miserable art and seek the truth elsewhere.[1]

Paracelsus launched a one-man campaign against what he considered stagnant medical and surgical practices. When lecturing before a medical faculty, he showed his disdain by not wearing a scholar's robe but an alchemist's leather smock. In a complete break with academic pretense, Paracelsus refused to lecture in Latin, the language of the educated elite, and only used colloquial German. Some considered Paracelsus a madman as he went from city to city burning and condemning the books of his rivals. Whether chimera or clairvoyant, his commitment to discovering the truth through observation and research was unusual and enlightening.

Paracelsus's greatest scorn was directed at the Greek physician and philosopher of the second century AD, Galen: "I will tell you, one hair on my neck knows more . . . and my shoe-buckles contain more wisdom than . . . Galen."[2] The two men were each other's doppelgangers. They were gadflies, boastful, boorish, intemperate, unwilling to compromise, and led lives filled with conflict and wanderlust. They were also prolific writers and masterful at exposing "errors" and stirring debate.

Nowhere was this more evident than in Paracelsus's denunciation of the long-dead Greek's studies on anatomy. At the start of the Renaissance, Galen's influence was so powerful that when doctors began to routinely perform human dissections and discovered stark differences between his pronouncements and their observations, they were flummoxed. In the over one thousand years since his passing, it was either forgotten or overlooked that Galen's anatomical discoveries were based on ape and other animal dissections. Physicians, not knowing what to make of these discrepancies, even suggested that the inconsistencies were visible proof that human anatomy had changed since the days of Galen. Paracelsus refused to accept such outlandish reasoning. He tried to convince everyone that Galen was wrong and human anatomy needed to be more accurately studied:

> [Surgeons] should know the make-up of man, where the bones and other structures lie and their relation to each other. If you do not know these things, how can you diagnose injuries or know how to put them right? It is not enough that you know the externals, you must know the internals better than the externals.... The surgeons must know human anatomy and not be like the barber or bather who knows no more than the butcher who cuts, trims and separates his meat.[3]

* * *

The growing interest in man's body was especially promoted by painters and sculptors; they gathered around anatomists who dissected human bodies. The artists sought greater realism in their depiction of the human form, and an understanding of bones, muscles, nerves, and deeper body parts afforded insight into proportion and structure. As early as 1490, Leonardo da Vinci planned an atlas of anatomical drawings and produced over 750 sketches of human anatomy (some contain anatomical errors based on Galen's musings), ranging from the fetus in utero to the smallest of blood vessels and everything in between. The untimely death of the anatomist that da Vinci worked with brought an end to the project before it could be published. Da Vinci's remarkable illustrations and notes were filed away and vanished from view. In the 1600s, almost six hundred of the surviving pictures were bound and ended up in the possession of the English Crown (where they remain as part of the British Royal Collection Trust).

Albrecht Dürer and Michelangelo also studied with anatomists. Dürer's work on human proportions, *Vier Bücher von menschlicher Proportion* (Four books on human proportion) was the first instance in which anthropometry (i.e., the scientific study of the measurements of the body) was used to illustrate human esthetics. As discerning as da Vinci, Dürer, and Michelangelo were as artists, they showed little academic interest in whether their observations matched the anatomical musings of Galen. Despite the discrepancies, their work fostered popularity in human dissection, especially as it related to Medicine. This interest was furthered during the fifteenth and sixteenth centuries, when Church officials reversed their long-standing ban against human dissection. As physician/anatomists increasingly collaborated with artists, the transition from the primitive illustrations of the medieval era to the realistic drawings of the Renaissance had an important impact on the development of surgery.

To the forefront of the revolution in anatomical studies stepped Vesalius with his celebrated treatise, *De Humani Corporis Fabrica Libri Septem* (On the fabric of the human body), one of the great treasures of Western civilization and among the most important books in the history of Medicine. Composed in 1543, when the author was twenty-nine years old, the *Fabrica*, with its blending of art, medicine, and typography, was a cornerstone of the Scientific Revolution and helped overturn the stifling dogma of Galenism by promoting the accurate study of the human body.

* * *

I met Walter on my opening day of medical school. There was no formal introduction, no handshake, no hello, no nod, just a frozen half smile. He was a short, wizened seventy-eight-year-old with thinning grayish hair, jug ears, a bulbous nose, and scruffy facial stubble. His teeth were decayed and his skinny arms and legs were set off against a protuberant abdomen. Walter had stubby fingers, enlarged knuckles, and nails that were splintered and dirty. His toes were no better off, curled and pushed to the side, ending in hornlike tangles. Walter's skin was hardened and wrinkled and covered with age spots, scars, and tattoos. It had a yellowish tint, as did the whites of his eyes. Physical appearance aside, Walter was special, for he was my cadaver.

For doctors-to-be, their first encounter with a cadaver (I had never seen a dead body before) can be a time of high anxiety. After all, to willfully take apart a human body is far from normal. From the psychological concerns that accompany the dismemberment of a human being to the distinctive odor of the chemicals that preserve cadavers—fruity and foul, somewhere between spoiled juice and stale urine (vestiges of the smell are imprisoned in my olfactory nerves)—medical students routinely name their cadavers as a way to deflect the strangeness of the situation. In Walter's case, a nickname was not necessary. A paper tag that provided his identity and told of his medical woes had been inadvertently left dangling from one of his toes. Walter was his real name and his life must not have been pleasant. He suffered from alcoholism, cirrhosis, emphysema, and heart disease and had died eight months earlier in one of Missouri's old soldiers' homes.

As disquieting as my first days in the anatomy lab were, I was enthralled with the structure of the body, its blueprint and its intricacies. Each detail of the human form, from the microscopic to the macroscopic, became familiar and known by name and touch. Every organ, every space, every tissue, was inspected and studied. I learned a new vocabulary of directional terms for the body: "medial" meant toward the midline and "lateral" away from the midline (e.g., the big toe is located on the medial side of the foot while the little toe is located on the lateral side of the foot). "Proximal" was toward the point of origin and "distal" away from the point of origin (e.g., the proximal end of the arm joins the shoulder while the distal end of the arm ends in the fingers). There were words for position; a body that is lying down is either "prone" (facedown) or "supine" (faceup). Even more bewildering, "right" and "left" were no longer my right and left, but Walter's right and left.

Beyond the fascination of learning the human road map and acquiring a new language, I enjoyed working with my hands and how competent they felt when holding a scalpel and scissor. For the surgeon-in-training, dissection of a human body provides an appreciation of three-dimensional anatomy unlike any other method of study. The thrill of integrating my fingers and brain became one of the driving forces that affirmed my decision to become a surgeon.

The anatomy lab was a large nondescript space with about two dozen metal tables on which the cadavers lay enclosed in plastic body bags. The professors and their assistants circulated through the room and guided us as we dismantled Walter.

Body cavity by body cavity, extremity by extremity, organ by organ, Walter slowly vanished from view and in six months he was gone.

In looking back, what impressed me about the experience, besides its inherent sanctity, was how my four-person dissection group examined the human body like Vesalius, over four centuries earlier. Distinct from pre-Vesalian dissections, there was no haughty physician sitting on high reciting passages from a codex overflowing with Galenic dogma, while an illiterate barber-surgeon dissected the cadaver. Back then, the discarded tissues were fed to a nearby pack of ravenous dogs. Since the pre-Vesalian doctor never deigned to move from his professorial chair and examine the organs on view, none of the assembled knew if what they were shown matched the reading.

Vesalius did away with this nonsensical approach to studying anatomy. He asserted that dissection had to be completed hands-on, by doctors themselves, a direct repudiation of the long-standing conviction that it was a loathsome task to be performed only by individuals from the lowest of social classes. How this maverick genius accomplished his objective is one of the most critical and engaging stories in the history of surgery.

* * *

Born in Brussels on New Year's Eve in 1514, Vesalius was a member of a well-to-do family who had extensive connections to the House of Burgundy and the Holy Roman Emperor's court, especially that of Charles V.* Vesalius studied medicine and surgery in Paris, where he listened to men who fully believed in Galenism; they relied on ancient handwritten manuscripts, rather than actual dissection, to teach anatomy. Frustrated by their ineptitude, Vesalius questioned the legacy of Galen and the manner in which anatomy was presented. In full scholarly revolt, Vesalius went about creating his own human road map. He searched graveyards for bodies and

---

* The Holy Roman Empire was neither "holy" (its leader was not crowned by the Pope) nor "Roman" (the territory was far from Rome). What began as a feudal monarchy during the Middle Ages became a complex of ever-changing lands centered on the Kingdom of Germany and Bohemia. It was an "empire" in name only because the territories it covered were mostly independent entities (duchies, imperial cities, principalities, and other types of domains) and the emperor was elected by the bishops, lords, magistrates, and princes of these enclaves. The Holy Roman Empire was dissolved during the Napoleonic Wars in 1806.

smuggled the decomposing remains back to Paris. When there was little of interest in the burial grounds, Vesalius visited the charnel houses, where bones exhumed from various cemeteries were collected. Working in private and mostly self-taught, he became highly skilled in human dissection.

Vesalius's efforts were interrupted by the outbreak of war between France and the Holy Roman Empire. As a citizen of the empire, he was compelled to return to Belgium, where he resumed his medical studies and briefly served as a surgeon in the army of Charles V. While in school in Leuven, he rummaged for bodies and bones in a field outside the city's gates, a place where executed criminals were left to hang and rot. Vesalius described how he once shimmied up a gibbet's wooden support, reached over its crosspiece, and hurriedly cut down a decaying corpse:

> The bones were entirely bare, held together by the ligaments alone.... I pulled off the femur from the hip bone. While tugging at the specimen, the scapula together with the arms and hands also followed, although the fingers of one hand and one foot were missing. After I had brought the legs and arms home in secret and successive trips (leaving the head behind with the entire trunk of the body), I allowed myself to be shut out of the city in the evening in order to obtain the thorax which was firmly held by a chain. I was burning with so great a desire ... that I was not afraid to snatch in the middle of the night what I so longed for.[4]

In 1537, after receiving his baccalaureate, Vesalius moved to Padua, where he believed there were more opportunities at that city's university for studying anatomy and obtaining a doctorate of medicine. His reputation must have preceded him because, within six months, Vesalius received his doctoral degree and was appointed to the faculty as professor of surgery, a position that required the teaching of anatomy. Vesalius's desire to demonstrate new methods of learning was apparent when he performed a series of cadaver dissections for the townspeople of Padua. Nothing that resembled Vesalius's style of study had ever been seen. The fact that the new professor rose from his seat to personally inspect and dissect the cadaver was highly unusual. Vesalius was Medicine's newest "all-in-one" anatomist, demonstrator, and dissector, and his "hands-on" principle remains his most lasting contribution to Medicine.

For his students, Vesalius located bones and internal organs by outlining their positions on the cadaver's skin and provided diagrams that explained structure and function. He made certain there was no disconnect between what was described and what was displayed. In 1538, he had six of his teaching illustrations published as woodcuts; *Tabulae Anatomicae Sex* are the earliest realistic anatomical illustrations specifically designed for physicians and surgeons-in-training. They were an immediate success, as shown by the numerous plagiarisms that soon appeared; in testimony to their popularity and being literally used out of existence, only two complete sets of the original prints have survived (one in the Bibliotheca Nazionale Marciana in Venice and the other in the Hunterian Collection at the University of Glasgow).

Vesalius's growing familiarity with human anatomy convinced him that many of Galen's assertions were incorrect; animal studies could not be substituted for human studies. "I am quite certain," he wrote:

> on the basis of the art of dissection as now reborn combined with a careful reading of Galen's works . . . that he himself had never cut open a human body and furthermore that, deceived by his apes . . . granted the infinite multiplicity of differences between the organs of the human and the simian bodies, he yet noticed none of them.[5]

As Vesalius grew more critical of Galen's failures, he prepared a new book on the complete human anatomy. For the first time, accurate drawings of the body were closely integrated with a written text. Vesalius's intent was to show the importance of observation-based dissections of human bodies and make the readers feel as if they were standing at his shoulder so they could see and replicate his methods.

Vesalius clearly believed the *Fabrica* would be a landmark in the history of Medicine; he paid meticulous attention to every detail of the book's making. He was surgeon-like with his dissections as he delicately stripped away tissue layer after tissue layer to reveal the underlying structures. Inch by inch, skin was flayed, bones stripped, muscles freed, and organs opened. Vesalius's exposure of human architecture through meticulous drawings was the Renaissance version of a modern CAT or MRI scan.

The brilliance of Vesalius lay not only in the precision of his dissections but also in his decision to enlist artists to produce illustrations based directly on his work. Never before had anatomical drawings been so accurately or straightforwardly linked with a descriptive text: Vesalius employed an elaborate system of cross-references between pictures and words. The illustrations were artistically beautiful (e.g., many were set against backgrounds of Paduan landscape), with innumerable anatomical peculiarities and variations.

Vesalius believed that Medicine should be viewed as a whole, another of his disagreements with Galen, who had called for the separation of medicine and surgery. Vesalius aired his concerns in the preface to the *Fabrica*:

> The art of medicine was torn in pieces long ago, when one of its basic instruments, the technique of surgery, fell into neglect and was, as it were, handed over to laymen and people with no knowledge of the discipline. . . . It is this low opinion that the common people have of surgery that is the main obstacle to our employing in this age the whole art of healing. . . . By this the whole of mankind (to put it bluntly) is the loser. . . . They have thus created endless toil for the most learned men . . . who endeavor to restore this part of the art to its former glory.[6]

Like most revolutionary works, the *Fabrica* attracted critics who railed at its defiance of Galenism. To these detractors, Vesalius responded with intemperate counterattacks. One year after the book's publication, whether due to professional frustrations or, perhaps, an incipient mental breakdown (he burned several unpublished manuscripts in public), a disillusioned Vesalius resigned his faculty position and became a surgeon to the court of Charles V and his son Philip II. No longer an academician but a full-time practitioner, Vesalius used the new position to further his clinical skills, particularly in surgery; among his successes, he completed a trephination of the skull on Philip II's son for bleeding in the brain secondary to head trauma suffered from a fall down a flight of stairs.

In 1558, Charles V died and Philip II, now King of Spain, transferred his court from Brussels to Madrid and invited Vesalius to accompany him. However, Spanish physicians turned on Vesalius, whom they considered a foreign upstart, especially when it came to his surgical ways. Conversely, Vesalius was angered when he learned that a Spanish anatomist had published a book that knowingly plagiarized the *Fabrica*'s text and illustrations. Several years later, a still angry Vesalius petitioned Philip II to allow him to leave the country to pursue outside ventures, including a possible return to his former academic position at the university in Padua.

In 1564, Vesalius departed Spain and set out on a pilgrimage for the Holy Land. Why he sought out Jerusalem is lost to history. Some have speculated that Vesalius had troubles with authorities of the Spanish Inquisition. Others say Vesalius attempted to dissect a presumably dead Spanish noblewoman who awoke at the first slice of her skin. Whatever the reason, the voyage was the last that Vesalius would take. During the crossing of the Mediterranean Sea, his ship encountered a violent storm and was left adrift with little food and water. Days later, the vessel was wrecked and Vesalius was washed ashore on the small Peloponnesian island of Zákinthos. There the not-quite-fifty-year-old succumbed to exposure and starvation. Alone and probably unknown, Vesalius, the individual who unlocked the door to human anatomy, was buried in what is now an unmarked grave.

Vesalius's contribution concerning the first of the four clinical fundamentals necessary to perform a safe surgical operation, an understanding of human anatomy, set a pathway toward the beginnings of modern surgery. At the same time, a contemporary of his was diligently at work resolving the second of the rudiments, the ability to control bleeding.

6.

TO STOP THE
FLOW

The wound that bleedeth inward is most dangerous.

John Lyly, *Euphues*, 1578

*Let us proceed with good method and good conscience in all our opera-
tions, which are of such great consequence, and not undertake them for
our profit but to aid the poor patients, using charity toward them.*

Pierre Franco, *Traité des Hernies*, 1561

A statue, special to the world of surgery, is located in the Plaza of Eleventh
November, the central square of Laval, France, a quaint town, two hundred
miles southwest of Paris. Pierre-Jean David (aka David d'Angers) fashioned a man
standing touching his goateed chin with his right hand, while his left arm falls
toward an arquebus (i.e., an early type of portable gun) and a stack of medical books
on which rest a collection of surgical instruments. When the monument was dedicated in 1840, flags waved under a blue sky, military troops paraded to the beat of
field drums, choirs sang, musicians played, and thousands of French citizens lined
the streets in an impressive display of gratitude and patriotism. Throughout the day,
civil authorities gave speeches, including a dithyramb that saluted the honoree as
"humble of heart, grand in genius," while scholars told of how by "the strength of his
spirit, the skill of his hands, the generosity of his heart, the height of his principles . . .
[he] could be the equal of the greatest and the best men whom the world had born."[1]

What makes this statue significant for surgeons, and why did thousands of citizens travel to Laval to show their appreciation of the long-dead honoree? The history of the sculpture provides answers. The monument was commissioned by the French government and paid for through donations from a wide array of individuals, ranging from Louis Philippe I, members of his Cabinet, fellows of the Royal Academy of Medicine, and faculty of the University of Medicine in Paris to thousands of ordinary folks. The citizens of France were honoring a surgeon who had died two hundred and fifty years before.

Ambroise Paré, born near Laval, was the most celebrated surgeon of the Renaissance. He severed the final link between the surgical dogma of the ancients and the scientific drive toward modernity. Moreover, Paré solved the crucial second element to surgery's development, the control of bleeding. Whether involved in the rigors of a military campaign, the business of a private surgical practice, or the intrigue of a royal court, Paré was set apart from his contemporaries by his everyday show of ingenuity, sensibility, and courage to act independently against existing doctrine.

Paré's influence on surgery went beyond "mere" technical achievements. He brought a paradigm shift in how surgeons think and act. Compassion and a respect for the healing power of nature were his hallmark. "Both God and Nature constantly remind the surgeon," wrote Paré:

> no matter how poor, in a given case, the prospect of a cure may seem, he should not for one moment cease doing his full duty; for God and Nature often accomplish what the surgeon believes to be impossible.[2]

Over a long and productive life, Paré became the most admired surgeon of his generation and was appointed surgeon-in-chief to four successive kings of France (Henry II, Francis II, Charles IX, and Henry III). If a pantheon existed to honor the surgical greats, a bust of Paré (along with one of Vesalius) would occupy its main apse.

* * *

There is little certainty about Paré's early years other than that his parents were poor and he was indentured to a series of barber-surgeons in the province of Maine (bordered by Normandy on the north, Brittany on the west, and the Loire River valley to the south). As to why barber-surgeons, an apocryphal story is that Paré's father was a barber-surgeon and valet to the Count of Laval and wanted his son to continue the family tradition. There might be some truth to this account because it is known that Paré's brother was a barber-surgeon and their sister was married to a Parisian barber-surgeon. What is indisputable is that in his late teenage years Paré moved from the countryside to Paris to seek further training. He attended lectures, performed autopsies, and served as an assistant to the barber-surgeons who worked at the Hôtel-Dieu, the large city hospital near the Notre Dame Cathedral on the Île de la Cité.

Paré's duties were ill defined, but surgical work in the early sixteenth century was generally mundane: blood let, fractures set, injuries treated, rotten teeth pulled, venereal sores cauterized, et cetera. Paré excelled and, after several years, he completed the training necessary for admission to the Guild of Barber-Surgeons. However, Paré postponed his request for membership, because he lacked the funds for the multi-day examination or even simple licensure fees. Instead, the twenty-six-year-old joined René de Montjean, a colonel-general of the French infantry, as his personal surgeon and trekked off to the battlefields of northern Italy.

War has always benefited surgeons. Battlegrounds, with their vast numbers and wide variety of wounded, provide intensive opportunities for the education and training of men who practice surgery. Paré, probably more than any other scalpel wielder of the Renaissance, gained his most profound surgical insights during the numerous armed conflicts that embroiled Europe. These struggles were politically convoluted and physically ferocious, particularly the series of Italian Wars between the kings of France and the emperors of the Holy Roman Empire that enmeshed many of the countries of western Europe along with the Ottoman Empire.*

---

* The Ottoman Empire was founded at the end of the thirteenth century in what is present-day Turkey. A century later, the Ottomans crossed into Europe and captured the Balkans, thus transforming their holdings into a transcontinental empire. In 1453, the Ottomans ended the Byzantine Empire with their conquest of Constantinople (the city would be renamed Istanbul). Over time, the empire became a multinational kingdom that included parts of central and southeast Europe, the Caucasus, western Asia, and North Africa and was at the center of relations between the Eastern and Western worlds for almost six centuries. The Ottoman Empire was dismantled following its defeat as a member of the Central Powers (Austria-Hungary, Bulgaria, and Germany) by the Allies (Britain, France, Italy, Russia, and the United States) in World War I.

* * *

When Paré left for the Italian War of 1536–1538, he joined an army without protocols for treating the wounded. This lack of concern was the era's putative military standard. If a solder was badly injured and no longer capable of keeping up with the army's movements, he was simply left behind to survive by his own devices. The absence of logistics occurred because Renaissance-era troops were controlled not so much by the mandate of a king but the direction of individual aristocrats, each with his own set of plans and clique of supporters who functioned as quasi-independent units. The consequence was an army that functioned more as a mob, characterized by its serpentine-like procession of often-drunken men marauding their way through the countryside with their arquebuses, cannons, lances, maces, and swords, accompanied by prostitutes, slaves, and a trailing parade of cows, goats, and pigs. In the middle of this chaos was Paré, a self-described "fresh-water soldier,"[3] a tyro with no actual experience treating battlefield injuries.

Shortly after French troops swept into northern Italy, Paré received a swift introduction to the horrors of war. At the siege of Turin, after riding what he described as "rough-shod over the dead bodies lying on the roadway," Paré came upon three soldiers in a stable who were horribly burned by gunpowder. A fellow combatant asked if anything could be done to save their lives. Paré's reply was a succinct: "No." Without betraying any emotion, the soldier took out his dagger and slashed his comrades' throats. A horrified Paré exclaimed, "You are a wicked man!" The soldier's reply was blunt and simple:

> I pray God that if it should ever be my fate to be situated as these three men . . . there may be somebody at hand who will do to me what I have just done . . . and will save me from a lingering and painful death.[4]

Within days of the mercy killing, Paré, the fledgling surgeon, was confronted with a large number of gunshot wounds that involved extensive burns and loss of skin, bone, and muscles. The general belief among Renaissance-era surgeons was that gunpowder was poisonous and any gunshot injury had to be immediately cleansed in a two-step process: cauterize the tissue with red-hot irons, then flood the area with a gummous-like mixture of boiling oil and herbs. The treatment was also used to staunch bleeding. Not only was the underlying belief in "poisoning by gunpowder" wrong, but the treatment produced unbearable pain and destroyed healthy surrounding flesh. As a novice, Paré initially accepted these notions and came to understand why cauldrons of scalding-hot oil of elders mixed with treacle, a molasses-like liquid, were always at the ready.

One day, the kettles ran dry. With him forced to take desperate measures, Paré's audacity and genius came to the fore. As the more experienced surgeons looked on with skepticism, Paré decided to forego trust in red-hot irons and boiling oil and concocted a salve meant to soothe a wound. He explains:

> At last, I wanted oil, and was constrained, instead thereof, to apply a digestive of yolks of eggs, oil of roses, and turpentine. In the night, I could not sleep in quiet, fearing some default in not cauterizing, and that I should find those to whom I had not used the burning oil, died impoisoned; which made me rise very early to visit them, where, beyond my expectation, I found those to whom I had applied my digestive medicine, to feel little pain, and their wounds without inflammation, having rested reasonably well that night. The others, to whom was used the burning oil, I found feverish, with great pain about the edges of their wounds. And then I resolved with myself, never so cruelly to burn poor men wounded with gun-shot. . . . See, then, how I have learned to dress wounds made with gun-shot, not by books.[5]

At a nascent stage in Paré's professional life, this singular display of resourcefulness marked him as special. Indeed, following the battles in northern Italy, an admirer remarked to de Montjean, "Thou hast a surgeon young in age, but he is old in knowledge and experience: take good care of him, for he will do thee service and honor."[6] In 1539, de Montjean died and a war-weary Paré returned to Paris. The money he earned on the battlefield enabled him to establish a private surgical practice and sit for the qualifying examination to the Guild of Barber-Surgeons. Paré's license was granted, and he married and settled down as a barber-surgeon at Pont Saint-Michel on the left bank of the Seine (an area adjacent to the present-day place Saint-Michel, sandwiched between the quai des Grands Augustins and rue de l'Hirondelle).

Three years later, war again broke out between Francis I of France and Charles V of the Holy Roman Empire. René I de Rohan, a viscount of lands in Brittany, implored Paré to join him in the conflict as his personal surgeon. Paré acquiesced and was shortly on the front lines in Perpignan, a southern French city near the Mediterranean coast and the border with Spain, when the Grand Master of the French Artillery was hit in the shoulder by a shot from an arquebus. Several surgeons tried unsuccessfully to locate the bullet. In frustration, the Grand Master demanded that Paré be consulted because, according to Paré, "he had known of my reputation in Piedmont [Italy]." Paré had the officer stand up and place his body into exactly the same position as when he was struck. "I found the ball in the flesh," related Paré, "making a little swelling under the shoulder blade. . . . I showed the other surgeons the place where it was and it was taken out . . . the honor remained with me for having found it."[7] As reasonable and straightforward as this maneuver was, the novel idea of reenacting an injury as part of a treatment plan brought Paré considerable acclaim.

When the fighting spread to Boulogne-sur-Mer on the north coast of France, Paré was redeployed. He had just arrived when asked to treat Francis de Lorraine II, Duke of Guise, who had been seriously injured by a lance. The weapon had pierced the skin above de Lorraine's right eye, glanced along his forehead bone, fractured the top of his nose, and continued under the skin to the left side of his face, where it exited below the left ear, near the nape of his neck. The blow was so violent that the shaft of the lance snapped in two, leaving part of the spearhead and several inches of wood firmly wedged in the bones of his face. None in de Lorraine's retinue, including his private surgeons, believed he could live. Even Paré was circumspect in his expectations. Yet, after several weeks of care, including Paré's forcible extraction of the embedded lance using a blacksmith's pincers, de Lorraine survived, notwithstanding a badly scarred face.

Although Paré had numerous surgical triumphs during his military service, de Lorraine's case was decidedly important to his career. The aristocrat was one of the most prominent individuals in France. His first cousin was Henry II, the future King of France, and as boys the two had been raised together. Subsequent to his recovery, de Lorraine was named the Grand Chamberlain of France, a position that made him an influential adviser in state affairs with daily access to the king. Paré's lifesaving treatment of de Lorraine brought him to the attention of the royal court and French nobility.

* * *

When the Italian War of 1542–1546 ended, Paré returned to Paris as a surgical superstar. He was invited to dine with one of the members of the city's Faculty of Medicine, to discuss his recent experiences with battlefield injuries. The physicians of the faculty were university educated in Greek and Latin and healed strictly through the use of herbs and medicines. They were pretentious and considered working with one's hands, vis-à-vis the members of the Guild of Barber-Surgeons or the College of Saints Cosmas and Damian, beneath their dignity and outside the whole of Medicine. However, during the opening decades of the sixteenth century, in an effort to further the scope of their authority, the physicians of the Faculty of Medicine signed contracts with members of the Guild of Barber-Surgeons in which the latter's right to practice surgery was formally recognized. The quid pro quo for the granting of "legitimacy" required the barber-surgeons to restrict their practice to the manual aspects of surgery and treat patients only when a member of the Faculty was present or had offered prior consent. In addition, barber-surgeons acknowledged the university-educated physicians as their superiors and consented to allowing them to proctor examinations for barber-surgeons wishing to obtain "master" status and membership in the Guild.

The barber-surgeons' rivals, the surgeons from the College of Saints Cosmas and Damian, were infuriated at this slight and began a lobbying effort to strengthen their credentials by obtaining full university privileges. Three decades later, Francis I somewhat honored their request and offered quasi-academic recognition that brought higher social status and the right to don a university gown. However, since the College of Saints Cosmas and Damian was still not considered a formal part of the University of Paris, its surgeons did not enjoy a standing commensurate with being on one of the school's senior faculties of law, medicine, or theology.

Paré was well aware of this political rancor, but over dinner with the member of the Faculty of Medicine the discussion was limited to observations about gunpowder, gunshot wounds, and his new treatment plan that used salves instead of red-hot irons and boiling oil. The physician listened and urged Paré to write of his experiences. This advice brought about the publication, in 1545, of Paré's first major book, *The Method of Treating Wounds Made by Arquebuses and Other Firearms*.

Words matter and, in their use, authors reveal themselves and their motives. Paré used his books as ploys to bolster his standing with the French aristocracy.

When *The Method of Treating Wounds* was first published, Paré dedicated it to de Rohan, whom he lavished with praise as *"trés illustre, et trés puissant"* ("very illustrious and very powerful").[8] Seven years later, when the work was revised, de Rohan suggested that Paré's career would be better advanced if the new edition was dedicated to Henry II. The suggestion proved prescient.

Although Paré was considered a barber-surgeon, his writings covered large segments of medicine, and his works, gossipy in spirit, illustrative by design, voluminous in amount, and influential in content, brought his knowledge and skills together. The common thread in his prose was a reverence for life and the belief that every human being deserved care and respect. This conviction is noted in Paré's oft-quoted expression of devotion and piety, *"Je le pansai, Dieu le guérit"* ("I dressed him, God healed him"). That he also interlaced his clinical discussions with stories from his personal life made his books not only educational but also entertaining and led to steady requests for them years after his passing.

In contrast with most other medical and surgical authorities who wrote only in Latin, Paré used the vernacular or everyday language of the masses, French in his case (he had no formal university education and little understanding of Latin). Over time, Paré's books were translated into German, Italian, and Spanish and reached a large audience of physicians and surgeons as well as common folk. An Englishman told of how surgeons throughout Europe "took no other course than that which was delivered by Paré . . . and they esteemed, and admired, and embraced his work alone, above all other books of Surgery."[9]

* * *

In 1552, during the Italian War of 1551–1559, Paré accomplished one of the great advances in the history of surgery. His efforts to have surgeons curtail the use of cauterizing irons and boiling oil to treat wounds had been only partially successful. When the injury was a simple through-and-through gunshot, with no bone involvement or major bleeding, Paré's method of applying a soothing salve worked reasonably well. However, if a bone was shattered along with loss of significant tissue, the standard treatment was immediate amputation. In removing a limb, especially at the level of the thigh, the greatest technical difficulty involves the effective arrest of bleeding from the many large blood vessels divided at the stump. When there is a continuous torrent of blood and no ability to control the hemorrhage, the anatomy is obscured and completion of the amputation becomes a challenge. To contain the bleeding, surgeons had little choice other than to sear the raw amputation stump with red-hot irons and immerse it in a kettle of boiling oil. The pain was terrible and, after a few days, the scab often broke loose and bleeding renewed, which necessitated another round of cautery and oil. The situation was further complicated because without an understanding of germs or antisepsis, wound infections set in, which, combined with the bleeding, left patients in grave danger.

Faced with the problem of uncontrolled bleeding in amputations, Paré sought alternative ways to staunch the hemorrhage. He read of the Greeks' and Romans' use of ligatures to tie small and medium-sized blood vessels, a technique that had been abandoned centuries before. Paré gave it further consideration and worked out some practical details for their application with large blood vessels, including the design of a forceps-like instrument called the *bec de corbin* (crow's beak), a predecessor to the modern hemostat. The device could grasp the severed end of an artery or vein away from the surrounding tissues in which it was imbedded. Once the blood vessel was steadied, a ligature was easily tied around it.

When French troops sieged Damvillers (a village located near the city of Verdun in northeast France), an officer was shot in the leg by a culverin, an early version of the musket. The damage was extensive and Paré was summoned. "I had to finish cutting [it] off," explained Paré, "which I did without applying the hot irons." Several weeks later, Paré returned to Paris with his recovered patient. "I sent him to his house," explained Paré, "merry, with a wooden leg, and he was content saying that he had got off cheap, not to have been miserably burned to stop the blood."[10] This unassuming account relates how Paré solved the second of the four foundational elements needed to successfully complete a surgical operation, the control of bleeding.

*　*　*

The forty-four-year-old Paré returned to Paris a bona fide celebrity, sought after by patients and peers. His books were best sellers. He was admired as the discoverer of key improvements in surgical techniques. Henry II named him his personal surgeon. Paré and his wife—they had one daughter—became philanthropic with their new wealth and supported nieces and nephews as well as poorer families in their Pont Saint-Michel neighborhood. The Parés also purchased a large house at Meudon, then on the outskirts of Paris, which served as a warm-weather retreat with its arbor and courtyard surrounded by vineyards.

Despite the trappings of fame and prosperity, Paré was still treated by the physicians of the Faculty of Medicine and the surgeons of the College of Saints Cosmas and Damian as a poorly educated and upstart barber-surgeon. This professional insult demeaned Paré's achievements and position in French society. The members of the College of Saints Cosmas and Damian soon realized that not having the nation's most powerful and renowned knife bearer on their roster was a public relations fiasco. Not only would Paré's membership bring prestige to their organization and help the College in its long-standing battles with the physicians, but his lobbying efforts on behalf of surgery could help them as much as it did the Guild of Barber-Surgeons. Conversely, Paré understood that to become a member of the College of Saints Cosmas and Damian was to gain a social standing that he did not have as a barber-surgeon.

In 1554, despite the College's statutes that required incoming candidates to have a university education, along with a knowledge of Latin, the directors agreed to forego these requirements and allow Paré to take their entrance examination. During the Latin-based test, Paré gave what was described as "feeble answers, most inelegantly worded." Nevertheless, he was granted his diploma because, according to a contemporary source, "the King wished it."[11] The next day, a reception was held in Paré's honor attended by bishops, lords, physicians, surgeons, and other notables from Parisian society. Henry II was so pleased with the proceedings that he presented Paré with one hundred ecus (gold coins) in honor of his appointment.

The approbation that members of the College of Saints Cosmas and Damian hoped to gain through Paré's admission was immediate. Their rivals from the Faculty of Medicine were hesitant to criticize the king's desires and, for a while, the physicians lessened their public disapproval of surgeons. In turn, Henry II made certain that surgeons had a continuous supply of cadavers to dissect to further their study of human anatomy. Paré was among the first to take advantage of the king's decree and performed dissections for the public as well as his students. He was thoroughly convinced of the importance of understanding anatomy as a prerequisite to practicing surgery and planned to spend his leisure time working on a book on the subject. This timetable was speeded up when Paré was involved in one of the most interesting events in the history of surgery, remarkable for those who were involved in the incident.

In 1559, during a jousting match to celebrate the signing of a peace treaty between Henry II and his once enemy, Philip II, the Holy Roman Emperor, Henry suffered an accidental but devastating head injury. The wooden lance of the king's opponent struck his helmet, shattered into fragments, and impaled Henry II's right eye. Henry was examined by the court physicians who, in view of the ghastliness of the injury, had little to offer. Surgeons searched for retained wood splinters that were thought to have pierced the king's skull but were unable to locate any. Henry II's wife, Catherine de' Medici, ordered the execution of four criminals whose heads were experimented on by having truncheons thrust through their eyes and into their brains in an attempt to ascertain the course of the wood splinters. All to no avail.

Paré was summoned but declared the wound to be mortal. On the fourth day, Henry II became feverish, delirious, and his eye socket began to ooze pus. A distraught Philip II called for his personal surgeon and, shortly, none other than Vesalius arrived. Neither of the surgical greats knew each other. Vesalius concurred that Henry II would not survive. A week later, after suffering the agony of a spreading cellulitis of his face, left-sided body paralysis, and uncontrollable seizures, Henry II died. The autopsy, attended by Paré and Vesalius, showed a large abscess of the brain secondary to the original wound.

The nature of any interactions between Paré and Vesalius remains conjecture. Neither man wrote of their encounter. However, less than two years after the death of Henry II, Paré authored his definitive anatomical text, *Anatomie Universelle du Corps Humain* (Universal anatomy of the human body), in which the influence of Vesalius and his masterpiece, the *Fabrica*, is unquestionable. Throughout Paré's text are dozens of references to Vesalius's writing. Paré's illustrations, although not approaching the brilliance of those in the *Fabrica*, were clearly inspired by the drawings of Vesalius's artists. Because Paré wrote in French and not Latin, his *Anatomie Universelle* played a major role in bringing the anatomical and surgical ideas of Vesalius, who wrote in Latin, to knife bearers with less formal education, especially barber-surgeons.

* * *

After he had served in one military campaign after another, Paré's later years were devoted more to his family and his practice/writing. When Paré's wife died unexpectedly, he soon remarried and went on to have another six children, the last when he was seventy-three years of age. Despite the tumult in his personal life, Paré remained active and prolific:

> I am so determined not to hide the talent it has pleased God to give me in Surgery, which is my calling in this brief life," he wrote, "that the more my days pass away, so much the more I feel driven to work yet harder while they last, to help, if I can, those who shall have to do with me.[12]

In 1575, Paré authored his masterpiece, *The Complete Works of Ambroise Paré, Councilor and First Surgeon to the King*. This compilation of his writings, mixed with autobiographical musings, was so popular that four editions were printed during Paré's lifetime. Their publication also precipitated a literary brouhaha that became a surgical cause célèbre with charges made against Paré ranging from moral indecency to plagiarism. For reasons of jealousy, the Dean of the Faculty of Medicine maliciously attacked Paré. The dean, who had just completed a manuscript that included topics on surgery, found his volume totally eclipsed by the popularity of Paré's *Complete Works*. The dean and his allies sought revenge by invoking a decades-old statute that prohibited the publication of any medical or surgical book, in a language other than Latin, without the express permission of the Faculty of Medicine.

The dispute lasted for more than a decade, time enough for the four editions of *The Complete Works* to be published. In the end, little came of the dean's condemnations. Throughout this time, Paré fearlessly challenged the deep-rooted authority of the physicians on the Faculty of Medicine who wanted to keep surgery and its practitioners in a state of meek deference:

> For more than thirty years I have been printing my treatises on Surgery; which not only have been opposed by no man but were received by one and all with favor and applause; which made me think, if I gathered them together, I should be doing a thing very agreeable to the public. Which I having accomplished . . . [but] lo and behold, the physicians . . . have set themselves to obscure and quench them, for this sole reason, that I wrote them in our

mother-tongue, in phrases quite easy to be understood. The physicians feared lest all who should get the book into their hands would be advised how to take care of themselves in time of sickness, and would not be at the pains to call them in. [The physicians] were moved by willful hate, envy, and jealousy, to see Ambroise Paré in some reputation as a man well esteemed in his profession.[13]

* * *

The socioeconomic and scientific changes that occurred during the Renaissance provided surgeons with their first substantive opportunities to become respected members of the healing profession. Although scalpel wielders continued to be viewed skeptically by physicians, the surgeon's clinical skills could not be blithely dismissed. Nevertheless, surgeons were still severely limited by their lack of understanding of the principles of anesthesia and antisepsis. As for Paré, his achievements produced a renaissance in surgery. He was a visionary who saw broader and clearer than any of his contemporaries and established new benchmarks to relieve the suffering of the injured and sick.

It is apropos that the last recorded public sighting of Paré was during the Siege of Paris in 1590, when fighting between Catholics and Protestants brought hardship and starvation to the populace. On a warm August day, the eighty-year-old Paré was walking along the Pont Saint-Michel when he found himself in the middle of a crowd of people beseeching a Catholic prelate for food. The official appeared uncertain what to do. Paré spoke up. "For God's sake, Monsieur, give it to them . . . the cries of these poor people, which mount to Heaven, are like warnings that you are responsible to Him."[14] This was Paré at his instinctual best, empathetic and pious.

Four months later, Paré died. He was buried in the nave of the Church of Saint André-des-Arts (near the present-day place Saint-André-des-Arts). In 1794, the church was torn down and his bones, along with others, were transferred to the municipal ossuary. No thought was given to singling out Paré's remains, which are lost among the millions of human bones that rest in the catacombs of Paris.

7.

THE CIRCLE

Nearly all men die of their remedies, and not of their illnesses.

Jean-Baptiste Poquelin (aka Molière),
Le Malade Imaginaire, 1673

A pitiful surgeon makes a dangerous sore.

John Marston, *The Malcontent*, 1603

In the sixteenth century, Vesalius and Paré created a revolution in anatomy and surgery: the former, by demonstrating that knowledge of human anatomy can only be gained through the hands-on dissection of cadavers; the latter, by showing how to control bleeding during an operative procedure. Their efforts fostered an environment in which individuals who had the courage to report findings at odds with accepted wisdom were no longer constrained by speculation and superstition. With the start of the seventeenth century, this spirit of inquiry and scholasticism brought about profound political and socioeconomic changes.

The seventeenth is best termed "the century of the mind." Parades of geniuses populated every discipline. Religion and philosophy had Descartes, Leibniz, Locke, and Spinoza; Rembrandt, Teniers, Vermeer, and Wren embodied the visual arts; music was represented by Cavalli, Monteverdi, Purcell, and Stradivari; and de Bergerac, la Rochefoucauld, Milton, and Pepys exemplified literature and the theater. In the sciences, Kepler, Galileo, Halley, and Newton explained the motion of the planets and laws of gravity as astrology gave way to astronomy; Beguin, Boyle, Sendivogius, and van Helmont transformed alchemy into chemistry; and Cavalieri,

Fermat, Huygens, and Pascal developed novel methods of numerical calculation to create modern mathematics and mechanics. Collectively, these men and their ideas supported the burgeoning Scientific Revolution. Experimentation and observation supplanted blind faith. The subjective became the objective as Galenism was shattered. A moment of truth was upon Medicine, one that had a crucial impact on the craft of surgery.

The man who introduced the new methods of scientific research was William Harvey, an English physician. He based his work on the anatomical studies of Vesalius and through dogged and sharp-eyed observations solved the most elusive and fundamental of the mysteries in Medicine: how blood flowed through the human body. It is hard to grasp the enormity of Harvey's achievement without recognizing the prevailing wisdom that his work struck down. Prehistoric humans undoubtedly realized that blood was in motion because, when they butchered a live animal, they saw pulsating arteries and oozing veins. Galen noted that a beating heart contracted in a staggered motion, which led to his hypothesis that two types of blood, arterial (life-giving) and venous (nourishing), were involved in a to-and-fro action.

Galen's thinking still held sway through the beginning of the seventeenth century. He believed that blood was produced in the liver from digested food brought to it via the intestines. In actual fact, the constituents of blood, red blood cells, most white blood cells, and platelets are produced in the bone marrow, the spongy tissue inside the cavities of bone. Galen stated that the dark red blood coming from the liver flowed through the veins of the body and was responsible for factors related to growth and nutrition and that this venous blood was consumed in its travels. He further maintained that the right side of the heart did not pump blood but was a specialized segment of the venous system with one major function, to convey nourishment to the lungs. Galen also hypothesized that a portion of the venous blood from the right side of the heart seeped across invisible openings in the septum, the muscular dividing wall between the right and left sides. On the left side of the heart, the venous blood that oozed through the septum mixed with "spirit-filled" air from the lungs and was transformed into bright red life-sustaining arterial blood. The arterial blood, warmed by the body's natural heat, left the heart and pulsed along the arteries where, in a tidal-like action, it provided vitality to the tissues and was eventually depleted and did not recirculate.

Galen's model was highly imaginative and wildly inaccurate but remained the archetype of the human cardiovascular system for nearly one and a half thousand years. He had no understanding of the true movement of blood and how it coursed from the right side of the heart to the lungs, where it gained oxygen, and then circled to the left side of the heart to be circulated throughout the body before returning, deprived of oxygen, to the right side of the heart.

The solution of the mystery of circulation was left to Harvey, a scholar who had a deep understanding of the history and literature of the subject. From Hippocrates to Galen, he knew these men, their writings, their successes, and their failures. Mindful of past inaccuracies, Harvey used human dissection, reasoned experimentation, and mathematical analysis to show that the heart is a complex, muscular pump and propels blood continuously through the vascular system in a circle-like fashion. In 1628, when Harvey authored his *Exercitatio Anatomica de Motu Cordis et Sanquinis in Animalibus* (Anatomical studies on the motion of the heart and blood in animals), it was as important an event to the future of Medicine as the printing of Vesalius's *De Fabrica*.

*   *   *

If a man is judged by his appearance and personality then Harvey was an also-ran. Stout and swarthy with an abruptness and testiness that exasperated his colleagues, he offset his eccentricities with sheer brilliance. Harvey's father was a prosperous merchant and his son was well educated. In 1588, the ten-year-old Harvey was sent to the King's School at Canterbury, where students lived a monk-like existence and were encouraged to converse only in Greek or Latin. Five years later, Harvey enrolled at Gonville & Caius College, a constituent unit of the University of Cambridge, and his interest in Medicine was soon piqued. Six decades earlier, John Caius, a respected anatomist and founder of the school, had roomed with Vesalius when the two men studied Medicine in Padua. Through Caius's auspices, Elizabeth I granted the faculty at Gonville & Caius the right to anatomize two executed criminals each year. These dissections were carried out in front of the student body. Thus, by the time of Harvey's graduation in 1597, he had received considerable introduction to the nuances of human anatomy.

Harvey sought out the best university to obtain his medical degree; the one in Padua was his first choice. He was admitted to the Universitas Juristarum, the more selective and influential of the two sections that made up the University of Padua. The school had an air of intellectual freedom and sophistication that was unmatched elsewhere. Academic standards were high, religious tolerance flourished, and the spirit of Vesalius, seen as rigorous inquiry, was pervasive. The presence of Galileo, professor of mathematics, added luster to the faculty; his lectures took place in the *aula magna* adjacent to the school's anatomical theater. That the older Italian influenced the younger Englishman seems logical since Harvey later employed advanced arithmetic formulas in calculating the heart's volume and output. These computations were among the most persuasive of his arguments that proved blood circulates and the beating heart is its driving force.

Harvey's intellectual growth flourished in the academic and social freedom of Padua. He stood out academically and was elected Councilor for the English Nation, a ruling body that represented the non-Italian students in their dealings with the administrators of the university. Harvey's interest in anatomy strengthened and he enjoyed a close friendship with Fabricius of Aquapendente, who held Vesalius's old position as professor of anatomy. Fabricius's confirmation of the presence of one-way valves in the veins and their role in directing blood back to the heart would play a significant part in Harvey's subsequent research. In 1602, Harvey graduated as a Doctor of Medicine and received an ornate diploma inscribed with a flourish of encomiums that left little doubt about his talents:

> [Harvey] has conducted himself so wonderfully well in the examination, and has shown such skill, memory, and learning that he has far surpassed even the great hopes which his examiners had formed of him. They decided therefore that he was skillful, expert, and most efficiently qualified both in arts and medicine, and to this they put their hands, unanimously, willingly, with complete agreement, and unhesitatingly.[1]

Harvey returned to London and applied for membership in the Royal College of Physicians. This was a key affiliation because that society had sole responsibility for credentialing physicians who wished to practice in the city. He was told that admission to the College was confined to graduates of English universities, but those who received a medical diploma from a foreign institution would be granted a license if they produced an ad eundem degree from either Cambridge or Oxford (this is the honorary granting of academic standing from a university to an individual whose actual work was done elsewhere). Harvey re-enrolled at Cambridge and, in

1604, received a medical diploma (ad eundem). That same year, Harvey married the daughter of the physician to James I, who was recently crowned king following the death of Elizabeth I.

Whether this was more a marriage of convenience than of love remains uncertain. The couple was childless and virtually nothing is known about Mrs. Harvey, who died more than a decade prior to her husband. What is apparent is that less than three years after the wedding Harvey was named a full Fellow of the Royal College of Physicians. In addition, he sought and received a difficult-to-obtain position on the staff of St. Bartholomew's Hospital after letters of recommendation were presented from James I. One year later, Harvey was appointed its physician-in-chief.

There is no denying that Harvey was a talented self-starter. He was so admired that aristocrats flocked to his office, including the Lord High Chancellor, Francis Bacon. In only a few years, Harvey was named court physician to James I and his heir Charles I. But an important question remains unanswered: What role, if any, did nepotism play in Harvey's initial success as a practicing physician? After all, one of his close friends described Harvey as "hot-headed," an impatient individual who did not suffer fools gladly. These are not the character traits that endear a physician to his patients. Even more disconcerting is what this same acquaintance said about Harvey's clinical acumen:

> All his profession would allow him to be an excellent anatomist, but I never heard of any that admired his therapeutique ways. I knew severall practisers in London that would not have given 3 ducats for one of his bills.[2]

Favoritism or not, Harvey's middling work as a physician should not be conflated with his astounding accomplishments as a researcher. During Harvey's early years of practice, no one knew that he was investigating the action of the heart and the movement of blood. He was an unrevealing man with no close friends who secreted himself in his laboratory for hours at a time. Year after year, unaided, Harvey dissected all manner of land animals and sea creatures. His medical sleuthing brought him to a conclusion that no man before had ever reached: the beating heart was an architecturally complex organ and its jerky pulsations drove the blood through the vessels of the body. Arteries were outgoing, veins were incoming, and the flow of blood through this closed-loop system was repeated indefinitely and curtailed only by death.

* * *

De Motu Cordis is a physically unimpressive book, five and one-half by seven and one-half inches, seventy-two pages in length, printed on paper of such poor quality that, over a four-century process, most existing copies are deteriorated with age-related browning ("foxing" is the term) and spotting. In his masterpiece, Harvey accurately described, for the first time, how the heart with its four chambers works. When relaxed between beats, the right atrium is filled with deoxygenated blood returning from the body through two large veins, the inferior and superior vena cava, while the left atrium is filled with oxygenated blood coming from the lungs via multiple pulmonary veins. Once both atria are full, they contract and force blood into their respective ventricles. The ventricles then undergo their own vigorous contraction that propels blood out of the right side into the pulmonary artery, which feeds the lungs, and from the left ventricle, through the aorta, to be distributed via the arteries.

For Harvey, a single word, "circle," defined as movement in a circuitous loop back toward a common starting point, encapsulates his years of research and pervades his writing. With neither a beginning nor an ending, the notion of a circle and its unbroken continuity was the anatomical model Harvey referred to when he explained the circulation of blood:

> I began to think whether there might be a movement, as it were, in a circle. Now this I afterwards found to be true; and I finally saw that the blood, forced by the action of the left ventricle into the arteries, was distributed to the body at large, and its several parts, in the same manner as it is sent through the lungs, impelled by the right ventricle into the pulmonary artery, and that it then passed through the veins and along the vena cava, and so round to the left ventricle in the manner already indicated. This movement we may be allowed to call circular. . . . By this arrangement are generations of living things produced.[3]

As much as the physical description of the anatomy of the circulatory system turned Harvey's doubters into believers, there was also his use of quantitative data to prove his thesis. He showed that the volume of blood made it physically impossible for the body's fluid to do anything other than return to the heart by the venous route. Since with each beat the human heart pumps between 2 and 3 ounces of blood (an observation Harvey made from cadavers) and, on average, it beats seventy times per minute, then in one hour it pumps over 10,000 fluid ounces or approximately eighty gallons (a gallon contains 128 ounces) of blood. The resulting amount of blood leaving the heart in a twenty-four-hour period exceeds an extraordinary eight tons (a gallon of blood weighs 8.85 pounds), far more than what a human being could meaningfully produce or metabolize. As Harvey pointed out, if the blood did not circulate in a self-contained circuitous system, then the body would explode from the increasing pressure of fluids with nowhere to go.

What Harvey could not explain was how the arteries and veins were connected to one another to complete the circular pathway. He was unable to visualize the capillaries, the arterial-venous go-betweens, because they were microscopic sized. Proof of their existence would wait several decades until the microscope was invented.* Instead, in the simplest of demonstrations, Harvey showed that some type of physical link between the arteries and veins had to be present. He placed a strap at the elbow just tight enough so that arterial blood could pass toward the forearm and hand, but venous blood could not flow back beyond the tourniquet. As the veins bulged with returning blood, Harvey explained that a yet-to-be-discovered pathway allowed the blood to pass from arteries to veins. Moreover, the swollen veins protruded farthest where unidirectional valves were located. As his mentor Fabricius had demonstrated, it was these valves that guided the flow of blood back to the heart.

* * *

The history of surgery is marked by an interplay between practice and research. Prior to the Scientific Revolution, practice was the driving force, which meant that individuals who performed surgical operations (e.g., trephination for a hemorrhage on

---

* By the late seventeenth century, Galileo's telescope revealed the enormity of the universe and Anton van Leeuwenhoek's microscope exposed the invisible world. Although the ground lens had long been used as a magnifying glass, van Leeuwenhoek's research led to the production of microscopes with the power to magnify an image up to 266 times. Marcello Malpighi, an Italian biologist and physician, identified the capillary connections between arteries and veins and showed that the blood always moved within vessels and did not drain into open spaces. This observation provided the missing link in Harvey's theory and proved decisively how the flow of blood was circular in nature.

the brain or amputation of the breast for cancer) often did not understand the reason why the procedure was effective. This lack of knowledge continued until discoveries were made that explained the principles that underlay the success of the technique (i.e., bleeding caused life-threatening pressure on the brain, which trephination lessened by allowing the blood to be evacuated, or breast cancer spreads through several routes). Although advancements occur in either stage, the rapidity of progress is limited unless practice and research maintain relatively close pace with each other.

The significance of Harvey's research first became apparent when he pointed out its relevance to the time-honored tradition of bloodletting. Paré demonstrated how the deluge of blood that flowed during a surgical operation could be controlled by the use of ligatures and tourniquets. Harvey explained the physiological principles involved in their placement. Thereafter, when a surgeon tied off an artery or a vein, he knew the role the vessel played in the movement of blood. Furthermore, Harvey taught that the failure of blood to flow freely from an incised vein during a bloodletting session was due to the tourniquet being applied too tightly, thus impeding movement of blood to the arteries and, consequently, into the veins.

Bloodletting was among the era's most common surgical procedures and a source of considerable remuneration for surgeons. Once Harvey explained the circular movement of blood, the drawing of blood became even more popular. The enthusiasm for bloodletting centered on the ancient Greek and Roman conviction that the body's four fluids (i.e., blood, black bile, phlegm, and yellow bile) held one another in balance to maintain a healthy state; when an imbalance occurred, disease became present. Blood was considered the dominant force in triggering an unevenness because, more than the other fluids, it was deemed capable of prompt changes in setting and strength in response to noxious stimuli. Whether congestive heart failure, inflammatory bowel disease, or a wound infection, the presence of an ailment was reason enough to remove body fluids, especially blood.

People suffered needlessly as bloodletting was carried further than ever before. In an age when no one understood what it meant to measure blood pressure and body temperature or breathing and heart rates, the surgeons who performed bloodletting had no physiological parameters to prevent them from harming patients. There was no known estimation of exactly how much an individual should be bled to reduce bodily imbalances. It was not uncommon for bleeding to continue until swooning or fainting occurred, a supposed indication that the body's equilibrium was restored. This clinical outcome is among the absurdities of bloodletting because, for some patients, fainting is more a psychological than a physiological response. The very sight of a frightening-looking multi-headed, vein-piercing lancet had the same effect as siphoning off large volumes of blood.

From a modern medical viewpoint, the astonishing thing about bloodletting was not its wide appeal but that an individual's essential life force could be withdrawn repeatedly in massive quantities over brief periods of time. Patients were often bled 16 ounces a day seven days in succession (the average male human body contains 175 ounces of blood). Doctors bragged about extracting 70 or more ounces of blood at a time from patients who were particularly corpulent. In comparison, modern-day donors are allowed to give 16 ounces (one pint) of blood per session, with a minimum of two months between each donation. The regard for bloodletting remained deep-seated and it was practiced on individuals from all levels of society. Even Harvey had unremitting faith in the ancient system of care and used it extensively on his patients, including James I and Charles I.

Harvey's later years were spent in quiet adulation, surrounded by his books and friends. As Thomas Hobbes, a contemporary English philosopher, noted: Harvey was "the only one who conquered envy in his lifetime, and saw his new doctrine everywhere established."[4] In 1657, at the age of seventy-nine, Harvey suffered a stroke that resulted in aphasia, the inability to speak. He used hand gestures and implored an acquaintance to perform a bloodletting on the veins at the bottom of his tongue, in the hope it would return his lost voice. The phlebotomy did little good and Harvey soon died. His body was encased in lead, a Harvey family tradition, and buried in a church in Hempstead, England. There remains the man who solved the great anatomical mystery that held back the evolution of surgery, and ended one area of dogmatism and speculation in Medicine. Harvey's contribution along with the breakthroughs of Paré and Vesalius soon led to a series of triumphal sociopolitical events along with several astounding advances in surgical operative technique that curbed the surgeons' genuflections to physicians.

8.

EMERGENCE

'Tis the Chyrurgions praise, and height of Art,
Not to cut off, but cure the vicious part.

Robert Herrick, *Hesperides* ("Lenitie"), 1648

The egotistical surgeon is like a monkey; the higher he climbs the more
you see of his less attractive features.

Anonymous, based on a seventeenth-century English proverb

During the late seventeenth and early eighteenth centuries, centers of surgical excellence emerged in London and Paris. Although a wide sea channel, stretches of land, and differing languages separated the cities, their stories paralleled each other, underscored by important changes in the organizational structure of their surgical communities. The transformations came about as surgical know-how spread across borders in Europe, to be shared by the growing number of individuals who performed surgical operations.

Progress on the clinical side was largely driven by detailed studies of human anatomy that provided the first scientific foundations for a scalpel wielder's work; dissection of bodies afforded surgeons a familiarity with structure and function not previously known. Based on new insights, surgeons' activities widened beyond amputations, bloodletting, fracture fixations, and wound care. The performance of progressively challenging surgical procedures (without an understanding of anesthesia and antisepsis) became a mainstay of better educated and trained surgeons as they separated themselves from the poorly educated and itinerant tradesmen who also practiced the craft.

As to the organizational structure of surgery, the individuals who performed surgical operations began to be united by membership in well-funded and widely respected professional societies. From these economically and politically astute alliances, notably the French Royal Academy of Surgery and the London Company of Surgeons, arose an autonomous surgical profession and the beginnings of organized surgery.

* * *

Behind the stone and stucco wall of 5 rue de l'École de Médecine, a short street in the sixth arrondissement of Paris, is one of the least appreciated treasures in the world of surgery. The address is best known as the birthplace of Sarah Bernhardt (a plaque on the outside wall relates the actress's story), but for surgeons the relevance concerns a tall octagonal building, topped by a massive dome punctuated with eight broad windows and an adorning cupola. Bulky wooden doors guard the entrance to the structure's courtyard, above which sits a sign indicating that the complex is presently a division of the city's Sorbonne University, Sorbonne Nouvelle, also known as Paris III. The university's Institut du Monde Anglophone occupies the building where classes, ranging from art to economics to literature of the English-speaking world, are taught. Regrettably, there is no physical evidence to indicate that the eight-sided structure once housed the oldest surgical amphitheater in France.

The current occupants are unlikely to appreciate the historical importance of the building or the story of its past lives. A gray and red marker provides few details other than the years of its construction (1691–1695), the king who authorized its erection (Louis XIV), the names of the architects (Charles and Louis Joubert), its original use (an anatomical amphitheater), and that, starting in 1748, the building served as the home of l'Académie Royale de Chirurgie (The royal academy of surgery). What is not mentioned is the subsequent decades-long use of the amphitheater as the headquarters of the École Royale Gratuite de Dessin (Royal free school of art) or, beginning in 1844, its lengthy service as the offices of the Société de Biologie (Society of biology), a scholarly association of academics and literati.

The plan for an anatomical and surgical amphitheater took root in 1655 when, following several centuries of disputes, the surgeons of the College of Saints Cosmas and Damian and the barber-surgeons of the Guild of Barber-Surgeons settled their differences and merged organizations. The members of the two organizations had obvious economic and social incentives in agreeing to the union. In the mid-seventeenth century, the craft of surgery could not support more than a few practitioners who confined their clinical work to operative procedures, even in as large a metropolis as Paris. Surgical operations were crude and uncommon. Other than for the most straightforward of procedures involving the external surface of the body, surgery's reputation for complications and pain meant that few but the brashest operators performed and only the most despairing of patients underwent an operative procedure.

On a practical level, barber-surgeons commanded higher fees than their counterparts; through happenstance, the parish church (Saint-Sépulcre) that the barber-surgeons were affiliated with was patronized by wealthier individuals than the surgeons' church, Saint-Côme. What the barber-surgeon did not have was the elevated social status of an individual who was a member of the College of Saints Cosmas and Damian. Without the mix of the two—a remunerative clinical practice and social respectability—the viability of a surgeon's livelihood was seriously jeopardized. The conundrum was solved by the merger.

The growing political and socioeconomic strength of the new union alarmed the physicians of the Faculty of Medicine who worried about the loss of their centuries-old "control" of barber-surgeons and, indirectly, surgeons. The physicians' apprehensions were summarized in a revealing letter written by their chief administrator:

> We are now fighting with our barber-surgeons who are uniting with the surgeons of St. Cosmas, our ancient enemies. Those of St. Cosmas are miserable scoundrels . . . who have added the barber-surgeons to their cause, by having them share their halls and their pretended privileges. Are these surgeons of St. Cosmas not shocking? They had permission from the king about three hundred years ago to gather together. They claim from the word "license" that they were allowed to make masters in surgery who were ignorant of Latin and would not even know how to read or write. We do not attempt to prevent their being surgeons of St. Cosmas or that others join with them. We would only like to have a company of barber-surgeons, as we have had until now, which would be dependent on our Faculty, and would take every year an oath of fidelity in our schools before our Dean.[1]

Initially, the physicians prevailed in their attempts to constrain the surgeons and barber-surgeons. Legislation was passed that ordered the united surgical community to provide financial gifts, abide by vows of deference, and consent to clinical submissiveness to the Faculty of Medicine. However, the efforts to ensure that surgeons remained beholden to physicians were not easily implemented; there were simply not enough physicians to supervise the large number of surgeons and barber-surgeons. Moreover, physicians had no understanding of the technical aspects of surgical procedures and could not possibly guide the scalpel wielder through a case.

* * *

Beginning in January 1686, a series of events curbed the surgeons' kowtows to the Faculty of Medicine and advanced the development of their craft. Louis XIV, the Sun King, had been ruler of France for twenty-three years when he complained of a tender lump adjacent to his anus. Physicians were consulted and a wait-and-see approach was recommended. When the swelling reddened and turned more painful, members of the Faculty applied compresses of barley, beans, flax, peas, and rye, all marinated and boiled in an acid-like liquid. The treatment accomplished little. The inflammation enlarged and an abscess formed. The sore was lanced to let the pus out and the abscess cavity was filled with caustic substances, a process that caused the king much discomfort. Despite these treatments and additional lancings, applications of leeches, use of enemas and laxatives, plus cauterizations with red-hot irons, the abscess continued to increase in size, reaching three inches in width.

As weeks turned into months, Louis XIV fussed and fumed over the physicians' failure to provide him relief. Moreover, the abscess leaked large amounts of foul-smelling pus that forced the king to change his clothes several times during the course of a day. A despondent Louis XIV isolated himself in the palace at Versailles. By May, the king was passing fecal material through the abscess and his physicians suspected that the sore had developed into an anal fistula.* To confirm their diag-

---

* Within the muscular walls of the anus are glands that secrete fluid to lubricate the anal canal. If a gland is blocked (among the causes are chronic constipation, overuse of enemas, forceful anal sex, and poor personal hygiene), the buildup of bacteria and fluid creates a swelling. With nowhere to go, the fetid material usually extends outward toward the skin's surface in the form of an abscess. Sometimes the abscess leads to the creation of a track/tunnel that stretches from an opening inside the anus (nearby the affected gland) to one outside on the skin. This track is known as an anal fistula or fistula-in-ano. Gener-

nosis, they injected a decoction of red St.-John's-wort into the skin-side opening of the presumed fistula. The dye moved up what had become a track/tunnel and passed into Louis XIV's anal canal. According to an eyewitness, "The King went to the toilet seat, passing the red liquid into a basin [through his anus]."[2] It was evident that a large anal fistula was present (physicians could offer no further suggestions) and some type of surgical remedy was needed. Charles-François Félix, the king's chief surgeon, was summoned.

Félix had never performed an operation for anal fistula. He informed Louis XIV that several months were needed to better understand the disease and its surgical treatments. Félix read the many authors who dealt with the surgical care of anal fistula, as far back as the *Corpus Hippocraticum*. In addition, he arranged for indigent patients, who suffered from anal fistula, to be sent to a hospital where he could perfect his operative technique. Dozens of individuals were experimented on. Many died. After six months, Félix announced that he was capable of performing "*la grande opération*."[3] Not only had Félix become deft at the procedure, but he also had devised two instruments unique for the king's repair.

At 7:00 am on November 18, Louis XIV, accompanied by his mistress, ministers, two physicians, and four apothecaries, was placed facedown on his bed. A pillow was positioned under the king's stomach and his buttocks and thighs were held apart by the apothecaries. An almost three-hour-long operation ensued without anesthesia or antisepsis. To start, Félix positioned a custom-built three-pronged metal retractor deep inside the king's anus and spread it wide (the only source of illumination was a flickering candle). Once Félix visualized the fistula's orifice within the anus, he used a scalpel to enlarge the fistula's other opening on the skin. He then introduced "*le bistouri à la Royale*,"[4] his newly devised scythe-shaped surgical knife, through the skin and guided its curved blade along the fistulous track/tunnel, into the anus. With one adroit slice of the bistoury's razor-sharp cutting edge, Félix divided the tissue. He inspected the opened track/tunnel and, using scalpel and scissor, removed calloused and necrotic matter. Félix finished by packing the wound with linen soaked in olive oil and egg white.

---

ally, an anal fistula is not harmful but can be painful and a nuisance. It is even possible with a large fistula-in-ano that fecal content can pass through the tunnel. Modern surgical treatment involves cutting open the track as well as surrounding necrotic tissue. The wound is dressed with antibiotic-infused gauze and healing occurs from the inside out. Thus, the anal fistula is ablated.

The pain must have been terrible, but other than for an occasional, "*Mon Dieu!*" (My God!),[5] Louis XIV suffered in silence. Shortly after the operation, the king was bled to relieve any "humoral" imbalances that might have resulted from the operation. Several hours later Louis XIV met with his council, and the following morning he welcomed ambassadors to show that he had survived the procedure. Despite appearances, the king's recovery was difficult. In December, three additional operations were needed to remove pockets of inflamed tissue—each procedure was more painful than the previous. Nevertheless, by late January 1687 Louis XIV resumed his normal activities. He never suffered a return of his anal fistula.

All of France celebrated Louis XIV's successful operations and recuperation; 1686 was declared L'année de la Fistule (The year of the fistula). Fountains of wine flowed in the nation's cities as the king used these patriotic festivities to strengthen his rule, emphasizing his courage in the face of personal adversity. Similar to the Sun King, Félix also deserves the label of "courageous." There is little doubt that a failed procedure, including the death of the king, would have led to unpleasant consequences for the surgeon and his craft. Instead, an exultant Louis XIV, fit and pleased with the knife bearer's work, awarded Félix three hundred thousand francs plus a large estate on the outskirts of Paris and elevated him to the nobility.

The ennoblement of Félix placed him on the same level with the royal physician. More importantly, the fistula operation demonstrated the curative powers of the scalpel and caused a shift in how the public viewed the craft of surgery. Surgeons began to be perceived as knowledgeable and intelligent, thinkers, not mere knife handlers who cut human tissue by rote. Word of Félix's success spread throughout Europe and, in faddish imitation, people flocked to Paris and its surgeons for treatment of anal fistula, even when the disease was not present. From being overshadowed and scorned by physicians, French surgeons captured Medicine's spotlight and garnered public approval with a single decisive clinical triumph.

* * *

Several years prior to the cure of his anal fistula, Louis XIV had declared surgery "an art considered one of the most necessary in the state."[6] When the "art" cured his anal fistula, the king reasserted his respect for the craft by decreeing that the surgeons of Paris had his approval to build an anatomical and surgical amphitheater. Funds were raised, architects hired, and in 1695, after four years of construction, the eight-sided structure was completed (the building's steeped-bank seating accommodated 750 persons, each with an unobstructed view of the dissecting/operating table). In a sign of respect, the amphitheater's cupola was topped with a replica of Louis XIV's crown. Over the front door was a slab of black marble on which was engraved a lapidary couplet by Jean-Baptiste de Santeuil, a French poet:

> *Ad caedes hominum prisca amphitheatra patebant,*
> *Ut longum discant vivere nostra patent.*[7]
> The amphitheaters of old were opened to take men's lives,
> Ours is to preserve them.[8]

The amphitheater was the most evident sign of the growth in prestige and prosperity of the Parisian surgical community, a transformation that received notice in a popular guidebook to the city:

> Three or four years ago, the surgeons constructed at great cost a clean and spacious place for their work [dissections, lectures, and operations], where a large number of people could comfortably watch everything they were doing . . . one can say that these Parisian surgeons brought their art further than it had ever been before, as can be judged by the marvelous procedures that one can see them perform every day; this comes from the care and thoroughness with which they aim to perfect their profession . . . which allows them to be considered Masters.[9]

In 1699, Félix used his influence to have statutes enacted that furthered the unity of the surgical profession. He believed that the "craft-guild" approach impaired the training and organization of men who wanted to be surgeons. The new rulings compelled scalpel wielders to abandon their informal attitudes to education and regulation in favor of a centralized system of supervision controlled by a meritocracy of well-educated surgeons. The laws gave rise to an important change in the composition of the Paris surgical community; surgeons with a university background and understanding of science began to divorce themselves from less educated individuals, primarily barber-surgeons and illiterate tradesmen, who also wielded the scalpel.

The decline of the less educated knife bearers signaled a subtle but definite shift in the character of surgery, which reflected scientific advances during the Enlightenment. Proponents of the "new" surgery insisted that surgeons have an extensive knowledge of anatomy and apply their fresh knowledge to the clinical side of the craft. It was argued that an understanding of human structure along with other general principles were critical elements in deciding whether and how to operate. "The operation itself . . . is only one factor in the care of a disease," noted a respected surgeon:

> The knowledge of the case, the complications which follow, the treatment which must vary according to the nature of the disease and the differences in these complications—all these factors, don't they form the essential tenets of surgery?[10]

In 1743, the concept of the surgeon as a learned individual, a university-educated man of science, was bolstered when Louis XV (Louis XIV's great-grandson and successor) declared that surgery had been degraded by its alliance with a "*Profession inférieure.*"[11] He permanently terminated any relationship between surgeons and barbers, eliminated the term "barber-surgeon," and prohibited barbers from performing surgical procedures. In addition, Louis XV's declaration established new educational standards, including a requirement that future candidates seeking designation as a surgeon must study Latin and obtain a master of arts degree from a French university. The king further ruled that by expanding their educational credentials surgeons should no longer be viewed as subordinate to physicians. To reinforce his decrees, Louis XV endowed several teaching chairs in surgery. The Faculty of Medicine contested the authority of surgeons to teach without the supervision of physicians. Not only did the physicians lose the dispute, but also the king granted surgeons the additional right to organize a formal "school," the Royal Academy of Surgery, based at their new amphitheater.

The Royal Academy of Surgery was the forerunner of the politically judicious and science-oriented organizations from which the modern profession of surgery arose. The intent, according to the Academy's director, was to "establish Surgery upon Observations, Physical Experiments, and Experience."[12] A first of its kind surgical journal was created for members of the Academy to publish their clinical observations. The *Mémoires* became a storehouse of practical information and took what had been private knowledge and personal opinions and made them available to the at-large surgical community and public. Lengthy essays on operations for bladder stones, cesarean section, cataracts, cleft lip, gallbladders, and hernias filled the pages. Each article was reviewed and edited by a committee of senior associates. Autopsy findings complemented case histories and research on animals tested the value of a surgical procedure. Besides its scientific offerings, the establishment of the Royal Academy provided a fresh approach to efforts at socialization that afforded a sense of group identity and camaraderie for surgeons. With the Academy supporting their endeavors, along with administrative and managerial assistance regarding economic issues, surgeons sought professional and social acceptance, maintaining that surgery, with its own body of science, was no mere stepchild of Medicine.

* * *

Based on their technical prowess and organizational successes, French surgeons asserted leadership in European surgery. However, they had rivals across the English Channel who also staked out surgery's high ground, citing their own technical achievements as well as their advances in the education and training of surgeons. Despite conflicting opinions, the similarities between the two countries' claims and their evolution are striking. In mid-sixteenth-century London, two separate organizations controlled the practice of surgery, the Guild of Barber-Surgeons and the Fellowship of Surgeons. The "Guild" was busier and larger, and its own meeting hall was a valued asset. The "Fellowship" was a more select body of "educated" surgeons who enjoyed higher social standing. Members of the two groups constantly squabbled and claimed the right to regulate the other.

In 1540, the animosities were set aside when Henry VIII ruled that the Guild of Barber-Surgeons and the Fellowship of Surgeons were to be united and named the Royal Commonality of Barber-Surgeons (the term "barber-surgeons" was used in the title because they were the larger of the two groups). This mandate was an important milestone in the evolution of surgery in England and led to closer cooperation between the two organizations. The charter of the new organization stated that members who practiced surgery could no longer perform barber activities and that barbers should not undertake any surgical procedures except dental work. Several decades later, the organization's authority was strengthened when a bill was passed in Parliament that specified that no individual could practice surgery in London without the written approval of two members in the Royal Commonality. As a consequence, over the next century and a half what was renamed as the London Company of Barber-Surgeons controlled surgery in the metropolis.

At the end of the seventeenth century, despite an appearance of normalcy in the Company's day-to-day activities, the better-"educated" surgeons in the organization petitioned Charles II that their association with men who continued to perform mostly "barber" work was detrimental to their surgical practices:

> It is found by experience that the Union of the Surgeons with persons altogether ignorant of the Science of Faculty of Surgery (as the Barbers are) . . . doth hinder and not promote the order for which they were united.[13]

The king took no action and the rancor increased. In early 1745, the London surgeons again asked to be separated from the barbers. This time the scalpel wielders were better organized, politically stronger, and able to cite precedent from the year before in France when Louis XV terminated the relationship between Parisian surgeons and barbers. More importantly, similar to the French knife bearers who had Charles-François Félix of anal fistula fame and his political savvy to spearhead their drive for separation, English surgeons were now led by an audacious partisan, William Cheselden, a surgeon of international renown, who had extensive ties with members of Parliament.

* * *

Cheselden's career was noteworthy for the range of his clinical accomplishments as well as the diversity of his outside interests. He was an architect, artist, litterateur, photographer, pugilist, raconteur, and all-around bon vivant who mixed freely with the luminaries of eighteenth-century London society. Isaac Newton was a close friend, as were Hans Sloane, the founder of the British Museum, and Voltaire, the French writer. Queen Caroline, wife of George IV, was Cheselden's patient. Alexander Pope, the poet, was an active correspondent. According to the bard, Cheselden was the "most deserving man in the whole profession of Chirurgery and has saved the lives of thousands."[14]

In 1710, after a seven-year surgical apprenticeship, twenty-two-year-old Cheselden was admitted to the London Company of Barber-Surgeons and began to teach courses in human anatomy at the group's hall. At this early stage in his career, Cheselden tried to earn extra income by procuring cadavers for use in private demonstrations. When the administrators of the Company heard of this, they summoned Cheselden to a special meeting. He was told that obtaining fresh bodies from the public executioners and using the corpses to teach anatomy in his private residence conflicted with his public work at the Company.

Cheselden was an outstanding lecturer (he was the first to introduce the formal teaching of human anatomy in London as a prerequisite to the study of surgery) and his home-based lessons did draw students away from the lackluster talks at the London Company's headquarters. The officials directed Cheselden to curtail his clandestine demonstrations or risk expulsion from the Company. Afraid to lose his standing in the city's surgical community, a chastened Cheselden acquiesced. However, the show of pique on the part of the Company's elders exposed Cheselden to the unrestrained economic and political strength of the organization and what he came to regard as their intolerable restrictions on the practice of surgery. Decades later, this incident would play a major part in Cheselden's role in shutting down the London Company of Barber-Surgeons and permanently separating surgeons from barbers.

By the mid-1730s, Cheselden had achieved international surgical renown. He was considered that era's cleverest surgeon and wrote a textbook, *The Anatomy of the Human Body*, which went through thirteen English editions, two American editions, and one German edition and became the standard work on the subject for almost a century. Although he was skilled in all fields of surgery, it was one operation that most displayed the technical abilities for which he earned surgical celebrity: the removal of stones from the urinary bladder, known as lithotomy.

Up to the time of Cheselden, lithotomy was a gruesome procedure and sufferers from bladder stones only submitted to it when the agony of their condition made life insufferable.* The ghastly operation involved a deep and lengthy incision in the

---

* Bladder stones are hard masses of minerals that form in the bladder. It was more common in former times because of poor diet, chronic bladder infections, untreatable physical abnormalities of the urinary tract, and the general ill health of the populace; bladder stones the size of a chicken egg were not uncommon. In modern times, with changes in nutrition, it is unusual for bladder stones to form. When bladder stones are present, the symptoms may include severe lower abdominal and back pain, difficult or painful urination, and blood in the urine. The discomfort can also be accompanied by chills, nausea, and vomiting. Today, when a bladder stone is too large to pass naturally, a surgical procedure is performed that places a

perineum (the area between the anus and scrotum or vulva), the passage of a metal rod through the penis or vagina into the bladder to serve as a guide, and the extraction of the stone with a forceps inserted through the incision and pushed into the bladder. The whole process often took more than an hour, and without anesthesia, plus the always-looming problem of infection, it was a horrific ordeal.

Through extensive research on the anatomy of the perineum and lower abdomen, Cheselden revised the placement of incisions for lithotomy such that blood vessels, intestines, and the prostate were less likely to be injured. Utilizing these modifications, Cheselden was able to complete the operation in one to two minutes, compared with one to two hours, and reduced the complication rate from over 50 percent to under 10 percent. Cheselden's almost sleight-of-hand operative dexterity was astonishing and his ability to nimbly deliver a bladder stone within seconds of making an incision brought him worldwide acclaim. Surgeons flocked to London to watch him operate and, in 1732, Cheselden became the first foreigner elected to the French Royal Academy of Surgery. Modest in demeanor, Cheselden admitted he was always nervous before an operation and, for this reason, his only chance at success was to perform a lithotomy as swiftly as possible:

> If I have any reputation . . . , I have earn'd it dearly, for no one ever endured more anxiety and sickness before an operation, yet from the time I began to operate, all uneasiness ceased; and if I have had better success than some others, I do not impute it to more knowledge, but to the happiness of a mind that was never ruffled or disconcerted, and a hand that never trembled during any operation.[15]

In 1737, at the height of his career, Cheselden retired from active practice. Whether a form of generalized anxiety related to the performance of surgical operations compelled this decision is unknown. He obtained a lucrative sinecure at a London hospital for the elderly and served the remaining fifteen years of his life as a full-time administrator and occasional surgical consultant. It was during this decade and a half that Cheselden became closely involved in the political activi-

---

small tube with a camera into the bladder. The surgeon uses a laser or a mechanical device to break apart the stone and flushes the pieces from the bladder. If a bladder stone is too large to fragment, then an incision is made directly into the bladder to remove it.

ties of the London Company of Barber-Surgeons. He, like other English surgeons of prominence, chafed under a system that required their diplomas to be cosigned by barbers who lacked a university education and a detailed knowledge of surgical science. More to the point, Cheselden considered the alliance between surgeons and barbers antiquated and an impediment to progress. In early 1745, the surgeons petitioned Parliament for a formal and legal separation from the barbers. The barbers objected, requesting that the status quo be respected. Parliament appointed a committee under the direction of Charles Cotes to study the matter.

Cotes was a physician, a low-ranking member of the House of Commons, and the beloved son-in-law of Cheselden; he was married to Cheselden's only child. At the committee's hearings, surgeons claimed that the union with barbers was no longer conducive to the advancement of surgery or the development of a surgeon's technical skills. The barbers denied this but presented no reasonable defense other than to note that there had been only two instances in the past of London-based companies being divided, felt makers from haberdashers and apothecaries from grocers, both in the early seventeenth century. Witnesses were interviewed, documents reviewed, and the committee concluded that the surgeons' demands were reasonable. Subsequently, a bill passed both Houses of Parliament and, in mid-1745, the London Company of Barber-Surgeons was dissolved. Thus was born an independent Company of Surgeons, the forebear to the present-day Royal College of Surgeons of England.

Although Cheselden never directly acknowledged his role in these events, there seems little doubt that he was the key force in the drive for dissolution. After the inquiry, it became known that he paid 550 pounds to defray the costs to bring the legislation before Parliament. His motive was largely centered on his decades-earlier difficulties with the London Company of Barber-Surgeons, which had led him to believe it would be impossible to advance surgical education and training until surgeons and barbers were permanently separated. Four years after the split, Cheselden discussed his prior annoyance:

> And the rulers of the Barber-Surgeons Company . . . contrived a bylaw to prevent the knowledge of anatomy from spreading; cunningly foreseeing that the younger surgeons by that knowledge would advance too fast upon them. They made it a penalty of ten pounds to dissect a body out of the hall without their leave, which

was scarce to be obtained: and if anyone offended (as they call'd it) they were sure to be prosecuted. The improvements in anatomy and surgery since their restraints have been removed, will sufficiently convince the world of the unfitness of them.[16]

Moreover, how was it that Cotes, a political unknown, wrote the bill and was appointed chairman of a major committee of the Parliament despite the presence of several prominent statesmen on the commission (i.e., William Pitt the Elder, a future prime minister of Great Britain, Horace Walpole, the antiquarian and man of letters, and Alderman Gibbon, father of the renowned historian Edward Gibbon, author of the magisterial *The History of the Decline and Fall of the Roman Empire*)? In the case of Cotes and the passage of the legislation, Cheselden's wealth, prestige, and influence spoke volumes. He was a behind-the-scenes surgical powerbroker who manipulated the political process, ensured its favorable outcome, and, in so doing, redirected the future of surgery.

* * *

By the mid-eighteenth century, surgeons were no longer regarded as illiterate charlatans or roving quacks. Instead, scalpel wielders had become technical innovators and began to rise above their traditional social status as unlearned tradesmen. Nevertheless, surgical operations remained a relatively crude art despite an increasingly greater understanding of human anatomy. In particular, the abdomen and chest were never opened, nor were high-risk procedures like amputations or trephinations performed on a regular basis due to the problems of pain and infection. Yet the rising ladder of social respect that accelerated under the authority of Félix and Cheselden drew better-educated and more committed people to the field of surgery. Notwithstanding the appeal, surgeons needed to be regarded as skillful thinkers, not only inventive technicians. Absent was a satisfactory expansion of the craft's scientific possibilities, a crucial necessity to strengthen the already-ascending spiral of professional stature. It would take the efforts of a genuine surgical genius to fill this void.

9.

TRANSITION

He who reduces the province of a Surgeon to only the performance of operations, and consequently directs his attention in a transient and careless manner to the less splendid parts of his profession, may learn the art of mutilating his fellow creatures with ease and dexterity, but will never deserve to be treated as a good Surgeon.

John Pearson, *Principles of Surgery*, 1788

Many and great are the improvements which the chirurgic art has received within these last fifty years; and many thanks are due to those who have contributed to them: but when we reflect how much still remains to be done, it should rather excite our industry than inflame our vanity.

Percivall Pott, *Chirurgical Observations*, 1775

In every surgeon's life, there are noteworthy events that shape his or her professional behavior. These incidents can vary from the success of an operation to the stress of a malpractice suit. Among my career-defining moments was the initial time I was handed a scalpel and told I was in charge. A person can read and study and rehearse, but the first time you care for another human being by cutting him or her open is an extraordinary experience. For me, it proved pivotal to my future calling in more ways than one.

My road to captaining an operating room began at the end of my internship year when I was on rotation at a VA hospital in Boston. Stephen Preston, a twenty-seven-year-old Vietnam veteran and construction worker, came to the hospital's outpatient clinic for evaluation of a swelling alongside his pubic bone. The bulge did not bother him and was most conspicuous when he stood or coughed. I was staffing the clinic and took Stephen's history. His story was classic and his physical examination revealed the presence of a groin hernia. The attending surgeon agreed with my diagnosis and scheduled Stephen for a repair the following week.

The attending was an English expat, born near the woods of Nottingham, whose credentials were exceptional: medical school at the famed University of London and surgical training at that city's storied Guy's Hospital followed by a two-year fellowship at Harvard's Beth Israel Hospital. I enjoyed working with him and was pleased to learn that he had a keen understanding of surgical history and was aware of my interest.

I was on night call when Stephen was admitted for his hernia procedure. He was placed on the operating schedule for the following morning and I was assigned as first assistant. That evening, I read about groin hernias knowing the Englishman would shower me with questions concerning the anatomy of the lower abdominal wall and groin. In addition to understanding the relationships of that region's ligaments and muscles, I refamiliarized myself with the surrounding blood vessels and nerves as well as the course of the all-important vas deferens, the almost foot-long zigzagging, spaghetti-thin tube that transports sperm. The vas lies in the area of a hernia repair and, when it is inadvertently cut or mishandled, the patient can be left sterile; conversely, it is the vas deferens that is purposely cut and tied when a patient undergoes a vasectomy.

If understanding the anatomy and its myriad of terms weren't enough of a challenge, I also had to learn the various surgical options. The mid-1970s were an era before the use of sterile synthetic mesh was a routine part of a groin hernia repair. Instead, sutures were employed to stitch various tissue layers to close the hole. There was a diversity of operations with each offering a variation on the theme of what tissues should be brought together to provide the strongest repair. The techniques and their technical differences were distinguished by eponyms (i.e., the names of the surgeon who popularized the techniques), ranging from the Bassini and Halsted repairs, initially reported in the 1880s, and the Ferguson and Tanner operations of the first half of the twentieth century, to the McVay and Shouldice procedures of mid-century. After several hours of reading interrupted by the occasional surgical emergency, I went to sleep believing I was prepared for most questions.

The morning began with the usual amount of scut work involved with taking care of twenty or so pre- and postoperative patients. The Englishman asked if Stephen was ready for surgery (i.e., history and examination completed, blood work, chest X-ray, EKG, and urinalysis available, operative consent dated and signed, and nothing was taken by mouth after 10:00 pm). I answered yes. As the attending walked away, he casually looked over his shoulder and said, "You'll be in charge and performing the surgery. I'll see you downstairs." Almost a half century later, I can still picture that tall figure leaving the surgical floor. My heart raced, my mind numbed, and anxiety took over.

In the operating suite, the Englishman and I scrubbed our hands and arms with antiseptic soap. As I washed, I looked through a glass window into the operating room. I watched as Stephen was transferred from gurney to operating table and put to sleep. It was apparent that I was nervous because several minutes into the scrub, in front of everyone—anesthesiologists, nurses, and orderlies—I fumbled the scrub brush and dropped it on the floor, thereby breaking sterility and necessitating my restart of the entire process. The attending recognized my unease and attempted to calm me by starting a conversation about everyday events. Did I enjoy the residency? How was my wife? What pursuits did I enjoy outside the training program? How did I become interested in surgical history?

His reassuring presence worked; when I walked into the operating room my nervousness had lessened. Our talk quickly turned to the surgery of groin hernia. Where would I place the incision? What tissues need to be identified? Semiconfident and with scalpel in hand, I made a four-inch incision in Stephen's right groin. I painstakingly separated tissue layer after tissue layer. It was forty-five minutes of awkwardness, but the dissection was completed, the vas deferens identified, and the hernia weakness exposed. In discussing which repair I would recommend, the attending asked, "Do you know the differences between American-based and English-based operations?" I explained what I knew and we agreed on a procedure that combined elements from both. I asked for silk sutures and, after an additional forty-five minutes of awkwardness, the repair was completed. The skin closure was anticlimactic as I breathed a sigh of relief. Satisfied that the hour-and-a-half operation had gone well—I felt all thumbs—my mentor again turned his questions to surgical history.

"Did you ever hear of John Hunter?" he asked. My response was a simple, "No," followed by, "Why?" The Englishman explained that Hunter was one of the most illustrious men in the annals of surgery. "You should get to know him," he said. "Like me, Hunter studied and trained in London, albeit two centuries ago, and much of what surgery is today is due to his influence."

I discovered that Hunter had incredible intellectual breadth and that, due to his perspicacity, surgery ceased to be viewed as a mere technical mode of treatment and, instead, took its place as a division of scientific Medicine firmly backed by experimental pathology and physiology. Hunter's curiosity was limitless and his interest in the world around him insightful. He viewed things in ways not previously imagined and made others see their significance. Hunter was the crucial transitional figure in surgery who bridged the gap between the dogma and empiricism of the old order and the research and science associated with the upcoming methods of anesthesia and antisepsis. How this eccentric genius accomplished his successes and their impact on the development of the craft are among the pivotal tales in the history of surgery.

* * *

There are few celebrated surgeons who had a less promising start to their career than Hunter. As a child and adolescent, he was incorrigible and indifferent to the value of formal education; he dropped out of school at age thirteen. Having grown up on a farm in the southeast of Scotland, he preferred the freedom of the outdoors to the confines of a classroom. "When I was a boy," he wrote, "I wanted to know all about the clouds and the grasses and why the leaves changed color in the autumn; I watched the ants, bees, birds, tadpoles, and caddis worms; I pestered people with questions about what nobody knew or cared anything about."[1] Over time, Hunter's inquisitiveness concerning the mysteries of nature led to his remarkable abilities to observe and analyze and link sensible premises with logical conclusions. These attributes became the foundation of his talents as a research scientist/surgeon.

Despite Hunter's early efforts at self-education, he remained without discernible skills for any practical occupation. In 1748, with nothing to look forward to, the unemployed twenty-year-old sought career advice from his older brother William, a prominent physician in London. The contrasts between the two brothers were striking. William was refined, university educated, and one of England's leading anatomists and obstetricians. He was an articulate and effective public speaker, who was a member of numerous learned societies and enjoyed the admiration and friendship of eminent men, especially those in the artistic and literary worlds. Over the years, William was appointed Physician Extraordinary to Queen Charlotte of Mecklenburg-Strelitz, wife of George III, elected a Fellow of the Royal Society (the oldest national scientific institution in the world), opened a renowned school of anatomy and medical museum in Great Windmill Street, and authored a book that revolutionized the study of the pregnant female with its realistic depictions of a fetus in utero.

John was William's polar opposite. He was intolerant and outspoken, with a quickness to anger that remained lifelong. "John was a rough lad," wrote a biographer:

> His professional ethics were second rate, his contempt of empty dignities and humbug was shouted from the housetops, and he hated fiddlers, laced ruffles and Frenchmen.[2]

William was uncertain what to recommend to his brash sibling and offered him temporary work in the dissecting room of his anatomy school. To William's astonishment, John proved incredibly talented at preparing anatomical specimens. Not only was he gifted at dissection—John had exceptional manual dexterity—but he also demonstrated a remarkable sense of discipline and responsibility that he previously lacked. John labored from sunrise until sunset and undertook his anatomical studies with a determination that would characterize the remainder of his life's work. An impressed William soon appointed his brother as a full-time demonstrator of anatomy.

John lectured through the school year and, during the summer months when no teaching took place, began to study surgery with the distinguished Cheselden. William took pride in his brother's budding surgical career but was concerned about John's lack of education and sophistication; to be a surgeon of repute in eighteenth-century England required eloquence, refinement, and proper schooling. With this in mind, William insisted that his sibling enroll at Oxford to gain some polish. However, not even the gravitas of Oxford could reform John. "They wanted to make an old woman of me, or that I should stuff Latin and Greek at the University," he explained, "but these schemes I cracked like so many vermin as they came before me."[3] After two months, John was back in London. His lack of oratorical skills and his ill manners—a biographer wrote that he was "much addicted to swearing, and constantly interlarded his conversation with expressions of this sort"[4]—would plague him until his dying day.

In 1754, Hunter undertook a surgical apprenticeship at St. George's Hospital, and he was later appointed house surgeon, akin to today's internship/residency. But investigations into human anatomy and surgery were no longer enough. Instead, it was the mysteries of life itself that commanded John's attention. He believed that to fully understand the pathology and physiology of humankind, the entire world of land animals, sea creatures, and plants needed to be examined. One of Hunter's profilers explained:

> He clearly saw, that in order to obtain just conceptions of the nature of those aberrations from healthy actions which constitute disease, it was necessary first to understand well the healthy actions themselves; and these required to be studied, not in man alone, but throughout the whole animal series, and even to receive further elucidation by comparison with the functions of vegetable life. It was no less an undertaking, then, than the study of the phenomena of life, in health and disease, throughout the whole range of organized beings, in which Hunter proposed to engage; an undertaking which required a genius like his to plan, and from the difficulties of executing which, any mind less energetic, less industrious, and less devoted to science than his own would have shrunk. . . . He appealed directly to Nature herself, and rested nothing upon the facts related by others, until, by the evidence of his own senses, he had ascertained their truth.[5]

Hunter's calling card became the study of comparative anatomy. Animals and plants of every sort were dissected to understand their similarities and differences. He went so far as to contact the keeper of wild beasts in the Tower of London for the animals' bodies after they died and made similar arrangements with circus owners and individuals who maintained private menageries. In his spare time, Hunter walked the botanic gardens of London and nearby towns to gather exotic plant specimens.

He drove himself tirelessly and the strain took its toll. First, there was a severe attack of pneumonia followed by symptoms of phthisis, better known as tuberculosis. With him weakened and barely able to function, his family urged him to abandon the putrid air of the dissecting rooms and seek healthier surroundings. At the time, England was entangled in the Seven Years' War, a massive global conflict that involved Great Britain, Portugal, and Prussia aligned against France, the Austrian-led Holy Roman Empire, Russia, and Spain. Through family connections, Hunter received a commission as an army surgeon. He served for four years at Belle Isle, a small island off the coast of France, as well as on the contested frontier border between Portugal and Spain. Even with his busy life as an army surgeon, Hunter found time to continue his research on animals and plants. In 1763, when the Seven Years' War ended, Hunter returned to London with over two hundred animal specimens pickled in alcohol, plus a vast collection of various body parts of soldiers—intestines, shoulder and thigh bones, and skulls fractured by French musket balls—who died in combat.

* * *

In London, Hunter established a surgical practice, but his patients were few in number. Financial strains were eased by Hunter's half-pay army allowance and a small side income derived from teaching anatomy and operative surgery. However, the practice of surgery became subordinated to his scientific investigations; throughout his professional life, he devoted the bulk of his money to research projects. Hunter might take a day occasionally to deal with an interesting surgical case, but treating commonplace diseases was, to him, irksome. "Well, Lynn," Hunter would tell his assistant as he went off unwillingly to see a patient, "I must go and earn this damned guinea, for I shall be sure to want it tomorrow."[6]

Within two years, Hunter managed to accumulate some savings and bought several acres of land on the outskirts of London and built a house and created a menagerie. It was there that his studies in comparative anatomy began in earnest and where his eccentricities flourished. Everyone who passed by the compound's black iron gates stopped to stare. Four massive stone carvings of lions guarded the double flight of steps that led to the front door over which hung the gaping jaws of a long-dead crocodile. On the sides of the house were giant pyramidal collections of shells that concealed entrances to subterranean chambers. Nearby was a conservatory where he kept dozens of beehives. The chimneys were topped by lightning conductors, invented by Hunter's friend Benjamin Franklin. But it was the surrounding backyard, as described by one of Hunter's biographers, that surely drew the greatest attention:

At the east end of the grounds was an artificial mound of earth, having an opening in its side, which led into three small vaults or cellars beneath it. . . . This mound was the "Lions' Den;" here he kept such animals as were most dangerous. In a field facing his sitting-room was a pond, where he kept for experiment his fishes, frogs, leeches, eels, and river-mussels; and it is said the pond was ornamented with the skulls of animals. The trees dotted about the grounds served him for his studies of the heat of living plants, their movements, and their power of repair. He kept fowls, ducks, geese, pigeons, rabbits, pigs, and made experiments on them; also, opossums, hedgehogs, and rare animals—a jackal, a zebra, an ostrich, buffaloes, even leopards; also, dormice, bats, snakes, and birds of prey. . . . Thus, the house was beset on all sides by strange creatures, and witnessed a vast number of experiments on the living and dissections of the dead.[7]

With the house and menagerie completed, Hunter began the scientific investigations that brought him international acclaim. Among the earliest studies was one on himself. A year after moving into his new home, Hunter was exercising when he tore his Achilles tendon, the tough band of fibrous tissue that connects the calf muscles to the heel bone. Typical of his genius at using every opportunity to make observations and offer analyses, Hunter studied how his own Achilles tendon healed while he experimented on dogs by cutting their tendons and sacrificing the animals at various stages of their recuperation. He showed that tendons heal through the formation of a strong scar-like substance that joins the severed ends.

* * *

Hunter was brilliant but not always right. This is seen when he served as his own research subject in one of the most extraordinary self-experiments in the whole of Medicine: he infected himself with venereal disease in an attempt to prove that gonorrhea (aka clap) and syphilis (aka pox) were separate manifestations of the same illness (which they were not!). Like most doctors of his day, Hunter recognized that the two diseases were transmitted by sexual contact. Little else was understood even though gonorrhea and syphilis were among the constant companions of the population. Remedies abounded, from balms to pills and potions; any and everything was tried but with limited success.

Hunter's belief that gonorrhea and syphilis were caused by the same agent or toxin was based on the long-established attitude that two diseases could not exist in an individual at the same time. Hunter knew that the clap and pox had different symptoms and thought gonorrhea represented the local expression of the disease while syphilis emerged once the illness spread throughout the body. Since the ever-curious Hunter could rarely resist the challenge of studying an ailment ripe for scrutiny, he determined to inoculate a person with gonorrhea and monitor him for the onset of syphilis. If, as Hunter postulated, symptoms of gonorrhea were followed by symptoms of syphilis, then the two diseases were one and the same. Contrariwise, if no suggestion of syphilis emerged, then they were separate entities. What he needed was an individual willing to be infected and a donor with severe enough gonorrhea to provide the sickening pus.

Not surprisingly, the search to find a suitable volunteer proved fruitless. Hunter then made an expeditious and pragmatic decision: he would serve as the experimentee. Hence, in the spring of 1767, Hunter smeared a lancet with gonorrheal pus from one of his patients and inoculated himself by puncturing the foreskin and head of his penis. Within days, a gonorrhea-like discharge oozed from Hunter's urethra. Two weeks later, a syphilitic chancre appeared on his prepuce. Hunter was ecstatic. As far as he was concerned, the experiment was decisive; the two illnesses were one, merely appearing in different states in the human body. "[The research] proves that matter from a gonorrhea will produce chancres," wrote Hunter, "and opens fields for further conjectures."[8] There was one major flaw—Hunter's findings were erroneous. He did not know that the anonymous penis he used as a source of gonorrhea also harbored syphilis. Hunter had unintentionally infected himself with both diseases.

Despite this faux pas, Hunter's determined approach to research and his voluminous publications helped bring the previously mechanical art of surgery and its technical concerns within the aegis of scientific Medicine. He showed that the practice of surgery could not be based upon clinical experience alone; surgeons required knowledge of pathological and physiological principles if the craft was to reach its full potential. The "how-to" of cutting bones, flesh, and organs could no longer be the sole interest of individuals who titled themselves surgeons. Knife bearers had to reorient their thinking and also pay attention to the manner in which the human body responded to disease and injury.

* * *

In 1771, Hunter married Anne Home; she was fourteen years his junior. By all accounts, the marriage was a happy one even though it appeared a mismatch. She was attractive, charming, and extroverted. He was aloof, bald, disheveled, and overweight. Few wives would put up with such a husband's oddities, let alone the persistent offending aroma of his collection of animals. Nonetheless, John could be a fascinating and stimulating individual, whose gentle side was brought out by Anne. Four children were born, but two died as infants. Neither the surviving daughter nor son had children of their own (whether they had congenital syphilis, passed from John to Anne to them, that left them sterile is an open question).

It was around the time of his marriage that honors and recognition began to come John's way. He was elected a Fellow of the Royal Society, named to the full-time surgical staff at St. George's Hospital, and received membership in the London Company of Surgeons. In 1776, George III designated Hunter his Surgeon Extraordinary, followed by appointments as surgeon-general of the army and inspector general of regimental hospitals. Hunter was now the nation's most esteemed surgeon and enjoyed great popularity along with a sizeable practice.

The astounding achievements of Hunter are even more remarkable given his two-decade-long saga of declining health. Shortly after his marriage, he suffered an attack of angina pectoris, a disorder marked by severe pain in the chest that often spreads to the arms, shoulders, and neck, caused by an inadequate supply of blood to the heart. From then on, he suffered more bouts of increasing frequency and severity. He never fully understood their etiology but came to recognize the role of his own emotions in initiating an episode. Still, Hunter remained unable to control his temper or step back from a simple slight. In a memorable quip, conspicuous for his self-awareness, tempered by a confessed lack of self-restraint, Hunter explained, "My life is in the hands of any rascal who chooses to annoy and tease me."[9]

Intimations of mortality or not, Hunter threw himself further into his research. He enlarged his menagerie and eventually dissected over five hundred different varieties of living creatures. From the smallest insect to the largest animal, there was little that escaped Hunter's knife and scissor. In 1783, he obtained the most sought-after specimen of all, the fresh corpse of Charles Byrne (aka O'Brien), an almost eight-foot-tall Irish giant. The towering Byrne was a local celebrity when a flimflam artist convinced his parents that the teenager could be their ticket to fame and fortune if they allowed him to be exhibited as a freak curiosity. Byrne and his hustler companion spent several summers touring county fairs, outdoor markets, and town theaters. Onlookers were eager to buy tickets to see the human colossus and the promoter was convinced that even larger crowds and greater financial rewards awaited the duo in the metropolis of London.

Byrne's companion/impresario placed advertisements in the city's newspapers: "IRISH GIANT, to be seen this, and every day this week, in his large elegant room, at the cane shop, next door to late Cox's Museum . . . Hours of admittance every day . . . at half-a-crown each person."[10] All seemed well as Byrne became the talk of the town. Members of the nobility, including King George and Queen Charlotte, made their way to view the boy giant. Journalists described the "elegance, symmetry, and proportion of this wonderful phenomenon in nature,"[11] while gossips speculated on Byrne's love life and sexual prowess. On the latter hearsay, a discomfited Byrne declared himself a "perfect stranger to the rites and mysteries of the Goddess Venus."[12]

Given Hunter's interest in anatomical oddities, he was among the first to pay half a crown to scrutinize Byrne. Hunter became obsessed with possessing the boy's body for his collection; the skeleton of a human giant would be the showpiece of his growing assemblage. The wait for Byrne's demise did not take long. Hunter's clinical acumen led him to discern that Byrne was not a healthy individual. "He stoops, is not well shaped, his flesh loose, his appearance far from wholesome . . . his voice sounds like thunder, and he is an ill-bred beast,"[13] wrote one of Hunter's friends. Byrne's disease, childhood acromegaly or gigantism, is caused by a benign tumor of the pituitary gland that secretes excessive amounts of growth hormone, resulting in coarsened facial features, disturbed heart function, enlarged feet and hands, and a gravelly voice.

As months passed, London's obsession with Byrne faded, as did the revenue he attracted. His erstwhile handler abandoned him and Byrne's ill health was further compromised by his habit of drinking large amounts of gin and whiskey daily. Because of Byrne's chronic drunkenness, shows had to be canceled, which, in turn, increased his drinking. By the spring of 1783, a debilitated Byrne appeared a dying man. He was not quite dead when London's surgeons began to haggle over who would get the corpse for dissection. A journalist declared:

> there have been more physical consultations held, than ever were
> convened to keep Henry the Eighth in existence. The object of these

Aesculapian deliberations is to get the poor giant into their possession; for which purpose they wander after him from place to place,
and mutter more fee, faw, fums than ever.[14]

Hunter was the most eager of the pursuers. He sent one of his employees on a
hide-and-seek mission to trail the invalid colossus in case he died suddenly. The spy
was no supersleuth, and Byrne discovered that the great surgeon wanted to anatomize him. Like most Londoners, Byrne feared the era's body snatchers—men who
prowled the cemeteries and churchyards nightly in search of fresh-buried corpses
and sold them to doctors—and dreaded the thought of being dissected. He sought
comfort in further bouts of drinking, which soon led to his death.

Hunter's scout learned the name of the undertaker whom Byrne had previously
asked to prepare his body for burial. A secret meeting was arranged between the
scalpel wielder and the mortician. After several hours of negotiations, the two men
agreed on a price to obtain the corpse—like many undertakers, this one, for the right
fee, colluded with body snatchers and their clients. In the heat of a summer's evening,
Byrne's coffin was opened, his body removed, and its weight replaced with pave-
stones. Hunter and his crew made a hasty retreat to his home, where Byrne's corpse
was immediately dissected. The body parts were immersed in a massive kettle of boiling water, separating flesh from bone. Hunter had his trophy but, for many years, kept
the existence of the giant's skeleton concealed from even his closest friends. But the
saga of Byrne's remains did not end on that dark night in a cauldron of boiling water.

It was Hunter's intention that when he died his massive grouping of almost
fourteen thousand specimens would be sold to the nation for a museum of natural
history. He valued the collection at seventy thousand English pounds and considered
the anticipated income his family's inheritance. However, the cash-strapped British
government showed no interest in investing in what many considered a scientific
boondoggle. Hunter's family was left in financial ruin. Not until 1799 did politicians agree to purchase the collection, but at the fire sale price of fifteen thousand
pounds. The specimens and preparations were placed in the care of the Company of
Surgeons (soon renamed the Royal College of Surgeons) and became the nucleus of
one of the great museums of comparative anatomy, osteology, pathology, and natural
history in the world. Byrne's reconstructed skeleton remained the College's famed
attraction, visited by scores of kings, queens, and other nobles and tens of thousands
of commoners.

The Hunterian Museum and the Royal College of Surgeons are located at Lincoln's Inn Fields, a large public square in London. During the Blitz the building was badly damaged by incendiary bombs and three-quarters of Hunter's collection was incinerated. Fortunately, prior to the attack Byrne's skeleton was secreted away for safekeeping. Following the war and the rebuilding of the College's headquarters, Hunter's showpiece resumed its place of distinction in a glass case in the middle of the museum. Recently, a public campaign has been mounted to end to what many consider the inappropriate and unethical display of Byrne's remains.

*   *   *

The later years of Hunter's life were a busy mixture of hospital work, scientific research, and teaching responsibilities. "As to my business, it is very nearly what I want, because it very nearly gets me what I want; beyond which I have no ambition," he wrote a friend:

> As to my studies and teaching, I am following my business for my students, pursuing my comparative anatomy . . . making experiments upon animals and vegetables . . . while all these concurring circumstances go on, I must continue to be one of the happiest men living.[15]

Hunter was considered a surgical educator without equal. He was argumentative and an iconoclast, but those close friends and young surgeons whom he drew around were privy to an alluring genius, a prophet of the coming science. To be part of Hunter's inner sanctum with its thought-provoking atmosphere of new ideas, shocking discoveries, and unusual theories was to have a ringside seat to the English Age of Reason. It was life on Medicine's new edge—adventurous, exhilarating, terrifying but always stimulating—shepherded by an individual considered the archetype of a surgeon/scientist. It is hardly possible to trace the evolution of any subject within surgery (e.g., aneurysm, artificial respiration, blood coagulation, hemorrhage, inflammation, shock, transplantation, and wound care, to cite a few) and its scientific underpinnings without coming across the name John Hunter.

Hunter's prediction as to how his life would end came true in the boardroom of St. George's Hospital. He had told an acquaintance that his chest pains were increasingly severe and the slightest provocation triggered them. "One of these days, and not long first," explained Hunter, "you will hear that I have dropped down dead."[16] A week later, during a debate over the qualifications of students who had applied for surgical training at St. George's, the end came. As Hunter championed their admission, he was cut off and challenged by one of his colleagues. Hunter's anger surged. He spoke a few words and suddenly stood up from his chair and rushed out of the boardroom in a seeming rage. This was no fury of emotions. Instead, Hunter was gasping for air and staggered into an adjoining room. There he collapsed lifeless into the arms of a bystander. Hunter's body was autopsied, which confirmed a diseased heart, and then placed in the burial vaults of the church of St. Martin in the Fields in Trafalgar Square. Six decades later, as Hunter's reputation flourished, he received state honors at a second funeral when his remains were reinterred in the north aisle of the nave at Westminster Abbey, near those of Ben Johnson, Sir Isaac Newton, and, afterwards, Charles Darwin and Stephen Hawking.

* * *

Stephen Preston left the Boston VA hospital three days following his hernia operation. His recovery was uneventful and he returned to work four weeks later. As for me, I received my evaluation one month after rotating out of the VA. "Excellent report," wrote the director of the residency program, "only weakness among many real strengths is technical ability. This will improve as you work on it." I was far from being the surgeon I wanted to become, but with over four more years of surgical residency in front of me, I assumed, correctly, there was time enough to work on my technical skills.

PART III

REVOLUTIONS

10.

PAIN-FREE

*Other discoveries and inventions have indeed been revolutionary in
their results for social advancement and comfort; but anesthesia outranks
them all, in its combinations of kindness and power at a point of
unutterable need.*

Frederic S. Dennis, *Congress of Arts and Science*, 1904

Any fool can cut off a limb; to save one is a true scientific triumph.

George Ryerson Fowler, *Annals of Anatomy and Surgery*, 1881

Most professions have a watershed moment, a time after which things will never be the same. For surgery, its turning point began in 1846 with the discovery of anesthesia and ended in 1867 with the development of antisepsis. The availability of anesthesia and antisepsis to control pain and infection—the last of four crucial fundamentals essential for the performance of effective and safe surgical operations (the first an understanding of anatomy and the second the capability of controlling bleeding)—dramatically transformed the experience of patients. Yet the introduction of these two epochal innovations was contentious, marked by profound debates concerning life, death, suffering, and the very nature of human existence.

Until the mid-decades of the nineteenth century, surgery endured as a limited craft. Pain and the always-looming problem of postoperative infection constrained the surgeon's reach. The deep-rooted image of the brutal and unfeeling

"Sawbones"* was fading, but the gamut of surgical operations remained narrow, mostly bloodletting, amputation, drainage of abscesses, extraction of rotten teeth, and setting of fractures. Some knife bearers, led by individuals like Hunter's disciples, attempted bolder and more dangerous operations, but the new surgical techniques were constrained by an ever-present reality of life, the unavoidable presence of pain. Despite the speed and finesse of a surgeon's scalpel, discomfort made surgical procedures unbearable and the bleeding and tissue damage brought deadly infections.

The torment that patients suffered was awful and the sounds of their screaming echoed through operating rooms. In an all-too-common theme, diaries, newspapers, and periodicals were filled with compelling accounts of surgical operations that attested to a patient's anguish. "When the dreadful steel was plunged into the breast—cutting through veins—arteries—flesh—nerves—I needed no injunctions not to restrain my cries," wrote the novelist Frances Burney (aka Madame d'Arblay) concerning her mastectomy. Burney, who had been Keeper of the Robes for Charlotte of Mecklenburg-Strelitz, George III's queen, described being conscious through most of the procedure:

> I began a scream that lasted unremittingly during the whole time of the incision—and I almost marvel that it rings not in my ears still! So excruciating was the agony . . . oh heaven—I felt the knife rackling against the breast bone—scraping it![1]

* * *

---

* "Sawbones" is a slang term used to describe a surgeon. The expression is often tied to the United States Civil War and the ubiquitous use of amputations and the sawing through bones as treatment for extremity injuries but, in fact, predates this era. Instead, the gruesome-sounding nickname was in use in Great Britain by the 1830s, heralded by Charles Dickens's employment of it in his 1837 novel, *The Posthumous Papers of the Pickwick Club*. In chapter 29, referring to several "nice young men belonging to one of the liberal professions," Dickens writes: "There's a couple o' Sawbones down stairs. A couple of what! exclaimed Mr. Pickwick, sitting up in bed. A couple o' Sawbones, said Sam. What's a Sawbones? inquired Mr. Pickwick, not quite certain whether it was a live animal, or something to eat. What! don't you know what a Sawbones is, Sir? enquired Mr. Weller; I thought everybody know'd as a Sawbones was a Surgeon. Oh, a Surgeon, eh? said Mr. Pickwick with a smile."

Throughout the preanesthetic era, scalpel wielders demonstrated an intriguing attitude toward surgical discomfort. Pain—whether inflicted by man or nature—might have been considered an everyday part of life, but surgeons avowed that it also served a protective role by sustaining a patient's vitality while his or her organs were under the threat of exhaustion due to the strain of an operation. This conviction was encouraged by religious leaders who argued that surgical pain should be regarded as a blessing from the Almighty and represented a challenge for the faithful to be Christ-like in their suffering. "The life of a person in good health is almost entirely barren, and that of one in sickness may be a continual harvest," wrote an influential prelate in the early seventeenth century. "It is on this account that we must have patience not only to be sick, but to have the sickness God wishes, in the place where He wishes, among the person whom He wishes, obeying the physician in each and everything."[2] By embracing the religious perspective and linking it to the surgical view, individuals who performed surgical operations maintained that a patient's suffering had a greater purpose and should be considered an essential part of healing.

Despite these fixed attitudes, the need to control pain became paramount as surgeons extended the assortment and complexity of operations. Since classical times, doctors had attempted to alleviate surgical pain, albeit with minimal success. The Greeks and Romans relied on alcohol and opium as well as marinated mandrake root as analgesics. By the Middle Ages, soporific sponges were recommended. These were sea sponges soaked in concoctions of hemlock, henbane seeds, ivy, mulberry juice, poppy, and wine that were inserted into or covered the mouth and nostrils of the patient. However, similar to other supposed painkillers, they did little to mitigate the discomfort associated with a surgical operation.

In the late eighteenth and early nineteenth centuries, the work of Franz Anton Mesmer led to the concept of mesmerism-induced painless surgery, a form of hypnosis. He was a quack who became a highly regarded faith healer. The German doctor's supposed powers were built around a bewildering pseudoscientific doctrine based on his "discovery" of a universal magnetic fluid. Mesmer believed that every human had magnetic fluid coursing through his or her body. Health resulted when an individual's magnetism was in balance while illness came from a lack of proper magnetic flow. Mesmer also preached that stable magnetism could alleviate surgical pain.

Mesmer enthralled his clientele with his imagined power to "magnetize" objects with a special wand aided by the combination of candles, incantations, incense, and music, all of which generated a form of mass suggestion. So powerful was Mesmer's control over his patients and his supposed ability to redirect their magnetic fluid that it was not uncommon for them, most often female, to be overtaken by violent convulsions accompanied with prolonged outbursts of sighing or weeping. This necessitated their being moved to a separate "crisis" room where he attended the women in private, a practice that led to raised eyebrows.

Mesmer's ideas were little more than hocus-pocus, but he stumbled on something that played a role in the history of surgical anesthesia as well as the practice of psychology. It was not Mesmer's correction of magnetic fluid imbalances that supposedly cured individuals. Instead, it was his ability to bring about a suggestive mental state in which illnesses, often of a psychological nature, could be treated. Mesmer's techniques, shed of their abracadabra appeal, became the forerunner to modern hypnosis; he is the individual whom the verb "mesmerize" is named after.

As word spread of Mesmer's work and knowing that some of his patients demonstrated diminished levels of consciousness during his séances, surgeons experimented with the idea of mesmerism-induced painless surgery. Knife bearers in England and India reported some "successful" trials, but in truth, mesmerism was slow to act, unpredictable, and useless in emergency surgical situations. The technique was eventually abandoned. Surgeons were forced to come up with other ways of easing surgical pain. A scalpel wielder in London designed a metal apparatus to compress a patient's limb prior to amputation, thus diminishing the extremity's sensibility by pinching its nerves so they could no longer communicate pain signals. Patients complained equally about the agony of the compression compared with the pain of the operation. Other techniques, including acupuncture and bleeding a patient into a faint prior to the operation, were tried but failed.

The effort to conquer surgical pain was at a standstill. "To escape pain in surgical operations is a chimera which should no longer be looked for in our day," wrote a well-known Parisian surgeon. "A cutting instrument and pain, in operative medicine, are two words which never present themselves, one without the other, in the mind of patients, and it is necessary for us surgeons to admit their association."[3] The overwhelming risk of mortality from infection and the patient's reluctance to endure pain caused surgical procedures to remain a last-ditch effort in a surgeon's armamentarium. The beginnings of surgical anesthesia needed advances in chemical practice and theory before the first reliable anesthetics could be available.

*   *   *

During the final decades of the eighteenth century, experiments in chemistry and the properties of gases led to the discovery of chloroform, ether, and nitrous oxide (aka, laughing gas). Humphry Davy, a young English chemist, who had served as an apprentice to an apothecary, investigated whether these new gases, particularly nitrous oxide, could be used to treat tuberculosis and other diseases. While doing experiments on animals and himself, Davy noticed that inhaling nitrous oxide gas brought on a sense of intoxication and giddiness and sometimes a momentary lapse into unconsciousness. He speculated about his research:

> As nitrous oxygen in its extensive operation appears capable of destroying physical pain, it may probably be used with advantage during surgical operations in which no great effusion of blood takes place.[4]

Little was understood about the physiology of respiration, and without a basic understanding of breathing Davy as well as other scientists were concerned that too long an exposure to nitrous oxide would not only lead to a manner of sleep but also bring about death by suffocation. There the cautions remained, for not one surgeon paid the slightest attention to his suggestion about the relief of surgical pain.

By the 1830s, interest in the effects of inhaling nitrous oxide as well as other gases on humans had spread beyond researchers and scientists. Word broadened to the public about the pleasant outcomes that came when dabbling with these aromatic and colorless compounds; from euphoria through lethargy and finally sleep, the consequences of breathing their vapors were powerful. Within a decade, ether gas parties and laughing gas frolics had become the craze as soused individuals, having lost all inhibitions, amused themselves with the gases' enjoyable effects. Still, the users of ether and nitrous oxide rarely pushed themselves to the point of unconsciousness. Lay individuals, similar to scientists, feared that prolonged exposure to the gases would lead to breathing distress and death. Temptations to use either compound to bring about insensibility for medical or surgical treatments were strictly avoided. No one recognized how the gases' intoxicating charms would lead to one of Medicine's holy grails, surgical anesthesia. That was until several dentists in America realized the significance of insensible sleep as a means to perform painless tooth extractions.

* * *

Situated in the West End neighborhood of Boston is one of the most eminent medical institutions in the world, Massachusetts General Hospital. It is the oldest and largest teaching facility of Harvard Medical School and the third general hospital to be opened in the United States. Founded in 1811, the original two-story Classic Revival–style rectangular building was fashioned out of white granite from a nearby quarry, highlighted by a massive Ionic portico at the center of its facade. Alongside the top portion of the portico is a square attic story with four brick chimneys crowned by a windowed dome that served as the ceiling of a surgical amphitheater.

For over two centuries, medical and surgical breakthroughs at Massachusetts General Hospital have transformed Medicine's landscape—thirteen Nobel Laureates trained or worked there. The surgical innovations have been especially impressive, including the initial organized use of antisepsis by a hospital in America (1876), one of the first employments of the X-ray in the United States (1896), recognition of the nature and surgical treatment of appendicitis (1896), and the earliest successful replantation of a severed limb (1962). One breakthrough, however, stands above all others, the first public demonstration of surgical anesthesia in the world (1846).

The discovery of surgical anesthesia is America's greatest contribution to the art of healing and one of its most important gifts to the whole of mankind. The suddenness of the leap in knowledge was shocking. One evening surgical anesthesia did not exist and the following morning news of its discovery spread throughout the land. "No single announcement ever created so great and general excitement in so short a time," wrote an eyewitness to its first use. "Surgeons, sufferers, scientific men, everybody, united in simultaneous demonstrations of heartfelt mutual congratulation."[5] The story of this momentous event that took place in Massachusetts General's surgical amphitheater, now celebrated as the Ether Dome, is one of cajoling, chance, and conniving.

* * *

At a time when the public lecture was part of America's democratization of knowledge, itinerant "professors" of chemistry and physics traveled the country's byways speaking on the wonders of electricity or the qualities of gases, especially nitrous oxide. Enthusiastic citizens lined up to listen and have a sniff or two of laughing gas, hoping to achieve a high as their friends chuckled at their antics. In early December 1844, one smooth-talking showman appeared in Hartford, Connecticut, and announced, with much ballyhoo, that an evening talk and grand exhibition of nitrous oxide gas would be held at the city's Union Hall. The advertisement in the *Daily Courant* promised forty gallons of the substance and eight strong men sitting in front-row seats to prevent injury to any participants. "The entertainment is *scientific* to those who *make* it scientific," promised the lecturer. "I believe I can make you laugh more than you have for six months previous."[6]

Among those who purchased a twenty-five-cent ticket was Horace Wells, a twenty-nine-year-old dentist. Ambitious but anxious and depressive, he watched as one of the partakers jumped wildly about the stage and plowed knee-first into a large wooden bench. The young man was injured enough to bleed but seemed unaware of his wound until the effects of the gas had worn off. The incident did not go unnoticed by Wells, who immediately deduced that a tooth might be painlessly pulled while a patient was under the similar effects of laughing gas.

Wells arranged to have the "professor" visit his office the following morning and administer the nitrous oxide to himself. After Wells took a few whiffs, one of his dental colleagues used forceps to extract a bothersome molar. "We knew not whether death or success confronted us," wrote the friend. "It was terra incognito we were bound to explore—the result is known to the world."[7] Wells awoke within minutes and, tasting blood in his mouth and feeling the space where the tooth once resided, supposedly exclaimed, "A new era in tooth-pulling! It is the greatest discovery ever made! I didn't feel it as much as the prick of a pin!"[8]

An ecstatic Wells had the "professor" show him how to prepare the nitrous oxide gas. One month and about a dozen patients later, Wells was satisfied that the vapors could be used safely. In January 1845, seeking fame and fortune, Wells journeyed to Boston to reveal his findings to William Thomas Green Morton, his former practice partner. Wells hoped that Morton's familiarity with the city's medical elite would lead to a public demonstration of painless tooth pulling: Boston was a center of medical leadership in America with an admired hospital, prominent medical school, and well-respected journalists.

Morton, at the age of twenty-seven, was a self-taught dentist and as much a bottom-line businessman as a budding researcher. He enjoyed a relatively successful dental practice but had a checkered past. Gossip was rampant about drinking problems, bankruptcies, and reports that he had been circumcised in a failed attempt to marry a wealthy Jewish woman and welched on the surgeon's seventy-five-dollar fee. Mindful of the tittle-tattle, Morton decided to attend lecture courses at Harvard Medical School to improve his dental skills and enhance his professional qualifications as well as his public standing. This was not unusual; through much of the nineteenth century dentistry was considered part of a physician's overall work. Those individuals who practiced dentistry but were not medical doctors had little legal or social accountability and were viewed as uneducated tradesmen.

While at Harvard, Morton studied with various members of the staff at Massachusetts General Hospital, in particular its somber professor of surgery, John Collins Warren, one of the country's leading surgeons. Founder of the American Medical Association (AMA) and the *Boston Medical and Surgical Journal* (the forerunner to today's *New England Journal of Medicine*) and author of the country's first textbook on surgical oncology, Warren represented a trusted name in the chaotic world of mid-nineteenth-century American Medicine. Morton also befriended Charles Jackson, an eccentric but highly regarded Harvard Medical School graduate, who served as his private tutor for instruction in medical chemistry. Jackson was outspoken and quick-tempered, but his knowledge of the basic sciences was superb.

Shortly after arriving from Hartford with news of his successful tooth extractions, Wells met with Morton and Jackson and discussed his concept of painless dentistry. "[The two] expressed themselves in the disbelief that surgical operations could be performed without pain," Wells later claimed. "Both admitting that this *modus operandi* was entirely new to them."[9] After mulling over the situation, Morton introduced Wells to Warren, who invited the dentist to demonstrate his discovery to a group of Harvard medical students.

It was to be an exciting day for the future physicians, and one of the young men even volunteered to have an annoying tooth pulled. According to an observer, Wells explained that he had made a discovery that would "prevent pain in the extraction of teeth" and "in all surgical operations."[10] The dentist prepared his equipment, administered the gas, picked up forceps, and grasped the student's molar. Suddenly the supposedly anesthetized patient groaned loudly. The implication was clear as pandemonium ensued. Spectators erupted into waves of catcalls and laughter. Several hollered that the entire spectacle was "a humbug affair."[11] In his anxiousness, Wells had not administered enough nitrous oxide. For the hapless dentist, it was too much to bear. The disgraced Wells fled the room. He returned to Hartford, not a prize-winning inventor but a vanquished risk taker. Within months, Wells had placed his house and dental practice up for sale as he fell victim to a severe depression.

Despite Wells's debacle, Morton realized the potential of his ex-partner's idea and took up the cause of painless dentistry. He was concerned about the reliability of nitrous oxide and, on the suggestion of Jackson, began to experiment with ether. The chemist had previously suggested that Morton use the compound in its liquid form as a local application to decrease a tooth's sensitivity. Jackson also described the stupefying effects of inhaling ether's vapor, though he advised combining it with atmospheric air to lessen the chance of deadly consequences.

Armed with this counsel, Morton spent almost two years perfecting his inhalation techniques and learning about the nature of the substance. He added oil of orange to mask ether's distinctive scent and devised an elaborate glass and metal contraption to administer the vapors. Morton was not simply inventing painless dentistry; he was pursuing the far larger and prestigious prize of pain-free surgery. By the fall of 1846, Morton was ready to publicly demonstrate the results of his experiments. He visited Warren, who agreed to help his former student. Shortly, Morton received a letter inviting him to come to Massachusetts General Hospital to "administer to a patient, who is there to be operated on [by Warren], the preparation which you have invented to diminish the sensibility to pain."[12]

On Friday, October 16, 1846, with the seats of Massachusetts General Hospital's surgical amphitheater filled to capacity, a nervous and tardy Morton entered the room's side door and was met by Warren. "Well, sir!" said the surgeon somewhat brusquely. "Your patient is ready."[13] Morton turned and looked at Gilbert Abbot, an asthenic appearing man of about twenty-five years of age, who suffered from a congenital tumor of convoluted and enlarged blood vessels under the left side of his jaw. After saying a few reassuring words, Morton positioned the mouthpiece of his newly designed breathing apparatus and told Abbot to take some deep breaths. Within minutes, Abbot was asleep. Morton stepped toward Warren and told him it was now *his* patient who was ready. The excitement in the amphitheater was like an opening night on Broadway as the smell of orange-scented ether filled the room and the crowd held silent with all eyes fixed upon the surgeon's every move.

Warren picked up a scalpel and made a three-inch incision through Abbot's skin. For twenty-five minutes the spectators watched in stunned disbelief as Warren performed pain-free surgery. The young patient did not budge as the older surgeon cut away an annoying tangle of fragile blood vessels. In Warren's biographer's words, the operation required "a protracted dissection among important nerves and blood-vessels . . . [and] the effect of the agent was made perfectly distinct to [Warren's] mind."[14]

Whether the men in the room realized they had just witnessed one of the most important events in human history is unknown. Warren looked over his audience and slowly and emphatically uttered what became five famous words: "Gentlemen, this is no humbug."[15] There was silence and then the slightest of murmurs. No one knew what to say. No one knew what to do. Warren turned to the awakening patient and repeatedly asked him whether he felt anything. The answer was an unbelievable, "No!" Warren explained: "[Abbot] said he felt as if his neck had been scratched but . . . he did not experience pain . . . although aware that the operation was proceeding."[16] There are moments in the history of the world when time seems to stop and everything changes. This was one of those instants.

The following morning, the *Boston Daily Journal* carried a short account of what had occurred under a bold headline, "SUCCESSFUL OPERATION."[17] "[Morton's] preparation," the reporter explained, "affords the surgeon the means of doing his work freed from all interruptions on the part of the patient, and gives him facilities for performing operations in the most expeditious manner."[18] Four weeks and several successes later, the crucial first announcement to the profession of the invention of surgical anesthesia was published in the *Boston Medical and Surgical Journal*:

> It has long been an important problem in medical science to devise some method of mitigating the pain of surgical operations. An efficient agent for this purpose has at length been discovered . . . of what now promises to be one of the important discoveries of the age.[19]

The news was electrifying and spread rapidly on the nation's burgeoning telegraph system. A steamer soon left Boston for Liverpool and carried with it letters from American surgeons attesting to the success of ether anesthesia, along with copies of the *Boston Medical and Surgical Journal*. Within weeks, a London surgeon prepared to do an amputation and skeptically announced to a crowd of students, "Gentlemen, we are going to try a Yankee dodge for making men insensible." Twenty-six seconds later, the patient's bloodied and sawn-off leg lay on the floor.

The scalpel wielder faced the students and conceded, "This Yankee dodge, gentlemen, beats mesmerism hollow."[20] "Good News from America! Hail, happy hour! We Have Conquered Pain," cheered the *People's London Journal.*[21] Within three months, ether anesthesia had been used in Austria, Germany, and Russia, and an American physician/missionary even employed it in China. Speed was no longer a knife bearer's sine qua non.

The benefits of ether anesthesia might have been incontrovertible, but many doctors claimed difficulty in administering it—too small a dose caused patients to be excitable and struggling and removed any sense of decorum. "[I] would think twice before I consented to inhale," wrote Charlotte Brontë, the famed English novelist and poet. "One would not like to make a fool of oneself."[22] Refusal due to an individual's unease was one thing, but concern that ether anesthesia actually jeopardized lives led doctors to fear its role in surgery. The editor of the *New York Journal of Medicine* warned:

> Serious and almost fatal consequences have followed the inhalation of it . . . which render it (when administered judiciously) a limited, dangerous, and uncertain preparation. . . . We are sorry to see many of our brethren, at home and abroad, stooping from the exalted position they occupy in the profession, to hold intercourse with, and become the abettors of, quackery in any form.[23]

There was also the challenge of personal rivalries and regional distrusts among America's physicians. "We are persuaded," wrote a doctor:

> the surgeons of Philadelphia will not be seduced from the high professional path of duty, into the quagmire of quackery by this will-o'-the-wisp. . . . We express our deep mortification and regret, that the eminent men, who have so long adorned the profession in Boston, should have consented for a moment to set so bad an example to their younger brethren as we conceive them to have done in this instance. If such things are to be sanctioned by the profession, there is little need of reform conventions, or any other efforts to elevate the professional character—physicians and quacks will soon constitute one fraternity.[24]

And there were the condemnations of self-righteous individuals who believed that the miseries of daily life were punishments from God and should be taken away only by the Almighty. "Anaesthesia is of the devil," declared the first president of the American Dental Association:

> It forms a servant we should deal very cautiously with. For my own part I could not conscientiously use an agent that would bring my fellow-man so near to the point of the separation of body and soul.[25]

* * *

It took a decade or so for patients' and surgeons' attitudes to change. During that time, the availability of ether and soon chloroform significantly increased the frequency of surgical operations; chloroform became the anesthetic of choice because it was more potent, less irritating, and much safer. "There has been a general rush towards the operating room, such as the world has never seen," commented a surgeon. "Great numbers of cases were successful . . . and this gave an *éclat* to the subject, and induced a confident state of mind in patients."[26]

The growth of anesthesia and increase in surgical operations were greatly influenced by events in Europe's Crimean War* and America's Civil War. The outbreak of the Crimean conflict caught the combatants unprepared and they had to take drastic measures to transform the fighting capabilities and medical care of their forces. At a time when disease, exposure, and malnutrition accounted for a disproportionate number of casualties, Florence Nightingale, an English nurse, revolutionized the

---

* The Crimean War (1853–1856) was contested on the Crimean Peninsula, a landmass jutting south from present-day Ukraine and almost completely surrounded by the Black Sea. The political background of the conflict concerned the decline of the Ottoman Empire, which led France and Great Britain to fear that Russia would pursue an expansionist policy and seek to control the Black Sea and its trade routes. Combat ensued when the English and French attacked Russia's stronghold naval base at Sevastopol, a city on the southern fringe of Crimea. Following a year-long siege, including a major battle at Balaklava (commemorated by Alfred Lord Tennyson, the English poet, in "The Charge of the Light Brigade"), the Russians abandoned Sevastopol. When Austria threatened to join the British/French/Ottoman Empire alliance, Russia accepted peace terms and the Treaty of Paris was signed.

care of wounded soldiers, which led to substantial improvements in battlefield medicine.

At the same time, the use of anesthesia became extensive. A war correspondent reported that Russian doctors "performed every operation with chloroform no matter how trivial it might be"[27] while French physicians employed it over twenty-five thousand times. A decade later, a report on surgical care during America's Civil War revealed that anesthetics were used "in no less than eighty thousand instances . . . and the inestimable value of the use of anaesthetics in military surgery will hardly be denied at this date."[28] Thus, the two wars served as mini-campaigns for the promotion of anesthesia, underscored by the surgeons who returned from the fighting and endorsed its safety to civilian populations. The conflicts also furthered the development of anesthesia by demonstrating that knife bearers could not be solely responsible for administering an anesthetic; an extra person, an anesthesiologist, was required for its proper dispensing.

With the patient's physical distress less of a concern, the psychological, social, and technical aspects of what occurred in an operating room were transformed. Scalpel wielders, who previously raced through operations under difficult circumstances—marked by the thrashing of an unanesthetized patient—could take their time and complete procedures theretofore impossible. Operations that once relied on sleight-of-hand dexterity, exemplified by Cheselden and his sixty-second extraction of bladder stones, were replaced by procedures based on more precise and thorough approaches. For patients, thousands of years of thinking about pain were torn asunder as scientific research brought fresh advances. "The creation of pain by any operation can only be regarded, at the present time, as both unnecessary and injurious," railed a surgeon. "As [etherization's] safety has been widely tested, philanthropy and that desire to ameliorate the sufferings of mankind . . . demand that neither prejudice nor ignorance of its effects should longer prevent its employment by every operator."[29]

Inhalational anesthesia deadened pain, but it did not address the last barrier that hindered surgery from moving forward, infection. If anything, the availability of surgical anesthesia worsened the problem. Since pain no longer impeded surgeons' technical capabilities, they performed increasingly complex and invasive procedures that reached deeper into the body. The consequence was greater tissue damage and blood loss, which led to overwhelming infections and mortality rates of 50 percent or higher. Until the challenge of uncontrollable postoperative sepsis could be resolved, surgery's development remained at a dead end.

*　*　*

As for Morton and his discovery, he was enough of an entrepreneur to understand that the only way he could secure financial recompense for his efforts was through a government-issued patent. When government officials assured Morton that rights were available, the dentist looked to strengthen the application through association with a well-known person. He chose Jackson and, in November 1846, federal authorities issued Patent No. 4848 to both Morton and Jackson in a ninety/ten split, respectively. Within days, Morton was selling rights to anyone hoping to cash in on the expected boom in painless surgery.

The temperamental Jackson grew jealous of Morton's higher stake and sparked a mad race for greater equity and official recognition. During these years, the French dominated the world of Medicine and investigators who wished to establish priority in a discovery used the Académie des Sciences in Paris to arbitrate such issues. Jackson sent a letter to French authorities claiming to be the sole originator of anesthesia. At the same time, a discouraged Wells also decided to seek his claim to anesthesia fame. When Morton realized that Jackson and Wells were courting the all-important French recognition, he issued a sixty-page treatise that outlined his justifications for rights to the discovery. In a Solomonic compromise, the Académie des Sciences awarded a joint prize for discovery to both Jackson and Morton: Jackson for his "observations and experiments on the anesthetic effects produced by the inhalation of ether" and Morton for "having introduced this method into surgical practice in conformity to the [*d'apres les indications*] instructions of Dr. Jackson."[30] Wells was never in the running.

The split decision only heightened animosities and forced Jackson and Morton and their supporters to seek a more definitive answer from the United States Congress. When members of Congress reached a compromise settlement, cries on the House floor of, "A bargain! A bargain!"[31] squelched the agreement. Each side accused the other of backroom political shenanigans that negotiated away potential profits. During another congressional session, a House committee decided that Morton deserved the credit for discovering surgical anesthesia and awarded him $100,000. The Senate disagreed and referred the anesthesia question back for another round of inconclusive hearings. And so it went, month after month, year after year, through countless arguments, hearings, and thousands of pages of sworn testimony. In the end, Congress never determined whether it was Morton, Jackson, or even Wells who discovered surgical anesthesia.

Wells was the first of the three to stop fighting. He succumbed to his worsening depression after the Académie des Sciences rejected his claim. Wells abandoned his family and headed to New York City, where he tangled with prostitutes and ended up in the infamous Tombs prison. In January 1848, Wells's existence came to a dismal end. The originator of nitrous oxide anesthesia stuffed a silk handkerchief doused with chloroform into his mouth and slit an artery in his thigh with a razor.

Morton and Jackson's feud extended past Wells's death. Once it became known that Morton's anesthetic agent was not a novel substance but common ether mixed with perfume, attempts to enforce the patent proved difficult. Morton's obsession with his fiduciary rights consumed him. He abandoned his dental practice, became destitute, and lived off the largess of friends. Jackson countered Morton's arguments with uncompromising antagonism. As late as 1858, a story in the *New York Times* noted that "the old triangular [anesthesia] war, from every corner, is waged with more vigor and bitterness than ever . . . the public has never yet agreed to which of the three claimants thanks are due."[32]

A despondent and paranoid Morton died of a stroke in 1868. Five years later, Jackson also suffered a stroke with resultant brain damage including the inability to understand or express speech. His family had him committed to the McLean Asylum for the Insane in Massachusetts, where he lived out the final seven years of his life. Death provided an ironical final chapter to the Morton/Jackson dispute. These bitterest of rivals were buried only yards apart in the Mount Auburn Cemetery in Cambridge, Massachusetts.

Anesthesia proved invaluable for decreasing pain and allowed surgeons to complete prolonged operations. But it would take another momentous breakthrough to clear away the final dilemma that haunted surgery: infection. The hurdle that was postoperative infection, its cause and lethality, remained a mystery. Answers were many, but none proved correct until a surgeon in Scotland made an insightful observation about wounds, infections, and a newly discovered form of life, germs.

11.
THEY'RE ALIVE

A good surgeon operates with his hand, not with his heart; though he knows well at the same time, in his heart, that for one moment of suffering he gives years of life and health.

Alexandre Dumas père, *Memoirs of a Physician*, 1847

Evils that former generations of surgeons deplored, but could not effectually combat such as, septicemia, pyemia, hospital gangrene, and erysipelas, have been much abated, as a direct consequence of a clear understanding of their essential nature and causation.

Arpad G. Gerster, *The Rules of Aseptic and Antiseptic Surgery*, 1888

Progress in surgery was at a halt. Surgeons understood the human road map and how to manage blood loss. They could bring an individual to insensible sleep safely while he or she was undergoing an operation. The scalpel wielders' technical wizardry dazzled the public. Surgeons had become showmen and surgery a spectacle. Nevertheless, far too many surgical procedures ended in the death of a patient. The culprits were overwhelming postoperative infections accompanied by their deadly warning sign, pus. This circumstance was all too common and the presence of pus was accepted and expected. Pus was termed "laudable"* and its existence regarded

---

* The phrase *pus bonum et laudabile* ("good and laudable pus") was first used in the early Middle Ages, although it arose from observations made by the ancient Greeks. Followers of Hippocrates believed that pus was an essential and welcomed element of a healing wound. Purportedly, pus was a result of spilled

as an indication a wound was healing properly, a notion that turned into surgical dogma. However, beginning in the late eighteenth century, as more technically advanced surgical techniques were devised and greater numbers of surgeons were trained, the challenge of postoperative infections became increasingly problematic.

Viewed through the distance of historical inquiry, it is easy to downplay what was an issue of terrifying consequence until slightly over a century ago: the tragedy of relatively healthy individuals, especially those in need of simple procedures, turned into surgical horrors as rampant wound infections sapped their life. Tens of thousands of innocent mothers and fathers and sons and daughters were dying for ostensibly no reason. The problem was that no one understood what an infectious disease was or how it was transmitted.

The surgeons' descriptions of this frequent clinical situation were invariable. On the third or fourth postoperative night, the patient's fever—which was as much anticipated as the creamy pus that filled the wound—shot suddenly higher while the tissue around the incision matched the ancient Greek Celsus's four signs of an emerging infection, "heat, pain, redness, swelling." The danger signal was sounded even though its pathogenesis, the biological cause of an illness, was not understood.

Surgeons were divided in their thinking. Some believed the difficulties were attributable to overcrowded and dirty hospitals where malodorous halls and walls produced a setting for diseases to spread easily. Others alleged that wounds became inflamed and pus filled when their raw surfaces were exposed to decaying matter transmitted through the air via noxious vapors. There were additional farfetched

---

and spoiled blood and, like any offensive humor, needed to be expelled from the body. From the perspective of a time before antibiotics, antisepsis, or an understanding of what was an infection, the idea of pus as "laudable" seemingly made sense. The principle of laudable pus remained unchallenged until the late Middle Ages when surgical scholars, led by Theodoric and de Mondeville, questioned the importance of pus in a wound. Despite their reasonings, the view that pus was a necessary component of healing was so ingrained any alternative ideas were largely discredited. As late as the mid-nineteenth century and the American Civil War, accounts of extremity amputations still noted how a "stump looks much better; granulations more fluid and healthy; discharge more laudable," only to find, days later, that the "stump has refused to heal . . . there being no prospect that it would ever become useful, the [remaining] leg was reamputated" (G. A. Otis and D. L. Huntington, "Wounds and Complications," *Medical and Surgical History of the War of the Rebellion*, part 3, [Washington, DC: Government Printing Office, 1883], 2:861). Not until the latter part of that century would research on bacteria and antisepsis lead to the recognition that pus was the sign of an infection, not a factor to be praised. By the first decade of the twentieth century, the concept of pus as laudable was eliminated from the surgical literature.

theories, but the speculation always assumed that diseased tissue had lost vitality, which led to putrefaction (better known as decay) and a debilitated and dying patient. A London surgeon provided an eyewitness account of these tragic situations:

> You are sensible, from the violence of the fever and the swelling of the limb, that mischief is going on within. The dry skin, the parched mouth, the thumping pulse, the restlessness and delirium, continue for some days, and there is a blackness round the wound threatening gangrene . . . the great wound begins to suppurate [to form pus] and opens very wide, the whole limb swells to an enormous degree. . . . You are careful to dress the limb every morning, and perhaps to clean it also a little in the evening. By regular washing and wiping with the moist sponge, you prevent those smells which depress the patient's spirits . . . you should be careful to have the windows open and the room ventilated, to change the linens, to make your patient wash his face and hands with cool vinegar and water, and when the matter [pus] is very profuse, to have the room fumigated with vinegar. . . . Often it happens, from the destruction of parts, or the unhappy circumstances of the patient, that all your cares are unavailing! Every time you examine the limb, you make discoveries of more extensive destruction, you find the whole limb swelling every day more and more, you find the matter running profusely from the openings . . . and the suppurations extending from the ham to the heel with intolerable fetor [a strong, foul smell]. . . . You find that you are no longer able to support the patient's health, that repeated attacks of diarrhea and fever have reduced him to extreme weakness; the wan visage, the pale and flabby flesh, the hollow eyes and prominent cheek bones, the squalid hair, the long bony fingers and crooked nails, the quick, short breathing, and small piping voice, declare the last stage of debility! The natural powers are then sunk so low, the appetite for food, and even the desire of life so entirely gone, that we would believe the patient past all help.[1]

An evil-sounding colloquialism was applied to this and other similar dreadful conditions, "blood poisoning." The phrase first appeared in 1847 when a physician described the existence of "several varieties of blood poisoning" and noted how they differed "materially in their appearances, course, and results."[2] Today we know that blood poisoning has nothing to do with an actual poison. It is not even a true medical term. Instead, the catchall idiom implies danger and for good reason: its name refers to the presence of bacteria in the blood or bacteremia. In its most aggressive manner, bacteremia can progress rapidly to a serious generalized sepsis and end in a fatality. Think of the modern-day disorder known as flesh-eating disease (in surgical parlance, necrotizing fasciitis) that results in the destruction of body tissue and often leads to shock, amputations, organ shutdowns, and death. Its nineteenth-century counterpart was a loathsome mass of human decay that went by the businesslike nom de guerre "hospital gangrene"; surgeons and patients lived in fear of its arrival. Similar to flesh-eating disease, hospital gangrene destroyed any tissue in its path, creating a rotting stink that permeated hallways and gagged the throats of nurses, patients, staff, and surgeons. The disease was so infectious that, once one case appeared, the whole ward was likely to be affected.

The deadliness of blood poisoning was among the reasons why the recognition of bacteria and an understanding of antisepsis proved more important to the development of surgery than the introduction of anesthesia. There was no argument that the relief of pain permitted a surgical operation to be conducted in a more efficient manner. Haste was no longer a prime concern. But the availability of anesthesia did not get to the root of the problem that held back surgery, infection. If anesthesia had not been discovered, surgical procedures could still be performed, albeit with much difficulty. However, without antisepsis, surgical operations often ended in death rather than pain. Clearly, surgery needed both anesthesia and antisepsis, but in terms of overall importance, knowledge of bacteria and how to control their behavior had a greater singular impact.

*   *   *

Surgical infections were tragic and scientific explanations were needed. The answers came primarily through the research of two geniuses. They were men who saw things that other individuals did not: Louis Pasteur, a French chemist, and Joseph Lister, an English surgeon. Pasteur's discoveries changed Medicine in many ways, but it was their relevance to wound infections that had the greatest impact on the development of surgery. He was born in the Jura, an area of lakes and mountains in eastern France.

In his early twenties, Pasteur moved to Paris, where, in 1847, he graduated from the renowned École Normale Supérieure, having submitted two theses, one in chemistry and the other in physics.

Pasteur was a lifelong academic and laboratory enthusiast; he was not a physician. Early in his career, his reputation as a brilliant chemist was established when he showed that the shape of molecules distinguished living from inanimate things. Pasteur's appointment as dean of the science faculty at the University of Lille,* at the northern tip of France, led to further research into the divide between biological and chemical processes. He was asked by a local winemaker to investigate the wine-manufacturing process because large numbers of his vats had soured. Pasteur set up a makeshift laboratory, including a microscope, in the winemaker's cave. To Pasteur's astonishment, he discovered that alcoholic fermentation involved living microscopic structures he called bacteria and concluded they were responsible for the spoilage. His further studies showed that similar microorganisms were also present in rancid butter and sour milk.

Pasteur's findings were earth-shattering. His critics acceded to the existence of microorganisms in various fermentable substances, but Pasteur's suggestion that they were a newly discovered form of life was beyond comprehension. His detractors asserted that the microorganisms generated spontaneously. Pasteur, who was no shrinking violet when it came to the defense of his scientific research, was adamant that these tiny creatures were alive, floated through the air on dust particles, and had living parentage. Life, he asserted, did not arise out of mere matter and the concept of spontaneous generation was a scientific hoax.

As Pasteur's research programs and professional life flourished—in 1867, he was appointed chair of organic chemistry at the Sorbonne—he undertook a series of experiments to silence his faultfinders. Pasteur had discovered that when bacteria were exposed to extreme temperatures they were destroyed, a technique that led to the process of Pasteurization, whereby foods are treated with heat to eliminate or inactivate dangerous microbes. For his research, he boiled broth to rid it of any microorganisms and create a sterile brew. He then placed the mixture in two different

---

* It was at the University of Lille that Pasteur voiced one of the most famous quotes in the annals of education and science: "*dans les champs de l'observation, le hasard ne favorise que les espirits préparés* (in the fields of observation, chance favors only the prepared mind) (*Oeuvres de Pasteur*, 7 vols., ed. Louis Pasteur Vallery-Radot [Paris: Masson et Cie, 1939], 7:131).

types of glass flasks; one had a straight open neck while the second had a swan or S-shaped neck that prevented dust and other flakes from touching the liquid. After several days of waiting, the broth in the open-neck flask was crowded with microbial life, while the brew in the swan-neck flask remained barren. This persuasive show of scientific proof demonstrated that the living organisms in the open-neck flask came from outside, on dust and other particles, rather than spontaneously generating; otherwise, the swan-neck flask would have also been swarming with microorganisms. This ingenious experiment and others to follow established what is considered a foundation of biological science: only life can produce life.

The bacterial contamination of beverages and food led Pasteur to speculate that the presence of microorganisms in humans might be a cause of disease. If fermentation and spoilage were connected through germs, could it be possible that putrefaction and infection were linked to bacteria? In late 1863, a Parisian surgeon authored a 750-page text, *De l'acide phénique*, in which he discussed Pasteur's ideas concerning putrefaction and bacteria as they related to human diseases. The following summer, a London knife bearer, who was the surgical consultant to Queen Victoria's household, addressed the British Medical Association and provided a lengthy review of Pasteur's work on germs. Similar to his French peer, the Englishman speculated about the bacterial origin of infectious diseases and wound suppuration:

> [By] applying the knowledge for which we are indebted to Pasteur
> of the presence in the atmosphere of organic germs which will grow,
> develop, and multiply, under favorable conditions, it is easy to un-
> derstand that some germs find their most appropriate nutriment in
> the secretions from wounds, or in pus, and that they so modify it as
> to convert it into a poison when absorbed—or that the germs after
> development, multiplication, and death, may form a putrid infecting
> matter—or that they may enter the blood and develop themselves,
> effecting in the process deadly changes in the circulating fluid. That
> these low forms of animal life may seriously affect the blood of the
> higher orders of animals, is clearly proved.[3]

Unfortunately, neither surgeon's ideas garnered much attention. Few scalpel wielders were intellectually ready to accept the fact that germs existed, they were living creatures, and they could harm patients. Besides, even if surgeons believed in the germ theory of disease, how could they control the negative effects of bacteria? Unlike Pasteur, who boiled liquids to destroy microorganisms, surgeons would not find it possible to heat a surgical patient to such an extent. Hence, no attempts were made to test the germ theory of putrefaction as it related to surgery.

That is until Joseph Lister, an English surgeon, combined Pasteur's discovery of bacteria with his own expertise in microscopy and knowledge of surgical wounds. The result was the greatest breakthrough in the history of surgery: antisepsis. How this insightful genius accomplished his discovery and secured the acceptance of antisepsis by a skeptical profession is among the monumental tales in surgery. As with other innovations that changed the course of human history, if a pantheon existed to honor the surgical greats who made critical breakthroughs, then Lister would sit with Hunter, Paré, Vesalius, Morton, Jackson, and Wells in the front row.

* * *

If ideal family circumstances existed in which a surgical mastermind was to be raised, then Lister grew up in them. His father was a successful wine importer and self-educated scientist who taught himself the essentials of optics and made innovations in lenses that transformed the microscope from a scientific curiosity to a formidable research tool. The work was important enough that he was awarded Fellowship in the Royal Society. Lister's mother was an elementary school teacher who self-schooled her children during their early years. His parents were Quakers with strong family ties. Quakerism, with its guiding principles of austerity, gratitude, and a resoluteness of character, was more than a religion—it served as a guide to their way of life.

Father and son were devoted to each other and there is little doubt that the senior Lister's interest in microscopy strongly influenced his offspring's early fascination with nature and Medicine. According to Joseph's biographer, he told his family, "when quite a child,"[4] that the practice of surgery would be his life's work. By Lister's early teens, he dissected farm animals, inspected their tissue under a microscope, and was conversant with and could draw many of the bones in the human skeleton.

In the fall of 1847, Lister enrolled at the medical school of University College in London. He had previously attended the undergraduate section for three years. In an interesting piece of surgical arcana, Lister was in the gallery, as a medical student-to-be, when the first operation under ether was performed in that city and the surgeon uttered his memorable words regarding the "Yankee dodge" and how it "beats mesmerism hollow."[5] Lister was eager to begin his medical studies, but his first year ended prematurely in an unexpected way. He resided in a gloomy boardinghouse ruled by a demanding fellow Quaker who allowed no downtime from the strains of schoolwork. Social engagements and friendships were eschewed while the religious teachings of Quakerism were emphasized. In the middle of this exhausting schedule, Lister suffered an attack of smallpox and returned to his classes before fully recovered. The result of the various stresses led to what was termed "a nervous breakdown." He grew restless, unfocused, and, perhaps, suicidal. In present-day psychiatric terms, the almost-twenty-one-year-old suffered an episode of acute depression.

At a time when there was limited understanding of mental illness and no antidepressant medications or electroconvulsive treatments, Lister's family prevailed upon him to leave school and remove himself from the environment that brought about the crisis. In late spring of 1848, Lister reevaluated his state of affairs while traveling around Great Britain, Ireland, and continental Europe. In July, his father wrote an insightful letter:

> I have compared [our cheerful parting] to the sunshine after a refreshing shower, following a time of cloud—and I trust the remembrance of our conversation may be permitted to dispel from thy thoughts, some phantoms of the dark—that thou wilt become fully aware of what is certainly true—viz. that the things that sometimes distress thee are really only the result of illness, following too close study . . . believe us, my tenderly beloved son, that thy proper part now is to cherish a pious cheerful spirit, open to see and to enjoy the bounties and the beauties spread around us: not to give way to turning thy thoughts upon thyself nor even at present to dwell long on serious things . . . do not consider thyself required to answer this which contains some things I should not generally advert to.[6]

Lister's mental collapse was the symptom of an on-and-off depression that he dealt with throughout his life. Moreover, the breakdown foreshadowed a change in personality from that of a relatively carefree youngster to a rather cold adult who had difficulty maintaining close interpersonal relationships. One colleague described Lister as always surrounded by a "cloud of seriousness" that "tempered all he did."[7]

Another labeled Lister as a "man of few words" with a "seriousness of purpose" evident in all his interactions.[8] This rigidity of personality might also be explained by a shyness and stammer that long plagued him.

Despite these somewhat off-putting personality traits, Lister was also viewed as a guileless, humble, and level-headed individual who showed unfailing sympathy for the afflicted. Surgeons might have disparaged his work on antisepsis, but none uttered a callous word about the man himself. Terms such as "courteous,"[9] "earnestness,"[10] "intellectual,"[11] and "modesty"[12] dot the biographies and reminiscences of Lister. His simple decency and dedication to his craft was particularly evident in his role as a teacher. An assistant recalled Lister's lectures as "peerless . . . contagious and inspired,"[13] notable for their practicality and wisdom.

* * *

In 1849, Lister returned to the University College medical school with a renewed passion for surgery. He received gold medals in comparative and pathological anatomy, honors in medicine and surgery, and perfected his skills in microscopy. In addition, he joined the school's debating club in an effort to overcome his stammer. In 1852, Lister was awarded his medical degree and, after passing qualifying examinations, received membership in the Royal College of Surgeons. For the next nine months, he served as a house surgeon, a position equivalent to the modern internship/residency. With no doubts clouding his desire for a career in surgery, Lister wrote to his parents:

> If the love of surgery is a proof of a person's being adapted for it, then certainly I am fitted to be a surgeon: for thou canst hardly conceive what a high degree of enjoyment I am from day to day experiencing in this bloody and butcherly department of the healing art. I am more and more delighted with my profession.[14]

By this time, Lister was twenty-seven years old and planned to travel through Europe to observe surgeons at work and then commence a private practice in London. However, his mentors suggested that he should first round out his studies in Edinburgh under the most renowned of the country's surgeons, James Syme, professor of surgery at that city's university. Within months of his arrival in the fall of 1853 Lister came to regard Syme as a trusted adviser and father figure, and later Lister would consider him a steadfast father-in-law. Lister's intended sojourn of several weeks turned into a quarter-century stay.

Despite the closeness of their relationship, there was no greater contrast in appearances and personalities than between Lister and Syme. The almost-six-foot-tall Lister was cultured and reserved, with an unflappable temper. He was fluent in French and German and measured in his choice of words. Syme was barely five and a half feet in height, with a headstrong self-confidence. His nickname was "the formidable,"[15] and the description was backed by a temper and tongue as quick as his mind. Yet Lister and Syme viewed themselves as complementary, evidenced by their deep admiration for each other. It was said that Lister was the only individual with whom Syme never quarreled.

Syme offered Lister a position as his first assistant. Two years later, Lister had so impressed Syme and others that, when he applied for an appointment as Assistant Surgeon to the Edinburgh Royal Infirmary and Lecturer in Surgery to the Royal College of Surgeons of Edinburgh there were no dissenting votes. In addition to caring for private patients and giving lectures, Lister began wide-ranging research that would lead to his momentous discovery of antisepsis. He speculated about putrefaction in surgical incisions and became convinced that the entity that caused the rotting of flesh was found within the wound itself.

Lister observed that putrefaction commenced in clots of blood located deep in an incision. The clots decayed, the rot spread to surrounding tissue, the four classical signs and symptoms of inflammation appeared (i.e., heat, pain, redness, and swelling), pus materialized, and the calamitous onset of blood poisoning was underway. Lister recognized this because his expertise with the microscope enabled him to scrutinize tissues, which led to his conviction that inflammation damaged the structure of tissues, disabled their function, and made them unable to fend off attacks.

Lister had been in Edinburgh six years, during which time he married Syme's eldest daughter, Agnes, and gained recognition as an up-and-coming scientist and surgeon. The summer of 1859 brought important news: the professor of surgery at the University of Glasgow suffered a paralytic stroke and the school was searching for a replacement. At the urging of Syme, Lister applied for and received the appointment. Syme's letter of recommendation described his son-in-law as having "strict regard for accuracy, extremely correct powers of observations, and a remarkably sound judgment, united to uncommon manual dexterity and a practical turn of mind."[16] By spring of the following year, Joseph and Agnes were settled in Glasgow, where, on her recommendation, his lecture hall was painted in the shiny chocolate browns and yellow creams that were the preferred colors of the day while the doors were turned green baize. Agnes would go on to play a critical role in Joseph's future successes as a research assistant and lifelong soul mate. The Listers looked forward to starting a family but remained childless.

When Lister was not busy organizing talks and tending to patients, he furthered his research into surgical wounds. Like all hospitals of that era, the Glasgow infirmary was filthy, poorly managed, and a breeding ground for pus-filled incisions and deadly infections. Lister believed that if he could clean the wards, his patients would not fall victim to inflammation and sepsis. Floors were swept, walls scrubbed, sheets changed, patients bathed, but to no avail. None of these measures lowered surgical mortality rates. Lister was flummoxed. Then, during the final days of 1864, the professor of chemistry at the university, who knew of Lister's interest in putrefaction and wounds, alerted him to recent papers published by Pasteur that showed how decay in food was caused by the action of microscopic-sized living organisms.

* * *

Lister pored over the articles, applied his skills in microscopy to studying bacteria, repeated Pasteur's experiments, and, in an aha moment, came to a similar conclusion as the Frenchman: it was invisible germ-laden dust particles falling into a wound that were the contaminating source of blood poisoning. Lister discovered that the same microbes were also found on the instruments, sponges, and towels used during a surgical operation and even on a surgeon's hands. He also came to the realization that an injury inflicted through a traumatic accident was already teeming with bacteria by the time the patient arrived at the hospital. Lister's inferences were incisive: a method was needed to prevent the introduction of germs into surgical incisions, and germs must be destroyed once they were in wounds. He also recognized that to prevent a wound from having contact with the air and dust particles was an impossible task. Instead, Lister settled on chemical-mediated antisepsis, knowing that Pasteur's method of destroying bacteria by excessive heat was not applicable to patients.

For a year, Lister experimented with a variety of chemicals but without success. In early 1865, his approach changed when he read a newspaper account of how engineers at a nearby sewage plant used carbolic acid (aka phenol, a derivative of coal tar) to reduce the smell of cesspits. Lister deduced that the carbolic acid killed the microorganisms in the refuse. He decided to employ the compound in his research on animals using dressings soaked in carbolic acid or simply pouring the solution directly into a wound. Convinced of carbolic acid's effectiveness in keeping bacteria at bay in an incision, Lister turned to human studies and the treatment of compound fractures. This type of injury, in which broken bone punctures the skin, had a high rate of infection because bacteria on the skin's surface gained access to deep tissues. That summer, Lister successfully used his new method:

> My house-surgeon, acting under my instructions, laid a piece of lint dipped in liquid carbolic acid upon the wound, and applied lateral pasteboard splints padded with cotton wool, the limb resting on its outer side, with the knee bent. It was left undisturbed for four days, when, the boy complaining of some uneasiness, I removed the inner splint and examined the wound. It showed no signs of suppuration, but the skin in its immediate vicinity had a slight blush of redness. I now dressed the sore with lint soaked with water having a small proportion of carbolic acid diffused through it; and this was continued for five days, during which the uneasiness and the redness of the skin disappeared, the sore meanwhile furnishing no pus, although some superficial sloughs caused by the acid were separating. But the epidermis being excoriated by this dressing, I substituted for it a solution of one part of carbolic acid in from ten to twenty parts of olive oil, which was used for four days, during which a small amount of imperfect pus was produced from the surface of the sore, but not a drop appeared from beneath the skin. It was now clear that there was no longer any danger of deep-seated suppuration, and simple water-dressing was employed. Cicatrisation proceeded just as in an ordinary granulating sore. At the expiration of six weeks I examined the condition of the bones, and, finding them firmly united, discarded the splints; and two days later the sore was entirely healed, so that the cure could not be said to have been at all retarded by the circumstance of the fracture being compound. This, no doubt, was a favourable case, and might have done well under ordinary treatment. But the remarkable retardation of suppuration, and the immediate conversion of the compound fracture into a simple fracture with a superficial sore, were most encouraging facts.[17]

Six and a half weeks after the wheel of a horse-drawn cart shattered James Green-lees's left lower leg, the eleven-year-old walked out of Glasgow's Royal Infirmary on his own two feet. This simple act ushered in the early modern era of surgery.

Further successes led Lister to extend the antiseptic technique from accident injuries to complex surgical operations. Time and experience brought modifications to his method. The caustic and irritating nature of carbolic acid was lessened by mixing it with boiled linseed oil or other substances. In addition, Lister began to not only use the carbolic acid mixture in wounds but also spray it into the atmosphere surrounding the operative table. He dipped his hands in carbolic, immersed his instruments in carbolic, and soaked his towels in carbolic. Confident of his results, Lister began to use a declarative and simple expression when discussing his research: "the element of incurability has been eliminated."[18]

One might think that the news of Lister's monumental breakthrough, first published in 1867, would have been received with great fanfare. However, much like the incredulity that followed the introduction of anesthesia twenty years earlier, the news of antisepsis was met with both indifference and opposition. Surgeons were baffled by the germ theory of disease, which was the foundation of Lister's system. They could not or did not believe in the existence of microorganisms as another form of life. Even when the presence of bacteria was accepted, they were deemed harmless contaminants and never the source of infection. Denials aside, it must have been a discomfiting and humbling task for surgeons to come to terms with the distressing fact that, since time immemorial, they had been inadvertently harming and killing patients by allowing incisions to be infected with invisible living organisms while filling with "laudable" pus.

Besides the human element of disbelief, there were also practical difficulties in evaluating Lister's technique. The system was complex and constantly changing; his skeptics characterized these adjustments as evidence that the method never worked. They did not view the modifications as part of the natural sequence of scientific investigation. As Lister's method grew more complicated, surgeons pointed to repeated failures, even when they supposedly followed his rules. The problem was that most scalpel wielders practiced a bastardized version, in which some aspects of Listerism were employed while various hard-to-break traditions were preserved. It was not uncommon for surgeons to assure that operative sites were carefully cleaned and even dip their instruments in a carbolic acid bath but refuse to scrub their hands or wash their blood and pus–stained operating frocks. Others sneezed over an incision or held scalpels and ligatures between their teeth, while professing to practice Lister-ism simply because they had sprayed the air in the operating room with carbolic acid. "I have felt that if the antiseptic treatment is to be of any use, it must be simpler than Mr. Lister has made it," declared a surgeon. "By his plan each patient requires five or ten times as much attendance as usual."[19]

In mid-1869, Syme suffered a debilitating stroke. Syme wanted Lister to suc-ceed him and that autumn Joseph and Agnes were again in Edinburgh. Lister un-derstood that because his antiseptic technique was often used carelessly, poor results needed to be explained and it was up to him to demonstrate the method firsthand. Lister's answer was to employ the Royal Infirmary as a training base where surgeons could personally observe his protocol; hundreds of scalpel wielders took advantage of the opportunity.

Lister also published scores of articles in the most prestigious of medical jour-nals. And he completed a series of what were regarded as crusades for antisepsis through the Continent. The surgeons, particularly in Austria-Hungary and Ger-many, embraced Lister and rapidly adopted his ideas. "The progress of Professor Lister through the university towns," wrote a medical reporter for the *Lancet*, "has assumed the character of a triumphal march ... with most enthusiastic receptions."[20] Banquets in his honor, with hundreds in attendance, were held in Berlin, Bonn, Munich, Halle, and Leipzig. In the latter city, the King of Saxony requested that an antiseptic-based operation be performed in his presence. Italian surgeons also con-firmed Lister's remarkable results and were soon followed by the French and Span-ish. But the tour's affirmations did little to change the opinions of the Americans and British who remained doubting.

*　*　*

By the mid-1870s, awareness of Listerian techniques had spread throughout the United States as antisepsis and the germ theory became the hot surgical topics of the day. In the spring of 1876, the debates reached a crescendo of sorts when one of the deans of American surgery penned an essay in which he praised the nation's knife bearers and quipped: "Little, if any faith, is placed by any enlightened or ex-perienced surgeon on this side of the Atlantic in the so-called carbolic acid treat-ment of Professor Lister."[21] This viewpoint was shared by others, notably Edward R. Squibb, the influential founder of E. R. Squibb and Sons, the forerunner to the modern pharmaceutical giant Bristol-Myers Squibb. "I confess to a strong prejudice, since first reading Mr. Lister's articles," argued Squibb, "against what I have regarded as a needless complication of a simple method. . . . Mr. Lister's honesty and earnestness grew into fanaticism, and led him to exaggerate and over-dose."[22]

America's knife bearers had split into rival camps and the challenge was how they responded to the issues this new style of surgical care posed to the profession. Were Lister's ideas truly groundbreaking? If so, how should antisepsis be implemented in a hospital or a surgeon's office? The tenor of the discussions changed when Lister was invited to participate in an International Medical Congress to be held in conjunction with the United States' Centennial Exhibition in Philadelphia's Fairmount Park. For Lister, his journey to the United States would be an exciting adventure. For Americans, the tour became a cultural milestone and a momentous event in the history of surgery.

In early August 1876, the Listers sailed from Liverpool on the SS *Scythia*. The ship was a showpiece of the Cunard Line, with elegant staterooms, richly decorated dining areas, watertight compartments, and a sophisticated steering apparatus. The newly built liner made trans-Atlantic travel faster (ten days) and safer than it had been. The Listers were seasoned travelers who looked forward to combining Joseph's professional activities with a sightseeing tour of America. Prior to heading to Philadelphia, they spent two weeks cruising up the Hudson River, visiting the Catskills, Albany/Saratoga, and Adirondack regions of New York, and crossing Lake Champlain, where they boarded a New York Central and Hudson River train that took them through Canada with stops in Québec City, Montreal, and Toronto. The Listers reentered the United States at Niagara Falls and rode the railroad's famous Water Level Route (this track followed rivers and had few significant grades) back to New York City.

When Lister arrived at the Centennial Exhibition in the first days of September, the fair was averaging nearly one hundred thousand visitors a day. It was an extravaganza of over two hundred buildings with tens of thousands of exhibits and the multicolored flags of nations waving everywhere, the grounds surrounded by a three-mile-long white picket fence. Lister was fascinated by the displays and, prior to the start of the medical meeting, spent a day touring the Exhibition's grounds. At noon on Monday, September 4, Lister led a parade of physicians into the ornate chapel of the University of Pennsylvania. The International Medical Congress was the first of its kind in America; almost five hundred physicians attended. The one hundred–plus talks included basic research, clinical studies, and historical and literary presentations. An extensive social program featured afternoon lunches and evening receptions as well as scores of private dinners. There was an on-site post office and rooms set aside for reading newspapers or just mingling. "Every arrangement," according to an eyewitness, "was convenient . . . there was no hitch, rub, or jar."[23]

When an announcement was made that Lister would serve as the Congress's president of the section on surgery, a round of "hearty applause"[24] filled the room. Despite the warm welcome and Lister's prominence, antisepsis and the germ theory were under assault. At the opening session, a physician gave a lengthy presentation on bacteria or what he termed "disease-germs." He was quick to note that there was no "satisfactory proof" that they were "necessarily connected" with any "infective diseases."[25] Speakers lined up to condemn all that Lister believed in. "Is it not to be feared that the particular treatment advised by Professor Lister," cautioned a cynic, "tends to divert the attention of the surgeon from other essential points?"[26] Things grew testier when a doyen of the older generation of America's knife bearers admonished Lister: "A large proportion of American surgeons seem not to have adopted your practice; whether from a lack of confidence or for other reasons, I cannot say."[27]

Lister was nonplussed. He was an experienced lecturer and, in two and a half hours of academicism and showmanship and one hour of answering questions, Lister explained the subtleties of his system, concentrating on the intertwined connections between dirt, germs, pus, and wounds. Without apologies, Lister acknowledged that his antiseptic scheme demanded scrupulous care. "It is the close attention to these minute details," he explained, "that renders this system so absolutely certain and safe in its results."[28] Wounds, he explained, should never be manipulated with unclean instruments or touched by unwashed hands or unbrushed fingernails. "If the surgeon's hands or an instrument are passed beyond the area of [carbolic] spray," he cautioned, "they must not be again brought near the wounds until they have been dipped in the [carbolic] antiseptic solution."[29] The Englishman's conclusions were profound: destroy germs on a surgical incision, prevent their access to the wound during the healing process, and pus will not form and infection is averted.

For some, Lister's talk was an unqualified success. A reporter called the lecture "the great event of the day,"[30] and another styled Lister among the "strongest of the foreign guests."[31] Several physicians spoke up and congratulated Lister on his work. "I am willing to accord to the antiseptic system . . . all or much that has been claimed for it,"[32] declared a healer from South Carolina. Another doctor acknowledged

Lister's inspiration and agreed that "perfect cleanliness is important in the treatment of wounds."[33] A surgeon from Ohio offered the most discerning praise: "Fellow surgeons, prepare for the revolution in our art. An antibacterial period is upon us."[34]

Lister's doubters, however, far outnumbered his supporters. Skeptics were upset over his long-windedness and the legitimacy of his research. "It was rather a doubtful thing for him to do," complained one eyewitness, "that is, if he were aware of the amount of time he was occupying."[35] "The hour being late," grumbled another nonbeliever, "I merely desire to point out a few facts which ... militate against the [germ] theory, as far as it claims that a certain class of minute living organisms ... are essential to disease-processes."[36] Others found Lister eccentric, an English oddball. One cynic went so far as to ridicule Lister by saying he had a "grasshopper in his head."[37]

Despite the less than enthusiastic reception, Lister was neither dissuaded nor upset. He was in America not only to sway the skeptics but also to see the country. Following the Congress, the Listers boarded a train and headed west to San Francisco. It had only been seven years since transcontinental tourism became possible, and train travel across the United States and its territorial areas still carried considerable risks—three months earlier George Custer and his army regiment had been annihilated in the eastern Montana Territory by Lakota and Northern Cheyenne warriors and later that fall ninety-two people would die when a train derailed on a bridge and plunged seventy feet into the Ashtabula River in Ohio. Nevertheless, Lister was a global adventurer and the opportunity to sightsee on a scale unimaginable in Europe was not to be missed. He would be the first surgeon of international repute to journey back and forth across the North American continent.

Ten days later, Lister and his wife arrived in California. They passed through Cheyenne, the capital of the Wyoming Territory, and Salt Lake City, a novel community headed by its founder, Brigham Young. For Lister, the Great Plains, the Rocky Mountains, and the West Coast were strictly about the views. The Listers returned east by way of recently burned Chicago and reached Boston, where he spoke to a class at Harvard Medical School.

The final destination was New York City. Lister agreed to perform a live demonstration of his antiseptic technique and, on October 10, stood in the Charity Hospital's surgical amphitheater on Blackwell's Island (now Roosevelt Island) in front of hundreds of onlookers. "I had no idea that I was to address so large a body of students," exclaimed Lister. "It is a most unexpected privilege."[38] Not only did the doctors-to-be watch Lister perform an operation under carbolic acid antisepsis (he drained a syphilitic abscess on a young man's groin), but a member of the audience "phonographically" recorded every word of the talk also. This is the earliest instance that a surgeon's lecture was documented live in America. What happened to the soundtrack remains a mystery.

Lister was his usual assiduous self. When a slight breeze from an open window blew his antiseptic spray away from the patient, Lister asked that the pane be closed. He used this episode to caution the students that minute attention to the details of the antisepsis routine was mandatory. After a give-and-take with the audience, Lister closed with firm counsel:

> Gentlemen ... open the abscess antiseptically; employ efficient antiseptic dressing, provide for the escape of [fluids] ... and the [pus] ceases from that time forward.[39]

Two days later, Lister and his wife boarded the SS *Bothnia* for a voyage back to England. A colleague reported that Lister "enjoyed his visit to America enormously" and was "glad he had undertaken it."[40] Lister's nephew described the tour as "one of the more important of what may be called [my uncle's] evangelistic journeys."[41] Although the drive toward antisepsis was not immediate, Lister's presence established a line in the sand between the surgically innovative and the surgically obsolete. Three years later, a surgeon noted:

> The Lister plan of the treatment of wounds has gained many advocates in hospitals in this [New York] and other cities. It is a matter of record that mortality, both in hospitals and private practice, has been greatly diminished since the antiseptic treatment of wounds has been adopted.[42]

* * *

Shortly after Lister's return to Edinburgh, he accepted a position as professor of surgery at King's College in London. Lister had long desired to return to England's capital, but he now had a specific reason, the continued resistance of the city's surgical community to his antiseptic system. Lister wrote a friend: "[My new appointment will] enable me to carry out . . . the thorough working of the antiseptic system with a view to its diffusion in the metropolis."[43] Similar to his schedule in Edinburgh, Lister gave two lectures a week that included demonstrations of his technique, while managing an active clinical practice. Unlike his talks in Scotland, which were crowded with enthusiastic students and supporters, the opposite was true in London—only a few disinterested men occasionally showed up.

Lister grew increasingly frustrated with his countrymen who continued to disparage his ideas. "It is no part of the business of the [English] surgeon to bolster up theories, be they good or bad, or to make facts rigidly conform to them,"[44] asserted a disparaging editorial in the *Lancet*. Similar to the Americans, one overriding reason explained why British surgeons were slow to acknowledge the germ theory of disease and the need for antisepsis. "The truth is, that this is a question in science rather than in surgery," explained a knife bearer in London. "While eagerly adopted by the scientific Germans . . . the antiseptic doctrine has never been in any degree appreciated or understood by the plodding and practical English surgeon."[45] Despite the initial pushback, by the early 1880s resistance in the British Isles to Lister's ideas faded and his teachings became part of everyday surgical practice.

In December 1892, Lister journeyed to the Sorbonne in Paris to attend a celebration of Pasteur's seventieth birthday. Over the years, the two men had become close friends and were regarded as the preeminent figures in science and surgery. Though he was only five years older than Lister, Pasteur was debilitated by a series of strokes. Lister delivered an address in French in which he expressed his deep gratitude and acclaimed the enormity of Pasteur's discoveries. "Thanks to you," said Lister, "surgery has undergone a complete revolution which has deprived it of its terrors and enlarged almost without limitations its power for good."[46] When Lister completed his remarks, Pasteur rose from his chair and, leaning on the arm of Sadi Carnot, the President of the French Republic, made his way to the podium, where he embraced Lister. According to the official record of the event, it was "like the living picture of the brotherhood of science in the relief of humanity."[47] Lister and Pasteur would never meet again.

In early 1893, Lister retired from his professorship. Several months later, Agnes and he were on vacation in Italy when she died from a rapidly spreading pneumonia. Lister lived another nineteen years, but his joie de vivre was never the same. Listerism had been accepted and he was celebrated as a surgical icon, but without his wife at his side the many accolades Lister continued to receive seemed empty in importance. These included honorary doctorates from the Universities of Cambridge and Oxford, the presidency of the Royal Society, and elevation to the peerage as Lord Lister of Lyme Regis, the first surgeon to receive such a title. His name was even immortalized with the invention of Listerine, a popular oral antiseptic. Lister died on a dreary morning in February 1912. A public funeral was held in Westminster Abbey, but his will specified that he be buried at West Hampstead Cemetery on the outskirts of London, next to his life's companion, Agnes.

* * *

By the end of the nineteenth century, the results of surgery were no longer left to chance. Surgical patients were more likely to leave a hospital alive than dead and with intact arms and legs. Knowledge trumped ignorance as meticulousness surmounted carelessness. Thanks to Vesalius and Paré, surgeons understood anatomy and how to stem blood loss. American dentists showed them how to control pain and an English surgeon discovered how to operate without causing infections. The four elemental barriers to successful operative surgery had been overcome and no part of the body was off-limits. No longer lauded solely for their dexterity and quickness, surgeons were increasingly admired for their cautiousness and discipline. Surgery was freed from its confining and primitive nest. Armed with containers of carbolic acid and ether, as well as an understanding of pathology and physiology, the emerging generation of scientific surgeons seemed capable of doing anything.

12.

SCIENTIFIC PROGRESS

The surgeon may harden himself whilst performing an operation, for he knows that he is acting for the good of his patient; but if we were intentionally to neglect the weak and helpless, it could only be for a contingent benefit, with an overwhelming present evil.

Charles Darwin, *The Descent of Man*, 1871

You cannot be a perfect doctor, till you have been a patient: You cannot be a perfect surgeon, till you have enjoyed in your own person some surgical experience.

Stephen Paget, *Confessio Medici*, 1908

I clearly remember the reprimand, terse but well meant. "Ira," said George Zuidema, the chairman of surgery at The Johns Hopkins Hospital, "a little less about the history of Hopkins and a little more towards your surgical work would be appreciated." He was correct. My interest in surgical history had grown considerably since my arrival in Baltimore, but the research and writing needed to take a backseat relative to my patient responsibilities. I heeded the chairman's counsel and renewed my efforts on the clinical side of surgery, but it seemed a Hobson's choice. For me, to be a resident at the renowned Johns Hopkins Hospital—one of the world's great medical establishments—and not be captivated by its history seemed almost sacrilegious. Indeed, in looking back at my life as a surgeon/historian, I have come to regard the transfer of my surgical training from Boston to Baltimore as my all-in-one exodus, hegira, and pilgrimage.

The Johns Hopkins Hospital was built on a thirteen-acre campus at the crown of what was then called Loudenschlager's Hill in East Baltimore. Because the site was away from a floodplain and housed a decaying and about-to-be-demolished general hospital/insane asylum, it attracted the interest of Johns Hopkins, a Baltimore banker and merchant, who bequeathed $7 million (approximately $180 million in 2022) for a hospital and university to bear his name. In May 1889, when the new hospital complex was completed, seventeen redbrick structures built in a Queen Anne style were situated pavilion-style around an open courtyard (they included an administration building, apothecary shop, bathhouse, dispensary, home for nurses, pathology building, and private and public patient wards).

John Shaw Billings, a distinguished surgeon and expert in hospital construction, designed the facility. A man with wide-ranging interests (his successful regulation of army hospitals during the Civil War established his career as a hospital architect), he had previously organized the Library of the Surgeon General's Office (precursor to the National Library of Medicine), managed the United States' Census Bureau's Division of Vital Statistics, supervised the 1880 census, and served as president of the American Public Health Association. Billings was later appointed director of the New York Public Library and planned its building on Fifth Avenue and 42nd Street, including placement of the iconic pink Tennessee marble sculptures of Fortitude and Patience, the lions that guard its front entrance.

Billings was an innovator and his ideas for The Johns Hopkins Hospital included central heating (the first in the nation) along with fully ventilated floors to allow the free circulation of outside air; in the late 1870s, when The Johns Hopkins Hospital was conceived, it was still believed that diseases were caused by stagnant "sick air" as well as poisonous vapors rising from the soil. His concern about the spread of disease was further allayed by having the inside ceiling and floor corners rounded to lessen the buildup of dirt. Billings also made certain that the gaslit buildings were prewired for the coming availability of incandescent electric lighting and rudimentary telephone service.

Presently, the Johns Hopkins Hospital complex contains over sixty buildings—some are specialty centers or mini-hospitals in their own right, including The Charlotte R. Bloomberg Children's Center, the Brady Urological Institute, Kennedy Krieger Institute, the Weinberg-Kimmel cancer center, and the Wilmer Eye Institute—although only three of the original redbrick structures remain. The most recognizable of the three is the four-story administration building with its centerpiece dome, spire, and eight-sided open rotunda. Since 1896, a ten-and-a-half-foot-tall Carrara marble Christ statue has stood in the rotunda and I, like thousands of residents before and after me, often rubbed the figure's toes for good luck.

Whether I was walking the hospital's corridors, caring for surgical patients, studying in the library, attending a lecture at the medical school, or pursuing a doctorate at the school of public health, the history of Medicine surrounded me. Above all, I learned that Johns Hopkins's bequest called for a close relationship, physically and philosophically, between patient care (embodied in The Johns Hopkins Hospital) and research and teaching (exemplified by the Johns Hopkins University School of Nursing [1889], the Johns Hopkins University School of Medicine [1893], and the Johns Hopkins School of Hygiene and Public Health [1916, renamed the Johns Hopkins Bloomberg School of Public Health in 2001], the three of which adjoin the hospital complex).

Hopkins's vision laid the foundation for a radical transformation in health care that brought about modern American Medicine through the alignment of clinical practice, education and training, and scientific research. This reformation was successful not because physicians and surgeons had fundamentally changed but because Medicine and its relationship to science had been irrevocably altered. Dogmatism, quackery, and sectarianism were no longer tenable within the confines of scientific truth. The foundations of surgery now rested on logical proof and technical expertise as the ascent of scientific surgery unified the craft and facilitated what had been an art to become a learned profession.

For over a century and a quarter, medical and surgical advances at The Johns Hopkins Medical Institutions have revolutionized health care—eighteen Nobel Laureates associated with the hospital and/or the medical school trained or worked there. The surgical breakthroughs have been particularly impressive, ranging from development of the radical prostatectomy (1903), the "blue baby" operation for congenital heart disease (1944), the nation's earliest male-to-female reassignment surgery (1966), to the first implantation of an automatic cardiac defibrillator (1980). Equally remarkable is the fact that many surgical specialties were initially formalized at Johns Hopkins, including gynecology, neurosurgery, orthopedic surgery, otorhinolaryngology, and urology. However, one series of groundbreaking contributions and the surgeon who made them stand above the others.

*　　*　　*

William Halsted's list of accomplishments seems endless: establishing the technique of local anesthesia; developing complex operations for breast cancer, groin hernias, goiters of the thyroid, and aneurysms of blood vessels; devising a method to suture intestines; introducing the use of sterile rubber gloves; and emphasizing the need for exacting techniques in the operating room, especially the gentle and tedious dissection of tissue. Beyond his scientific accomplishments, Halsted established the first surgical residency training program in the United States with the goal of creating surgical teachers, not merely competent operating surgeons. More than any other individual, Halsted set the tone for this most important period in surgical history. His work introduced a "new" surgery, based as much on an understanding of pathology and physiology as on know-how in anatomy.

Halsted's admirers termed him a "genuinely scientific surgeon," one who was "animated in high degree by the spirit of scientific inquiry."[1] As such, Halsted moved surgery from the heroics of the operating amphitheater to the quiet of the operating room and the privacy of the laboratory. Although other American surgeons had greater national and international reputations, his story is the most remarkable; noteworthy for the breadth of his achievements and their enduring impact on surgery, but heartrending upon realization that Halsted, while self-experimenting with cocaine for its use in local anesthesia, developed a lifelong drug addiction.

In 1892, Billings presented a report to the Board of Regents of the Smithsonian Institution on achievements in American Medicine. Asked to delineate the advances that highlighted the nineteenth century, he showed no hesitation:

> The most important improvements in practical medicine made in the United States have been chiefly in surgery, in its various branches. . . . I am glad to be able to say that the standard of acquirements in surgical education has been and is now rising, and our leading medical schools are now being equipped with buildings, with apparatus, with laboratories, and, most important of all, with brains, which enable them to give means of practical instruction equal to any to be found elsewhere.[2]

Billings described how Halsted and his acolytes were breathing scientific life into the halls of Hopkins as American surgery ceased to be a mere passive beneficiary of European surgical knowledge. Instead, surgeons in the United States staked their claim to international leadership and separated themselves from their old-world counterparts.

Halsted grew up in Manhattan and enjoyed a princely youth and early adulthood. His father was a well-to-do wholesaler of European dry goods and provided his son with the advantages that mid-nineteenth-century America offered its Anglo-Saxon upper class. Young Halsted had private elementary school tutors, attended boarding school at the Phillips Academy at Andover, and, in 1870, matriculated at Yale. Despite the excellence of his schooling, he was an indifferent student who received mediocre grades while pursuing social activities over academics. Why Halsted decided to study Medicine with its intensive schooling remains conjectural. He never provided answers, but his influential and strong-willed father was a member of the board of trustees of the College of Physicians and Surgeons in New York City (presently the Columbia University Vagelos College of Physicians and Surgeons) and his father's brother was a respected physician at the New York Hospital. Whatever the impetus, in 1874 twenty-two-year-old Halsted enrolled at the College of Physicians and Surgeons and transformed his academic lifestyle. Three years later, he received a medical degree with honors, ranking among the top ten in his class. Halsted obtained a prized internship at Bellevue Hospital, which was followed by a short stint as a fledgling surgeon at the New York Hospital.

The year 1878 was the middle of a medical renaissance in Europe. The basic sciences (i.e., bacteriology, embryology, histology, pathology, and physiology) were growing tremendously. Austro-Hungarian and German doctors had been the first to grasp their importance and were successfully integrating the sciences with clinical investigations. As the German-speaking empire grew, a great scholastic achievement came to fruition in the form of the richly endowed state university, academically diverse, highly organized, and packed with laboratories. The national accomplishments of these universities became international and, from 1870 through the beginning of World War I, the Austro-Hungarian and German schools were meccas for aspiring students from all over the world. In fact, the education of many American physicians, surgeons, and scientists was not considered complete until they had spent time at a German-language university. The attraction was inescapable and fifteen thousand American doctors undertook some manner of study in Austria-Hungary or Germany during those years. For individuals desiring a prominent career in surgery (assuming their personal finances were adequate), time spent in these countries was an absolute requirement.

Coming from a wealthy family, Halsted had the means to travel to Europe, and an intense atmosphere of scholasticism greeted him when he arrived in Vienna in November 1878. "What impressed me chiefly was the magnitude of the operations, the skill of Billroth and his assistants,"* Halsted wrote a friend:[3]

> I also sat upon the benches, often seven hours a day, listening to medical lectures, and was so impressed with the characters and lives of some of my teachers that I believed they represented all that was most advanced in medicine.[4]

After Vienna, Halsted's travels included stops in Berlin, Hamburg, Kiel, Leipzig, and Würzburg. By the time he returned to New York City in September 1880, Halsted had observed or worked with most of the giants of Austro-Hungarian and German surgery, men who were pioneers of modern surgical science.

The two years in Europe were Halsted's surgical baptism. He saw how great German surgeons literally bred more great German surgeons, and it was these men and their schools of surgery who offered Halsted the inspiration and philosophies he incorporated into his activities back home. The intellectually curious Halsted had a firmer command of scientific methods, a broader education foundation, and a more sophisticated outlook on Medicine than most of his peers. In Manhattan, Halsted became a whirlwind of activity as he joined numerous hospital staffs (i.e., Bellevue, Roosevelt, and the Charity Hospital), conducted daily teaching rounds, taught private classes in anatomy, and counted some of the most eminent names in New York Medicine among his closest friends. "Halsted," according to a contemporary, "was the most talked-of among the younger surgeons of that period in New York and many of the older ones shook their heads over his innovations."[5]

---

* Of Europe's many surgeons, the young Halsted was most interested in observing the celebrated Theodor Billroth, director of the University of Vienna's surgical clinic and father of modern abdominal surgery. Shortly after Halsted's arrival in Austria, he befriended one of Billroth's first assistants who gave him unrestricted access to Billroth's surgical wards. An early believer in antisepsis, Billroth performed a number of complex and landmark surgical operations including the earliest successful removals of the esophagus, larynx, rectum, and stomach for cancer. A genial and resourceful academician, he was widely published and established the first modern program of surgical training in Europe. In his private life, Billroth was a talented musician who patronized many of Vienna's composers, particularly Johannes Brahms, who dedicated his two string quartets (Opus 51) to him.

Several incidents epitomized Halsted's gumption. He came to favor Listerism while studying abroad and, thereafter, refused to perform surgical operations without proper sterile conditions. Bellevue's antiquated operating rooms did not fit his needs and the older surgeons refused to comply with his requests for remodeling. A rankled Halsted raised $10,000 from family and friends and erected his own operating room in a tent on the hospital's grounds. Halsted's surgical space had piped-in gas, hot and cold running water, apertures for light and ventilation, a central drainage gutter, and a maple floor "laid almost as finely as a bowling alley."[6] Inventive and practical was one thing, but Halsted was also bold and daring. In 1881, he made surgical headlines by performing the first emergency blood transfusion, under extraordinary circumstances. He was called to see his sister after she had given birth but was dying from blood loss. He withdrew his own blood, transfused her with it (Halsted had no knowledge of blood types, but fortunately, he and his sister were a suitable match), and then operated on her, in her home, on her kitchen table, to save her life.

Halsted approached his social life with the same fervor he gave to surgery. He was an integral part of Manhattan's Gilded Age party scene and fancied himself a "gay blade," that era's fashionable man-about-town, with a luxuriously furnished bachelor pad at Madison Avenue and 25th Street and membership in the nearby exclusive University Club. There were endless dinner parties, musical soirées, and open houses, all attended by a revolving group of young businessmen and professionals. One visitor recalled Halsted as a "model of muscular strength and vigor, full of enthusiasm and of the joy of life."[7] Halsted's career was on the fast track when, in late 1884, a series of scientific events forever altered his life.

In Vienna, a young Sigmund Freud authored a detailed review of the physiological effects of cocaine and its potential use in treating neurological diseases. He also noted the anesthetizing effect that the drug had when it was rubbed on or injected into the skin. At Freud's suggestion, one of his colleagues experimented with cocaine and discovered that applying drops of its liquid form would numb the eye. When these startling findings were discussed at a medical meeting, a visiting American physician reported them in a short letter to a New York–based medical journal. This information introduced the concept of local anesthesia to an American audience and influenced Halsted to commence his own investigations into the usefulness of cocaine in surgery.

*   *   *

Through experiments on himself, Halsted learned how to inject the drug to block various nerves and obtain local anesthesia. It was an impressive scientific achievement made all the more spectacular since he served as his own primary guinea pig. Unaware of cocaine's addictive properties, Halsted experimented with it freely; the indiscriminate use of cocaine was not yet regarded as a public health and social problem, nor was it illegal to possess the drug. Halsted found that when he injected himself it produced more than just an area of temporary numbness. There was a stimulating effect that increased his stamina, cleared his mind, and enlivened social encounters. Halsted sniffed cocaine at the theater, kept vials of it at his bedside, stored it in his office, and increased his self-experimentation. Within six months, he was drug dependent, acting irrational, and facing professional ruin.

Halsted had previously authored over twenty well-received medical articles when he attempted to write a report on his research with cocaine. The opening sentence, contrasted with his prior lucidity, rambled through 118 words and sixteen commas. "Poor health," admitted Halsted, "disinclined me to complete a somewhat comprehensible paper."[8] The article's syntax was embarrassing enough that, four decades later, when the Johns Hopkins Press published a memorial edition of Halsted's collective works, the editor decided to suppress the piece: "its republication is here omitted as this would require such reediting as is not deemed expedient."[9]

As the effects of his addiction worsened, Halsted was threatened with professional extinction. His attendance at meetings declined and, by mid-1885, Halsted was unable to deliver a series of lectures in competition for the chair of surgery at his alma mater. A colleague sensed the seriousness of the problem and convinced Halsted to join him for a "therapeutic" sailing trip to the Caribbean's Windward Islands (now the southern islands of the Lesser Antilles). With virtually no information available about cocaine addiction and little in the way of effective treatment, the voyage, in February/March 1886, was an unmitigated disaster; Halsted filched cocaine and alcohol from the ship's supply room. Halsted's companion despaired over his behavior and urged that he admit himself to a mental hospital. The seven months of treatment at Butler Hospital in Providence, Rhode Island, were inconclusive. During this time, Halsted's father pleaded guilty to embezzling business funds that included a dubious but uncontested loan of $24,800 to William (approximately $700,000 in 2022), sizeable enough for Halsted to maintain financial independence for many years.

In late 1886, following Halsted's discharge from Butler, he realized there was neither a personal nor professional future for him in New York. With his family in fiscal disarray, cognizant of his poor health and widening social embarrassment, Halsted accepted an invitation from his colleague/traveling companion, who had recently relocated to Baltimore to supervise the opening of The Johns Hopkins Hospital, to work in the institution's new pathology laboratory. Nonetheless, Halsted's attempt at what one historian labeled a "form of occupational therapy"[10] failed and he returned to the mental hospital for most of 1887.

The romantic tale of Halsted, an upstart surgeon wending his way through the chaotic world of 1880s American Medicine, seemed to have reached its end. But the unexpected happened during Halsted's confinement. He somehow managed to lessen his unrestrained abuse of cocaine and replaced it with a controlled addiction to morphine. Halsted's use of morphine was no less a habit and remained his lifelong nemesis, but through self-discipline he regained a measure of direction over his day-to-day existence.

*   *   *

In January 1888, Halsted returned to Baltimore and began to work again in the Johns Hopkins pathology laboratory and treat surgical patients at facilities throughout the city. Over the next few years, he conducted landmark studies on wound healing, the proper handling of tissues during an operation, the incorporation of antiseptic principles, and devised elements of the modern mastectomy and groin hernia repair. Halsted hoped to obtain a full-time position at The Johns Hopkins Hospital and, three months after its opening, an administrator wrote to a member of the medical staff: "Halsted (popularly known in hospital circles as Jack the Ripper), does nothing but operate the whole forenoon and it must be admitted with brilliant results."[11]

Halsted, the clinician, researcher, and surgeon, had returned, but these reincarnations were vastly different from what they had been. A change in his personality was obvious. Drug addiction had taken its toll and stripped him of his joie de vivre. The bold and risk-taking knife bearer was gone. Instead, there was an aloof and deliberate individual, who wielded his scalpel in a cautious and perfectionist manner. The outspoken scientist had turned into an obsessive and reclusive investigator, one who relished his privacy. When Halsted walked through the corridors of The Johns Hopkins Hospital, he characteristically lowered his head or turned away, so as to avoid any personal interaction. He appeared a lonely man always lost in thought. It was this Halsted, whom faculty members and students solemnly referred to as "the Professor,"[12] a persnickety, unapproachable surgical genius, who would change the world of surgery.

Halsted's search for perfection in his surgical work was mirrored in his personal life. In matters of dress and grooming, he remained fastidious but in an odd sort of manner. His shiny silk top hats or pitch-black derbies, impeccable cravats, hand-stitched gloves, English-made boots and shoes, and Parisian laundered shirts and suits were viewed as peculiar fashion statements in a hospital setting. The idiosyncrasies in his clothing and personality were also apparent in Halsted's married life. He wed one of his operating room nurses who was equally eccentric. Childless and reclusive, they had separate apartments in a sprawling three-story mansion and rarely interacted with each other. The couple went out of their way to avoid social gatherings and, if visitors came unannounced, the maid was instructed to inform them that the Halsteds were not home. It is not certain how aware Halsted's wife was of her husband's morphine habit. Their lengthy summer vacations (June through September) were spent at an isolated country house in the mountains of western North Carolina. However, Halsted often left, for weeks on end, to travel alone to see the eminent surgeons of Europe, especially the Nobel Prize winner Theodor Kocher of Switzerland.*

By early 1889, Halsted's rehabilitation convinced the trustees of The Johns Hopkins Hospital to appoint him to an interim position; they were unaware of his drug dependency. "Halsted is doing remarkable work in surgery," wrote a member of the medical staff. "I feel that his appointment to the University and the Hospital would be quite safe."[13] Despite Halsted's morphine addiction, he never experienced further mental deterioration and his academic career and private surgical practice took off. Three years later, the trustees made Halsted's appointment permanent by

---

* Theodor Kocher, the first surgeon to receive the Nobel Prize in Physiology or Medicine, pioneered studies in the pathology, physiology, and surgery of the thyroid. His award (1909) was significant because it underscored the legitimacy and importance that was attributed to surgical treatments by the opening years of the twentieth century. In 1871 Kocher was appointed professor of surgery at the University of Bern, and he remained there until his death in 1917. He was highly regarded for how he tediously studied surgical illnesses from their pathological/physiological aspects before applying surgical methods to their cure. Kocher proved a key influence on Halsted, who considered him a kindred spirit with his exacting techniques and assiduous approach to surgical operations, especially his gentle handling of tissue.

naming him surgeon-in-chief to the hospital. Over the coming decades, his legend grew and attracted worldwide attention.

Halsted conducted surgery as a form of scientific inquiry. He proved, to an often-leery profession and public, that the centuries-old grab-and-slash way of doing things was gone. Halsted banned quickness and roughness, replacing them with accurateness and thoroughness. His methods went beyond simple safety. His operations on the bile ducts, blood vessels, intestines, and thyroid restored form and function to as near normal as possible. During his thirty-year tenure, Halsted's methods earned the epithet "Halstedian techniques," which remains a widely acknowledged surgical imprimatur. With a bit of literary license, H. L. Mencken, the Baltimore-based critic of standards of taste and culture in the United States, described Halsted's ways:

> He was one of the first surgeons to employ courtesy in surgery, to show any consideration for the insides of a man. . . . Halsted held that if you touched an intestine with your finger, you injured it and the patient suffered. . . . That was new doctrine when he began. . . . He was gentle—and a little inhuman. He had to be because he was so sensitive.[14]

* * *

During Halsted's many trips to Europe, he could not help but notice the stark contrast between the American and Austro-Hungarian/German standards of surgical education. For an American knife bearer, attempts at formal training were a matter of personal will with little practical instruction. There were a few "teaching hospitals," but the American approach to surgical schooling consisted mainly of operating room work with little integration of the basic sciences. This style of learning could not keep pace with the rapid explosion in surgical knowledge and left the surgical trainee too inexperienced.

Halsted sought to correct this deficiency with a more rigorous and sophisticated post-medical-school surgical-training program. "We need a system," he told a group of doctors, "which will produce not only surgeons but surgeons of the highest type, men who will stimulate the first youths of our country to study surgery and to devote their energies and their lives to raising the standard of surgical science."[15] Halsted wanted to imitate in Baltimore the German-speaking university system of surgical assistantships. In that system, "assistants," the brightest medical school graduates, competed for hospital positions and, after many years and advancing levels of responsibility, the opportunity to serve as chief associate to a professor of surgery. The Austro-Hungarian and German assistantship programs were structured like a pyramid—every year less competitive assistants dropped out until only one remained.

Halsted designed his surgical internship/residency program at Johns Hopkins to be also based on increasingly complex clinical responsibility. The surgeons-in-training supervised those junior to them while Halsted demanded that these men spend years—upwards of a decade or more—surviving physical rigors, unrelenting competition, and, for many, financial hardship. Moreover, Halsted did not guarantee that participants could retain their status year after year. The trainees' motivation, besides a desire to acquire knowledge and skills, was the opportunity to have Halsted designate them as his house surgeon (in today's terms, the chief resident), a title considered one of the pinnacles of early surgical success. "These positions are not for those who so soon weary of the study of their profession," warned Halsted, "but it is a fact that the zeal and industry of these young assistants seem to increase as they advance in years and as their knowledge and responsibilities become greater."[16]

Halsted was resolute in his belief that talented surgeons begot talented surgeons. Of the seventeen men who served as Halsted's house surgeons, eleven implemented Halstedian residencies at other hospitals, from which another 166 of their own house surgeons graduated. Even Halsted's residents, who did not achieve the rank of house surgeon, profoundly influenced American surgery. Men in this group established the country's first residency programs in otorhinolaryngology, orthopedics, and urology. So fundamental was Halsted as American surgery's Adam that the methods and techniques of what became known as Halstedian-style schooling live on as the approach by which most American surgeons continue to be educated and trained.

In the latter years of his life, Halsted suffered repeated attacks of abdominal and chest pain, initially thought to be heart related but eventually diagnosed as stones in an infected gallbladder. In September 1919, one of Halsted's former chief residents removed his gallbladder. Three years later, the problem of stones returned along with the onset of jaundice. Another procedure was performed but was complicated by postoperative pneumonia and intestinal bleeding. In spite of repeated blood transfusions, Halsted expired on September 7, 1922. Following cremation, his ashes were placed in the family crypt in the country-like setting of Greenwood Cemetery in Brooklyn, New York. In an interesting aside, close by Halsted's grave lie several other prominent American surgeons including Valentine Mott, the country's most celebrated knife bearer in the mid-nineteenth century; J. Marion Sims, the developer of a surgical technique to repair vaginal tear complications of childbirth but who refined the procedure at the expense of enslaved and vulnerable black women; John Wyeth, Sims's son-in-law and organizer of the New York Polyclinic Graduate Medical School and Hospital and an early president of the AMA; Lewis Pilcher, founding editor of the nation's most influential surgical journal, the *Annals of Surgery*; Thomas Joiner White, one of the first African-American general practitioner/surgeons; and Mary Amanda Dixon Jones, among the earliest female obstetrician/gynecologists.

*　*　*

By the first years of the twentieth century, surgeons had transformed their craft into a profession thriving with self-confidence. The more aggressive manner in which knife bearers approached surgical diseases reflected their appreciation of the value of science to their clinical activities. Based on the work of individuals like Billroth, Halsted, and Kocher, surgeons demonstrated a confidence in their abilities to excise a disease at its root and cautioned that, without an operation certain surgical patients faced undeniable doom. Heralding their successes with novel procedures— such as those for appendicitis, breast cancer, hernia, intestinal maladies, and vascular conditions—surgeons extended their skills to illnesses previously considered outside their technical capabilities. "So well is this idea established in the popular mind," declared a surgeon in New York:

> that almost miraculous cures, daring ventures, and the boldest of procedures are scarcely looked upon as out of the range of ordinary expectation. There is now something so tangibly demonstrative in the recovery of desperate cases that no room is left for argument and no cause for doubt. The skillful hand, the accurate knowledge, and the

fertile resources of the surgeon, place his science nearly on the level of an exact one, enabling him not only to determine with almost unerring certainty the pathological condition of a given trouble, but to demonstrate its presence and overcome its otherwise mortal tendency.[17]

Despite their technical skills, clinical realities would soon provide a new challenge to the more invasive techniques of surgery. With their larger incisions, extensive dissections, and greater blood loss, surgeons unwittingly became their own worst enemies. Large numbers of postoperative patients continued to die and the cause(s) needed to be determined.

13.

THE SHOCK OF
TECHNOLOGY

Surgery, after all, is an affair of the spirit; it is a fierce test of a man's technical skill, sometimes, but, in a grim or long fight, it is above all a trial of the spirit; and there are few things that cannot be conquered if a man's heart is set on victory.

Berkeley Moynihan, *British Medical Journal*, 1923

I would like to see the day when somebody would be appointed surgeon somewhere who had no hands, for the operative part is the least part of the work.

Harvey Cushing, letter to Dr. Henry Christian, 1911

The catchphrase from the science fiction series *Star Trek*, "to explore strange new worlds, to seek out new life and new civilizations, to boldly go where no man has gone before," defined the mission of the starship USS *Enterprise*. The crew's journey into deep space was made possible through the crucible of mid-twenty-third-century science and technology. Analogous to the premise of *Star Trek*, the synergy between science and technology in the late nineteenth and early twentieth centuries enabled surgeons to go bravely into areas of the body previously unexplored. The nature of humankind, to discover and learn, to follow the impetus of curiosity and innovation, pushed knife bearers as they exploited the latest scientific marvels.

By its very nature, surgery is interventional, and the opening years of the twentieth century, filled with technologic wonders (e.g., automobiles, refrigerators, telephones, typewriters, et cetera), underscored that characterization. Painless and infection-free surgery, coupled with a preoperative diagnosis established by X-rays and the presence of electric lights to illuminate the operative field, offered far more to patients than the simple bandages and braces of times past. With the main barriers to surgical ingenuity and knowledge gone, the craft assumed the role of an influential and steadying force within the whole of Medicine—from 1890 through 1920, a time when the AMA was the most respected of the nation's medical organizations, eighteen of the thirty men who served as its president were surgeons.

The practical application of science and technology changed surgeons' expectations as much as those of the public. Surgery, which always had an overly dramatic role in the world of Medicine, could legitimately claim a capacity for healing that overshadowed the still tentative and inconclusive efforts of medicine. "The day may be early coming when there will be no opprobrium in surgery save ignorance of the proper methods and incompetency in execution," declared one scalpel wielder. "Though this day has not arrived, yet it is true there should be no compromise in completeness short of the limits of safety."[1]

Surgeons and their craft represented the adventurous spirit of the new century, the explorers of an uncharted frontier. Before long, surgical admissions far outnumbered medical admissions to the expanding hospital systems in Europe and North America. Two scientific/technologic innovations were largely responsible for these changes: the discovery of X-rays in 1895 and, by 1900, the widespread use of electric lighting.

*   *   *

In the mid-fall of 1895, Wilhelm Röntgen, a physics professor at Würzburg, Germany, was working in a darkened laboratory with an electron tube—a vacuum glass cylinder that blasted electrons from one electrode to another—when he observed a strange phenomenon. An invisible energy that radiated from the tube had penetrated layers of surrounding cardboard and produced a faint green glow on a nearby fluorescent screen. Röntgen experimented with other materials (e.g., paper, rubber, and wood) that he wrapped around the tube but found the X-rays (he termed his discovery "X-rays" because their composition was unknown) passed through all substances except for lead. The emissions also darkened photographic plates and, as an experiment, Röntgen had his wife place her hand between the source of the X-rays and a plate. To their amazement, the bones in her hand were distinctly outlined. The findings were so startling that Röntgen's report on "shadow pictures" soon appeared in a scientific periodical and, by early 1896, was translated and published in the United States.[2]

There is no overemphasizing the profound effect that the discovery of the X-ray had on the broadest range of human existence. The finding was a scientific bombshell that warranted interest from scientists and laymen alike. Newspapers and magazines printed stories, true and false, about the newly discovered rays. Women were cautioned that handheld X-ray devices could peer through their clothes. Men were warned that police would adapt X-rays to spy on nefarious activities. There was even the suggestion that X-rays might be exploited to see through walls into private spaces and spy on people's intimate activities.

Notwithstanding these unrealistic concerns, the opportunities for using X-rays in Medicine were immediately apparent and surgeons were the first to do so. Initially, the new tool was valuable in diagnosing fractures, locating bullets, and detecting other metallic objects in the body. Shortly, abnormalities like gallstones and kidney stones came under scrutiny. The availability of X-rays let the scalpel wielder have a better idea of what would be found when a patient's body was opened and how successful the operation had been after the wound was closed. To visualize a change in the internal landscape following the alignment of a broken bone or the removal of gallstones provided surgeons with immediate proof of the effectiveness of their treatment. So pronounced was the fascination with what became known as "radiographs" that a surgeon stated the obvious:

> The manifold uses to which Roentgen's discovery may be applied to medicine are so obvious that it is even now questionable whether a surgeon would be morally justified in performing a certain class of operation without having first seen pictured by these rays the field of his work, a map, as it were, of the unknown country he is to explore.[3]

Not only did the accessibility of X-rays change the definition of what constituted a successful surgical intervention, but also the physical presence of an X-ray apparatus lent an air of modernity and scientific progress that impressed patients and marked surgery as an up-and-coming profession. Within one year of Röntgen's announcement, X-rays were part of the generally accepted technology utilized by all surgeons as well as a matchless sign of their clinical authority. "No surgical consulting-room is fully equipped without an apparatus for X-ray investigation," declared one knife bearer. "It is as essential to the surgeon as the mirror to the laryngologist, or the stethoscope to the general practitioner."[4]

By 1900, the use of X-rays passed beyond simple demonstrations of skeletal abnormalities or detection of metal objects in the body. It became apparent that X-rays killed rapidly dividing cells, an observation that intrigued cancer researchers and brought about the beginnings of radiation oncology. Although surgeons would no longer be the only practitioners at the forefront of advances in radiology, their early appropriation of the new technology demonstrated that the X-ray machine was an indispensable medical and surgical device.

* * *

During the first decades of the twentieth century, surgeons moved away from so-called kitchen surgery, where patients underwent a surgical procedure in their homes, on their kitchen table, into newly built hospitals with operating rooms of spotless purity, around-the-clock nursing care, and capable surgical residents. The pragmatic realities of a surgeon's work changed as busy knife bearers found it costly and inefficient in lost work time to travel long distances to treat patients. The simple fact was that hospitals could afford expensive new technologies that made them the logical places to practice an increasingly complex and technically demanding craft. In what became a synergistic relationship, a growing surgical workload provided the financial basis for the rapid expansion of hospitals. For instance, at Pennsylvania Hospital in Philadelphia, one of the nation's largest, over eight hundred surgical operations were performed in 1899. This one-year total surpassed the number of procedures completed at that institution during the entire first half of the nineteenth century. In 1870, fewer than two hundred hospitals existed in the United States; by 1910, the number topped four thousand.

A hospital's employment of technology, particularly for surgeons, is best explained in one word: "electrification." Throughout the centuries, surgical operations were performed under less-than-ideal illumination using light from candles, fireplaces, kerosene/oil lamps, or sunlight. In an effort to deal with this difficulty, surgical amphitheaters were constructed with windows that faced southeast to afford as much daylight as possible; a cloudy or rainy day precluded any possibility of surgery. Even the use of highly polished mirrors to reflect light toward the operating table proved inadequate, as knife bearers complained about the color and quality of concentrated sunlight. Moreover, the slightest movement of personnel often created shadows or blocked the incoming sunshine. If surgeons were to expand their operative prospects and, at the same time, be able to visualize hard-to-see body parts, then a more constant, focused, and reliable source of light was needed.

Beginning in the late 1890s, the problem of ineffective illumination lessened as electric lights were installed in operating rooms. When lights were first developed, their presence represented more than illumination—they were a sociologic phenomenon that affected our daily existence. Lighting meant that small towns could be as sophisticated as large cities; lit theaters drew people to evening shows, lit playing fields allowed those who worked during the day to attend nighttime events, and lit homes led to more extensive family gatherings. Lights also kept criminals in dark places while the public remained safe. Even the tiniest of villages installed arc-light towers to illuminate their streets, turning their part of the world into a marvel of the industrial era. It was no wonder that people hailed the arrival of electric illumination with cannon fire, music, parades, shows, and ceremonial funerals for candles and lamps.

For surgeons, complicated and expensive lighting equipment was generally found in well-funded institutions. Hospitals went to great lengths to supply their surgical staff with the newest in electrical apparatus. "There is much to be said in regard to artificial lighting," wrote a hospital architect. "The lighting of the operating room needs careful study, both for day and for night."[5] He recommended three alternate ways to use electric incandescent lights in an operating room: a row of small fixtures around the perimeter or on the ceiling of the room; a swinging crane-like central light nicknamed the illuminator with a bowl-shaped reflector; or a fixture with multiple arms, devised to avoid shadows. The architect also cautioned that a large supply of hand-electric torches be stored at the nurses' station in case of a power failure.

Beyond the convenience of lights in the operating room, a hospital's pursuit of surgeons included the availability of electric batteries and electrified instruments. This was crucial for those who practiced ear, nose, and throat surgery, ophthalmologic surgery, and urologic surgery. The ability to peer into the tiniest spaces of the body required specialized equipment (i.e., otoscopes, laryngoscopes, ophthalmoscopes, cystoscopes, et cetera) and, without an adequate light source, the viewing was difficult. "I have no doubt that in the near future," wrote an ear, nose, and throat surgeon, "when electric lighting will have been adopted universally . . . electric-lamps for the laryngoscope will supplant all other sources of light."[6] Four decades later, an electrical engineer was even more laudatory: "I wish to assert that in all human history no lamp ever invented has contributed so much to the welfare of the race; has done so much to alleviate suffering and preserve human life, as the surgical lamp."[7]

Electricity became an essential element of Medicine. Dozens of companies sold lights for surgical instruments along with high-end batteries as advertisements for electromedical instrument manufacturers proliferated in medical and surgical journals. The electrical contraptions were expensive; a series of batteries mounted in an oak or mahogany cabinet, plus the dozens of electrode attachments for devices designed to visualize different parts of the body (e.g., bladder, ear, nose, rectum, throat, and vagina), cost upwards of $300 (approximately $9,000 in 2022 dollars). Busy surgeons found it most convenient and financially sensible to utilize a hospital's instruments. Major hospitals had the purchasing power for electric wiring, power generators, and sophisticated electrical equipment long before the average surgeon did.

*   *   *

Through the opening years of the twentieth century, the availability of technologic wonders like electric lights, X-rays, and other scientific marvels helped surgery reach a level of popularity and scope previously unimaginable. Knife bearers—exemplified by Charles and William Mayo, who turned a small clinic in Minnesota into a namesake surgical shrine, or Frederick Treves in London, renowned for his treatment of Joseph Merrick, the elephant man, as well as saving the life of Edward VII by removing his gangrenous appendix—were celebrities in their own right. Ambitious surgeons viewed themselves as more than highly skilled technicians. Now they could be thought of as courageous and progressive scientists who practiced the most exciting form of therapy that Medicine offered, surgery. The lifesaving possibilities of a surgical procedure were almost a foregone conclusion; a surgeon's recourse to his scalpel seemed reflexive and operations, heretofore unimaginable, became the norm. The body's untouched interior was there to be explored, mapped, and mined.

Various new procedures were tried as surgeons showcased the virtues of cutting and excising, of removing a disease at its core. "It appears to be pretty well settled that hardly anything is impossible of accomplishment when skill with the knife is called in question in battling with what were formerly considered to be incurable maladies," explained an American surgeon. "And truly, in comparing the present with the past, there is less room for exaggeration in this belief than would at first be supposed."[8] For some knife bearers though, their upbeat optimism turned into a fanatical enthusiasm.

At the turn of the century, William Arbuthnot Lane, a highly respected English surgeon, reported a supposedly new syndrome of severe unrelenting constipation that impaired quality of life. Lane opined that, in a sluggish colon, poisons were absorbed from ever-present fecal matter that created a condition he termed "autointoxication." Lane urged the drastic step of removing the entire colon, advice taken seriously by an unknowing public. His operative know-how was in great demand, and it is unlikely that any surgeon before or after him ever completed as many colon removals as Lane did. By 1915, his theories on the relationship between constipation and illness were deemed nonsensical and the Lane colectomy for intestinal stasis was relegated to the surgical dustbin.

In America, beginning in the late 1880s, Edwin Hartley Pratt promoted orificial surgery, a bizarre scheme to treat diseases solely through operations on the mouth, penis, rectum, and vagina. "A vigorous sympathetic nervous system means health and long life," explained Pratt:

> Bring me an individual with clean lips and nostrils and unobtruding tonsils; a rectum that presents neither piles, prolapses, fissure, or ulcer—an individual whose sexual orifices are smooth and free from all irritation; if it be a man, his foreskin shall be free, the frenum of sufficient length, the urethral passage smooth . . . if a woman, her hymen must be pale and atrophied, her urethra devoid of carbuncles and ulcerations, her internal and external os uteri reasonably patulous; bring such an individual and I will point to the same person and show you a human being whose digestion is good, whose sleep is sweet and restful . . . whose very existence is a constant source of uninterrupted delights. . . . What surgical interest have we in these facts? It can be told in just one sentence. The weakness and power of the sympathetic nerve lies at the orifices of the body. Surgery must keep these orifices properly smoothed and dilated.[9]

In Pratt's perverse view, problems such as anxiety, constipation, eczema, headache, insanity, insomnia, rheumatism, and tuberculosis could be treated with a surgeon's scalpel. Like any savvy promoter, he authored a lengthy monograph, *Orificial Surgery and Its Application to the Treatment of Chronic Diseases*, organized a specialty organization, the American Association of Orificial Surgeons, and served as editor-in-chief of the start-up *Journal of Orificial Surgery*.

The orificial philosophy attracted a large following of practitioners, who were, in every sense of the word, surgeons. They performed formidable surgical procedures, including abdominal and vaginal hysterectomies, repair of complicated cervical and perineal lacerations, circumcisions on adult men, and radical hemorrhoidectomies. It is impossible to accurately determine how many Americans fell victim to this unorthodox surgical philosophy, but with almost one thousand known practitioners, orificial surgical operations must have numbered in the tens of thousands.

Late-nineteenth- and early-twentieth-century American society was particularly prone to the establishment of unconventional medical practices and alternative therapies. It was the heyday of panaceas, patent medicine, pills, and powders. For almost three decades, the allure of orificial surgery and its eccentric measures was strong, but the onset of World War I and the growth of conventional surgical therapies brought an end to the aging population of orificial surgeons. Similar to other eccentric practices that occurred in American Medicine of this era, the long-forgotten, short-lived, and appropriately discredited movement of orificial surgery was more a symptom of the times than a competing effort to undo the parallel scientific evolution of surgery.

Apart from outrageous operations like colectomies for constipation or orificial repairs, the rapid growth in surgery came about due to a marshaling of organizational, scientific, socioeconomic, and technologic forces. However, a critical issue emerged from the growing number of bloodier and extensive procedures: an increasing number of postoperative deaths. This was mystifying, because knife bearers thought the widespread use of anesthesia and antisepsis would curb the high mortality rate already associated with surgical operations. Their thinking was correct in that fewer patients succumbed to postoperative infection, but another problem came to the fore, surgical shock.*

---

* Surgical shock is a critical condition brought on by a number of mechanisms; among them are acute loss of blood before or during an operation, serious traumatic injury, and overwhelming postoperative infections. Shock results in decreased blood flow through the body and failure of the circulatory system

By creating larger wounds, handling tissue roughly, and causing substantial blood loss, knife bearers unknowingly became their own worst enemies. "Deep mischief is lurking in the system," was how one surgeon described the situation:

> The machinery of life has been rudely unhinged, and the whole system profoundly shocked . . . there is not enough power in the constitution to reproduce and maintain it.[10]

Postoperative patients were dying and the etiology and seriousness of shock with its puzzling onset and myriad symptoms needed to be understood and managed to make surgery truly safe.

When surgeons first investigated the nature of shock, they were limited to what they observed; knife bearers lacked instrumentation to measure physiological parameters like blood pressure and temperature, nor did they understand their significance. Surgeons came to realize that shock usually appeared following a prolonged operation or a severe accident, especially when there was a significant loss of blood. Acknowledging the typical cold arms and legs and faint pulse of patients in shock, knife bearers found that when they examined the arteries of these individuals, the blood vessels were pliable and relaxed, as though the circulatory system did not contain enough blood to fill them. The recognition that shock was due to "missing blood" and how to treat the disorder was investigated by numerous researchers. The studies of George Washington Crile, who held the conviction, unusual for his era, that the surgical laboratory was an essential adjunct of the operating room, rose above the others.

* * *

There are few surnames in surgery as well recognized as that of Crile. He founded the Cleveland Clinic and the American College of Surgeons (ACS), had a lunar

---

to deliver oxygen and vital nutrients to organs, especially the brain, heart, lungs, and kidneys. The chief clinical features of surgical shock include low blood pressure, rapid breathing, fast and weak pulse, pallor, coolness of the extremities, decreased urine flow, and a change in mental alertness. The treatment involves keeping the patient warm, providing blood transfusions and other fluids intravenously, administering drugs to improve cardiac, circulatory, and kidney function, and curtailing the hemorrhage of blood.

impact crater and World War II Liberty ship named after him, designed the most widely used surgical clamp, the Crile "mosquito," and authored two dozen books, including the best-selling *A Mechanistic View of Peace and War*, which received a full-page review in the *New York Times*— "Dr. George W. Crile finds the man of today a red-handed glutton, whose phylogenetic 'action patterns' are facilitated for killing."[11]

In 1887, Crile graduated as valedictorian from the Wooster College Medical School (presently the Case Western Reserve University School of Medicine) and was awarded a highly sought-after internship at University Hospital (now the University Hospital Cleveland Medical Center). During his internship, Crile was in charge of treating a youngster whose legs had been crushed by a streetcar. Despite state-of-the-art surgical care, including amputation, stimulant drugs, and twenty-four-hour nursing, the boy went into shock and died. Crile was crestfallen, and from his exasperation emerged a lifelong commitment to investigate the nature of surgical shock.

Crile's interest led to his taking courses in experimental histology, pathology, and physiology at New York's College of Physicians and Surgeons. "As I look back," Crile later wrote, "I realize that aside from acquiring laboratory technics this trip to New York liberated me from much ignorance."[12] During the 1890s, Crile, who was the newly named professor of surgery in the Cleveland College of Physicians and Surgeons, furthered his research by working with the foremost physiologists and surgeons in London, Paris, and Vienna. Crile's investigations led to his first book, *An Experimental Research into Surgical Shock*, along with numerous invitations to speak before medical and surgical societies. "George W. Crile, of Cleveland," wrote a leading American surgeon:

> had been heard of as far west as Chicago within a few years of his [medical school] graduation. In 1890, those of us interested in organized medicine thought well enough of him to take a chance and to invite him to read a paper on "Shock" before the Chicago Medical Society. He came. He was a young man under thirty years of age, handsome as a prince, with an enthusiasm that fairly took our breath, and with a convincing manner that captivated us, old and young.[13]

Crile was viewed as a pioneer of science-based surgery as he united the research laboratory and the operating amphitheater. Initially, Crile investigated the use of stimulant drugs as a way to combat shock, but he found them ineffective and occasionally dangerous. Next, he turned to the intravenous administration of saline solution, but the positive benefits were fleeting and the negative effects of overloading the body with salt and water were treacherous. What became the most important outcome of these early investigations was Crile's recognition that the management of shock was largely a question of how to maintain blood pressure at normal levels.

Around this time, an Austrian physician identified the three human blood types, A, B, and O, and demonstrated that transfusion between persons with the same blood group did not lead to an adverse reaction. Based on these findings and the results of his investigations, Crile began blood transfusions in humans. "Judiciously employed," he wrote, "transfusion will surely prove a valuable, often life-saving, resource; injudiciously employed it will surely become discredited."[14] Crile's intrepid step was a milestone in the history of surgery and led, on the battlefields of World War I, to the first large-scale use of blood to treat shock.

* * *

The First World War began in the summer of 1914, following the assassination of the heir to the throne of the Austrian province of Bosnia by a Bosnian Serb nationalist. Within one month of the murder, Austria-Hungary declared war on Serbia, Great Britain declared war on Germany, Germany declared war on Belgium, France, and Russia, and Russia ordered a general mobilization of its populace. Europe was aflame and, for the first time in history, the mortality from battlefield casualties exceeded that from communicable diseases. News of the war's outbreak astonished most Americans. President Woodrow Wilson asserted that the United States would remain neutral. His sentiments lasted less than three years. In January 1917, Germany began unrestricted submarine warfare, and two months later three unarmed American merchant vessels were sunk without warning. In April the United States Congress declared war on Germany.

War has always posed moral dilemmas for surgeons. Scalpel wielders gain unparalleled clinical experience through incalculable human suffering while successful operations place soldiers back on the front to face injury once again. "The traumatic surgery of [World War I]," acknowledged a distinguished American surgeon, "has constituted a tremendous vivisection experimental laboratory in which not mice, nor rabbits, nor guinea-pigs, nor dogs have been the subjects of experiments, but human beings, the choicest young men of the civilized world."[15]

The war was a conflict of attrition with unrelenting bombardment and deadly new weaponry (e.g., flame throwers, poison gas, tanks, et cetera) that required the organization of sophisticated field hospitals to treat the massive number of casualties. The neurological nature of many of the wounds was devastating. They were related to the soldiers' habit of peering imprudently over the tops of the unprotected trenches only to be shot in the head. There were not just injuries from shell blasts and bullets, but other deadly conditions were frequent. Trench foot was ubiquitous, a painful condition of blue, cold, macerated-looking feet caused by long standing without a change of boots in the muddy trenches. As a result, extremity amputation was one of the most common operations. Tetanus was rife early in the conflict until an antitetanus serum became available. Enormous numbers of men were incapacitated by shell shock: pure psychological breakdown secondary to the tremendous strain of trench warfare and incessant shelling.

Surgeons, with their knowledge of trauma care, were the obvious choice to manage these problems and the facilities in which wounded soldiers were cared. Few knife bearers had the administrative genius, patriotic fervor, or professional credentials of Crile, who was appointed a major in the Medical Corps and senior consultant in surgical research. It was his idea to establish field hospitals based on America's university hospitals, and by war's end virtually every important medical school in the United States claimed its own battlefield facility. Hometowns sponsored them with pride. Local businessmen raised money to equip their units and women volunteered with the Red Cross to hand-make dressings, sheets, and towels.

The war provided thousands of doctors with a crash course in military medicine that catapulted surgical practice and the treatment of shock forward. "Every bed, every aisle, every tent, every inch of floor space was occupied by stretchers," wrote Crile. "The operating rooms ran day and night, without ceasing. I had two hundred deaths on one night in my own service. The seriously wounded piled up so fast that nothing could be done with them."[16] Most of the field hospitals and their casualty clearing stations contained "shock wards" where surgeons, physiologists, and other researchers worked together.* From this experience, protocols were established on

---

* Among the individuals that Crile worked closely with was Alexis Carrel, a French surgeon who was awarded the 1912 Nobel Prize in Physiology or Medicine for his studies on a technique to suture blood vessels. Similar to Kocher's 1909 Nobel Prize in Physiology or Medicine, Carrel's honor did much to corroborate the validity of surgery and its operations. Carrel was born in Lyon, but the majority of his experimental work was completed in the United States, where he was on the staff of the Rockefeller Institute for Medical Research in New York. Following World War I, Carrel's experimental activities concerned

how to manage surgical shock; knife bearers found the standards invaluable once they returned to their civilian practices.

The conflict also called attention to the importance of specialty practice to the future of surgical health care. Orthopedic surgery, neurosurgery, and plastic surgery were strengthened as stand-alone specialties as surgeons performed new and elaborate procedures on the extremities and joints, and the head and neck. The war also showed that strict practice standards had to be enforced if a physician was to be deemed a surgical specialist; at a time when the military wanted every doctor it could recruit, the army rebuffed over 50 percent of the supposed ophthalmologists and ear, nose, and throat specialists seeking enlistment because their clinical skills were second-rate.

*   *   *

The ascent of American Medicine to a position of international leadership began with the medical and surgical triumphs of World War I. Prolonged combat destroyed large swaths of the Continent and weakened many countries' financial standing and social cohesiveness. The number of European combat-related fatalities was staggering,* a whole generation of young men wiped out, dead, or broken and crippled. Deprivation was evident throughout the land. "There are only sad things to report," wrote the professor of surgery in Leipzig to Halsted in Baltimore:

> The saddest is that in each nation a few hotblooded politicians and radical nationalists exert more influence on the masses than 99% of the rational thinking intellectuals. . . . This stupidity de-

---

the transplantation of organs. In 1935, in collaboration with famed aviator Charles Lindbergh, he devised a machine to supply oxygen to organs removed from the body, thus opening the way to organ transplantation. When World War II broke out, Carrel returned to France as a member of a special mission for the French Ministry of Health. In 1940, following the Nazi occupation, Carrel became director of the Carrel Foundation for the Study of Human Problems, which was established by the French Vichy government, a Nazi puppet regime. Although Carrel was known to despise Hitler, the fact that he collaborated with the Vichy government made him suspect. In the repercussion that followed France's liberation, Carrel was accused of cooperating with the Germans. The foundation was closed and Carrel's health failed as he feared arrest as a Nazi apologist. Carrel died in November 1944 with a tainted reputation.

*   Austria Hungary, 1,016,200 dead and 3,620,000 wounded; France, 1,150,000 dead and 4,266,000 wounded; Germany, 1,800,000 dead and 4,216,000 wounded; Great Britain, 744,000 dead and 1,675,000 wounded; Italy 460,000 dead and 947,000 wounded; and Russia 1,700,000 dead and 4,000,000 wounded.

stroyed a nation which was capable to excel intellectually in any area for 50 years or more. . . . Our science is heavily threatened by poverty. Perhaps people will start writing poetry and philosophize again, at least they don't cost anything. Undoubtedly, technology, the natural sciences, medicine, and surgery are finished.[17]

A vacuum existed globally in surgical research and therapeutics. It was only natural and inevitable that surgeons from the United States, the industrialized country least affected monetarily, physically, and psychologically by the war (53,400 dead and 204,000 wounded), would fill this void. "There was never a war in which the medical profession received the authority and won the credit as it did in the last war," wrote a contemporary American observer, "and there never was a time when the medical and surgical profession had the honor and credit that it has today."[18]

Crile returned to Cleveland a war hero, decorated with the American Distinguished Service Medal, the Legion of Honor from France, and membership in Great Britain's Most Honourable Order of the Bath. He was promoted to brigadier general in the Army Reserves and resumed his professorship of surgery at Western Reserve Medical School, a position he held until his death in 1943. In an editorial that accompanied his obituary in the *New York Times*, the writer told of Crile's "restless imagination" and how "there was something about him that recalls the scientific romanticism of the Renaissance."[19]

Surgeons were about to convert their embrace of science and technology into economic power through higher incomes, legal power through management of hospitals, and professional power through specialization. The public had never experienced such a fundamental change in surgery, nor had knife bearers ever received such approbation. Surgery had taken on a modern-day look; knife bearers wore caps, gowns, masks, and rubber gloves, patients donned robes, operating tables were draped in cloth, and instruments were bathed in metal basins that contained new and improved antiseptic solutions. Everything was clean and orderly, with the conduct of the surgical operation no longer a haphazard affair. The craft was stronger than ever with a newfound enthusiasm and swagger as surgeons guided the rapidly changing world of American Medicine. With a spirit of radical intervention and perfectionist technique, surgery's outsized role would define and influence much of the nation's medical culture in the opening decades of the twentieth century.

PART IV

BAPTISMS

14.
MASS APPEAL

*Day after day the surgeon invades territory which the physician deemed
his own, and saves from pain and death the patient whom medical art
was impotent to help.*

Henry Maudsley, *British Medical Journal*, 1905

*A good surgeon is a good medical man who can cut. Most of the surgeons
have forgotten their medicine but go right on cutting.*

Martin H. Fischer as quoted by Howard Fabing,
Fischerisms, 1930

The decade following World War I, the "Roaring Twenties," was an exciting
and prosperous time for the United States. In the wake of Henry Ford's production of the Model T and the flourishing of oil companies, a web of highways
spread across the nation as the automotive and energy industries took hold. In 1927,
Charles Lindbergh's flight over the Atlantic Ocean from New York to Paris roused
the country and brought about the business of aviation. Bootleggers, flappers, and
speakeasies thrived despite a constitutional ban on the manufacture and sale of intoxicating liquor.

The American way of life appeared fundamentally secure when Herbert Hoover
was inaugurated as president in March 1929. However, the feelings of prosperity
belied an underlying reality. Inordinate speculation in stocks had created enormous
wealth on paper, but the optimism and financial gains of the bull market were tempered by warnings about excessive trading, especially for individuals who bought on

margin (i.e., the purchase of a financial asset using borrowed funds from a bank or broker). The cautions went unheeded and, in October 1929, panic selling occurred and the stock market suffered the "Great Crash." The ongoing crisis was exacerbated when Congress yielded to lobbying interests and passed legislation that implemented protectionist trade policies; the law raised tariffs on over twenty thousand imported goods. The effect on foreign trade was disastrous and, following retaliatory tariffs plus an unavoidable decline in industrial growth, the country was plunged into a crippling financial depression.

By 1931, tens of millions of Americans had lost everything. Banks failed, businesses closed, factories shut down, foreign commerce halted, and taxes could no longer be collected. The pressure for political change brought about the election of Franklin Roosevelt as president in 1932. Roosevelt would not be able to immediately reverse the depression, but during the first years of his administration recovery was pursued through large federal spending on projects such as the Civilian Conservation Corps, the Public Works Commission, and the Tennessee Valley Authority while Congress created the Federal Deposit Insurance Corporation, the Labor Relations Board, and the Securities and Exchange Commission and strengthened the Federal Trade Commission. In 1935, acting on Roosevelt's belief that the government should assure long-term economic security for the elderly, the poor, and the sick, Congress passed the Social Security Act.

* * *

Despite the decade-long financial downturn, continued progress in science and technology furthered surgery's development. The advancements were so pronounced that, by the mid-1930s, the foundation of basic surgical procedures on the organs in the abdomen, the lungs, and the brain was completed. These clinical successes bolstered the growing acceptance of surgery as a legitimate scientific endeavor, evidenced by the extensive use of the nation's most common surgical operations, appendectomy and tonsillectomy. The wide embrace of the two procedures occurred once doctors and the public accepted—as state-of-the-art medical thinking—the notion that deadly bacteria routinely lurked in the nooks and crannies of the appendix and tonsils. "It must not be forgotten," warned a throat surgeon, "that the tonsils ... afford nests for the reception and culture of micrococci that may give rise to serious trouble. These depressions are sometimes very deep, plunging down ... and form an ideal incubator for the development of micro-organisms."[1] The theory of "focal infection" and its lethal consequences became so ingrained that the rationale for removing the appendix and/or tonsils seemed to be the very existence of the organ itself.

More than any medical therapy, the removal of tonsils was considered a safe and simple surgical cure-all against many childhood and adulthood infections. The extent of this belief is evidenced in a survey of 1,000 school-age children for tonsillar problems in New York City in 1933. Of the randomly chosen youngsters, 611 had already undergone a tonsillectomy. The other 389 were evaluated by a panel of physicians and 174 were told they needed to have their tonsils removed. The 215 children with presumably healthy tonsils were assessed by a second group of doctors who felt an additional 99 needed a tonsillectomy. A third set of physicians evaluated the remaining 116 children, of whom 51 were recommended for removal of their tonsils. By the end of three different examinations, only 65 of the original 1,000 children had tonsils that were not recommended for excision.[2] Since it is now known that the tonsils and appendix aid in immune function—the theory of "focal infection" has long been discredited—the harm caused by the excision of millions of these healthy organs can only be imagined.

The unmitigated use of tonsillectomy was considered a triumph of early-twentieth-century Medicine and public health. However, as common as tonsillectomies were, no operation captured the public's appreciation of surgical savoir faire more than removal of the appendix. Appendectomies took the search-and-destroy mission for villainous bacteria deep into the inner recesses of the body. Surgeons dove fearlessly into the abdomen, located the problem appendix, and erased its existence. "Appendicitis, more than any other acute disease, interests all classes of the community," explained a surgeon:

> It is everywhere present; it is serious and alarming; it appears under many guises and passes through many phases; it calls for heroic treatment . . . and so has become a favorite theme of modern surgeons; about it have centered some of the most stimulating and vital surgical discussions of our times.[3]

The wholesale diagnosis of appendicitis and its management by appendectomy became a major factor in defining who was a surgeon. Treatment of the lowly and unassuming appendix transformed the way Americans doctored themselves—

appendicitis took on the moniker "America's disease" and appendectomy became "America's operation." Surgery moved center stage as surgeons oriented their practices around the new operation and hospitals adapted to meet the clinical demand. As an admirer of the surgical scene declared: "American surgeons have done more to show the importance of operative treatment of appendicitis than the rest of the world put together."[4]

* * *

For centuries, healers had misguided notions concerning bellyaches and their origins, but the appendix was rarely considered the source. A brief explanation of abdominal anatomy is in order. It is easiest to picture the abdomen or belly as containing two coexisting systems of organs. The first consists of the stomach, the duodenum, and the small and large intestines—the appendix is a wormlike appendage, usually three to four inches in length, whose base is attached to the beginning of the large intestine. The complicated process of digestion begins and ends within these structures, from the stomach, where digesting enzymes and acidic fluids convert raw food into a pulpy mix, to the large intestine and its task to reabsorb the water used in the course of digestion and store the remaining waste as feces before its expulsion through the anus. The second system of organs includes the gallbladder, kidney, liver, pancreas, and spleen, some of which support the process of digestion. The inside wall of the abdomen as well as certain of the organs are covered by the peritoneum, a veil of flimsy self-lubricating tissue that allows these structures to expand and contract smoothly against one another.

Doctors had long considered the ileocecal junction—where the end of the small intestine, the ilium, joins the beginning of the large intestine, the cecum—as the root of most abdominal evil. They had myriad expressions for problems in this area, but none of them amounted to anything more than semantic bunkum: cecitis, colic passion, ileocecal abscess, iliac passion, pericecal abscess, typhlitis, typhlenteritis, or the high-sounding perityphlitis vermicularis. The confused vocabulary indicated a lack of understanding, one that lasted through the ending decades of the nineteenth century.

In 1886, Reginald Fitz, a Harvard professor of pathological anatomy, turned Medicine upside down when he stated it was inflammation of the lowly appendix that caused many abdominal pains. The no-nonsense Fitz explained that he had observed hundreds of autopsies of persons who died in various stages of appendiceal disease and was convinced that the ileocecal junction was mistakenly vilified. Instead, the true culprit for much abdominal pain was the appendix and its disorders should be termed "appendicitis." He even went so far as to suggest that appendicitis was strictly a surgeon's disease:

> Its eventual treatment by appendectomy is generally indispensable. Urgent symptoms demand immediate exposure of the appendix, after recovery from shock, and its treatment according to surgical principles.[5]

Fitz turned appendicitis into a well-recognized pathological entity and laid the groundwork for the emergence of appendectomies as a common surgical necessity. Until the 1880s, entering the abdomen for any type of surgery was unthinkable with a death rate that approached 100 percent. By 1900, the availability of anesthesia and antisepsis and improved technical skills had decreased the mortality rate to below 5 percent. "Now there is no organ in the abdominal cavity that is not daily explored," proclaimed Samuel Hopkins Adams, the muckraking American journalist:

> Perhaps the most notable success is in appendicitis. Twenty years ago, the sufferer from appendicitis died—by another name, preferably "inflammation of the bowels" or "peritonitis." To-day, the death rate in the best equipped hospitals is not five per cent.[6]

Most of the organs within the abdomen are attached to their surroundings by folds of tissue that maintain their position. Without this measure of consistency, the surgeon's quest to cure disease would be difficult. The opposite situation exists for the appendix. It has no supporting scaffold, and while the base of the wormlike appendix is typically found at the beginning of the large intestine, the tip of the appendix can be variably located. Like a child playing hide-and-seek, it goes wherever it likes. The tip can be found upward toward the liver, downward into the pelvis, sideways into the middle of the abdomen, forward toward the abdominal wall, or stealthily tucked behind the large intestine.

The varying locations make the diagnosis of appendicitis a challenge. Patients with an inflamed appendix display countless warning signs depending on where its tip is located. As a result, when doctors relied only on observation and examination they easily confused appendicitis with less serious conditions. Many patients, who should have undergone an appendectomy, did not receive timely surgical attention and succumbed to a burst appendix. "I know of no operation," wrote a renowned knife bearer, "presenting more difficulties in its surgical technic and medical management than acute appendicitis, and there is perhaps no other surgical disease presenting so many complications."[7]

By 1920, American surgeons were performing appendectomies on 95 percent of patients admitted with a diagnosis of appendicitis. A decade later, surgeons were completing over one hundred thousand appendectomies annually. Hospitals prospered on the fees from appendectomy patients. Fledgling pharmaceutical companies developed antiseptic dusting powders, bacterial antitoxins, and protein-rich antimicrobial serums to treat the disease. "Better to take out a healthy appendix and have a patient recover," justified one surgeon, "than [to leave] a diseased one and have the patient die."[8]

The idea that it was worth the risk of performing an appendectomy on a questionably diseased appendix versus waiting for the organ to become severely inflamed reflected the public's support for the concept of "exploratory" surgery. I witnessed this firsthand in May 1967, when I was completing my freshman year at Union College in Schenectady, New York. One day for lunch, I wolfed down two large meatball submarine sandwiches. Three hours later, I, who was previously healthy, was at the school's infirmary watching the doctor slam his hand on a desk. "Young man," he exclaimed, "you have appendicitis and need to see a surgeon!" Before I knew it, I was in a knife bearer's office, where, after abdominal and rectal exams, he told me I needed an emergency appendectomy.

The passage of time has fogged my memory, but I know my parents were notified (they lived in New Jersey) and told to fly up. The operation lasted less than one hour. Two days later, I felt well and was discharged. When I saw the surgeon for my postoperative visit, he informed me that my appendix had been slightly inflamed. There was no discussion of a formal pathology report, not that I would have understood its relevance at the time. Today a pathological examination of any excised appendix is mandatory because only through inspection under a microscope can it be conclusively stated whether the appendicular tissue was diseased. The remainder of my recovery was uneventful and I've never experienced any difficulties from the operation—the other surgical procedure I've undergone was a tonsillectomy at the age of five. I recount this story for two reasons: first, to show that my appendectomy and becoming acquainted with nurses and surgeons was a crucial episode that fostered my early interest in being a scalpel wielder; and second, to illustrate, on a personal level, the ubiquity of appendectomies and tonsillectomies during much of the twentieth century.

Beginning in the 1920s, the United States was in the grip of appendiceal mania as talk about the appendix crossed over into popular culture. In *Arrowsmith*, Sinclair Lewis's 1926 Pulitzer Prize–winning novel about contemporary Medicine, he used the appendix to illustrate a doctor's fondness for his calling:

> Look here! Look here! See that? In the bottle? It's an appendix. First one ever took out 'round here. I did it . . . did the first 'pendectomy in this neck of the woods, you bet![9]

There were well-known musical ditties and poems:

> So, they turned the ol'-time doctors down, an' got a young
> chap, —well
> He knowed more new diseases than the dictionaries tell!
> An' though were poor an' humble the country run 'erbout,
> We kin have "appendicitis" now an' all the new things out![10]

And the United States Public Health Service sponsored a public awareness campaign:

> Don't gamble with appendicitis—don't use a laxative—call a doctor.[11]

Appendicitis assumed a firm hold on the imagination of the public and became a fashionable disease. "There is a well-marked appendicular hypochondrosis," explained one doctor. "Through the pernicious influence of the daily press, appendicitis has become a sort of fad, and the physician has often to deal with patients who have a sort of fixed idea that they have the disease."[12]

*   *   *

Although the safe performance of surgical operations had advanced, crucial medical instrumentation like blood pressure cuffs, electrocardiograms, pulse oximeters to assess oxygen levels in the blood, respirators, and thermometers had not been developed. Moreover, antibiotics, intravenous fluids, and oxygen masks were not available. The consequence was that even a supposedly conquered disease like appendicitis continued to pose risks. No one would learn that lesson harder than Rudolph Valentino, bon vivant, dancer, movie star, and poet. He was that era's unrivaled pop icon and sex symbol. Women swooned at the mere mention of his nom de guerre, the Latin Lover. Valentino seemed the epitome of life itself and his fans were shocked when, in mid-August 1926, newspaper headlines announced that the thirty-one-year-old entertainer "goes under knife . . . for appendicitis."[13]

For days, the nation's ears and eyes were focused on New York's Polyclinic Hospital as Valentino struggled against one postoperative complication after another. Initially, the public was assured by Valentino's surgeons that there was not much to be concerned about: "Mr. Valentino's condition is very encouraging and he is resting comfortably. He seems to be a little brighter and his condition is favorable."[14] What his fans were not told were the dire operative findings. Valentino's appendix was not the only problem: he also had a perforated stomach ulcer with half-digested food and gastric juice spreading uncontrollably throughout his abdominal cavity.

Gastric juice is extremely corrosive and meant to stay within the confines of the digestive tract whose specialized tissues are able to process the liquid's harsh nature. The difficulty comes when this juice leaks out of the stomach—usually from a perforated ulcer—and eats away the inside of the abdomen, literally self-digesting the patient's inner recesses. The result is peritonitis, a painful inflammation of the flimsy self-lubricating inner lining of the abdomen and its internal organs.

Valentino's problems were exacerbated by the fact that he had severe abdominal pain for several days before agreeing to be evaluated by a physician. When the actor was finally seen, the examination showed "board-like rigidity of the entire abdominal wall" consistent with a "rapidly spreading vicious peritonitis." An immediate operation was urged as "his only chance for life." The surgeons faced a stinking abdomen filled with yellow-greenish pus and yards of convoluted, inflamed beet-red intestine. Four hours later, they had removed Valentino's appendix ("[it] was acutely inflamed from a secondary infection"), repaired a hole from an ulcer in his stomach ("the tissue of the stomach for one and one-half centimeters immediately surrounding the perforation was necrotic"),[15] placed two rubber tubes through the actor's lower abdominal wall to drain fluid, and hoped for the best. In an era before there were recovery rooms or surgical intensive care units, the critically ill Valentino was transferred to a private two-room suite on the hospital's eighth floor.

Valentino recovered in his mahogany bed as the glamour of Hollywood and the silent screen descended on his room. Bouquets of flowers crowded the suite and overflowed into the hallway. Joseph Schenck, chairman of the board of United Artists Corporation (the company that held Valentino's contract), his wife, the actress Norma Talmadge, along with Gloria Swanson, arrived unannounced at the hospital but were told by the star's physicians that it would be inadvisable to disturb him. Telephone and telegram greetings arrived from John Barrymore, Charles Chaplin, Douglas Fairbanks, Mary Pickford, and Adolph Zukor. Major Bowes discussed Valentino's medical condition on the radio. Thousands of fans gathered in the streets outside hoping to gain a glimpse of the star, including one with a monkey who tried to sneak into the Polyclinic. A private detective was hired to guard the suite's entryway and intercept unauthorized visitors.

By the fourth day, the surgeons were pleased enough with Valentino's condition that they declined the use of Metaphen, a new powerful antiseptic sent by an admirer, and decided not to issue further reports unless things changed. "I have been deeply touched by the many telegrams, cables and letters that have come to my bedside," wrote Valentino. "It is wonderful to know that I have so many friends and well-wishers both among those it has been my privilege to meet and among the loyal unknown thousands who have seen me on the screen and whom I have never seen at all."[16] Schenck and Talmadge were allowed to visit. "He greeted me cheerfully," said Schenck. "'Hello, Chief. Can't you get me out of here?'"[17] The cheerfulness was premature.

Contrary to what present-day surgeons understand about placing the stomach and intestines at rest after a formidable intra-abdominal procedure, on the second day following his surgery Valentino was given chicken broth, French Vichy water, and peptonized milk for dinner. Oatmeal for breakfast was added the next morning. Each meal was followed by indigestion and abdominal discomfort. The necrotic stomach ulcer had not sealed and the ingested food and corrosive gastric juices continued to leak and rampage about Valentino's belly. In turn, virulent bacteria swelled their ranks and marched through his body as they devastated his immunologic defense mechanisms. Surgical shock set in. Valentino's team of surgeons tried their best, but the odds were stacked against them. Eventually, they declared that Valentino had only "a fighting chance."[18]

On day six, Valentino developed chest pain. Overwhelming sepsis took hold as pneumonia went about its deadly dance and shock set in. Valentino's temperature spiked to 104 and his breathing turned rapid and shallow. The actor struggled to catch his breath against the bacteria-laden fluid that swamped his lungs. Valentino's blood pressure dropped, his heart activity lessened, his kidneys shut down, confusion developed, coma ensued, and within twenty-four hours the era's greatest lover and matinee idol was dead. He is among a long list of famous American appendicitis victims, including George Bellows, Walter Reed, Daniel Patrick Moynihan, Frederic Remington, and Brigham Young.

In the days that followed Valentino's death, rumors spread that he had actually been poisoned by a jealous woman or shot in a quarrel. A story in *The Nation* gave voice to these revelations joined with a backhanded compliment to the surgeons. "Poor Rudy—the kid was knocked off," said the unidentified source. "Yuh can't tell me he died from those things the surgeons did—the whole thing looks fishy to me."[19] Not knowing who or what to believe, Valentino's fans were in a frenzy. Over one hundred thousand people lined the streets of Manhattan to pay their respects at his viewing, handled by the Frank E. Campbell Funeral Home, then at Broadway and 66th Street. Windows were smashed. Fans rushed in. "Thousands in riot at Valentino bier; more than 100 hurt . . . mounted policemen charge again and again in vain," ran a banner headline in the *New York Times*.[20] The turmoil died down once Valentino's body was taken by train to California and interred at Hollywood Forever Cemetery, where he remains today. In an interesting surgical-historical aside, the clinical findings in Valentino's case were so distinctive they received a modern eponym. Valentino's syndrome consists of pain in the right lower abdomen, mimicking appendicitis, but caused by gastric juice that leaked out of a perforated stomach ulcer and secondarily inflamed the appendix.

* * *

By the 1930s, surgical intervention of the abdomen was considered de rigueur* as surgeons turned their clinical and research skills to the two other major body cavities, the chest and the head. A surgeon in New York explained that just as the

---

* During the intra-war years, other notable operations on the abdominal organs included those for cancer of the colon, esophagus, pancreas, stomach, and rectum; ulcers of the stomach and duodenum; obstruction of the small and large intestines; and inflammatory bowel illnesses (i.e., Crohn's disease and ulcerative colitis).

abdomen could be safely explored, the interior of the chest should be similarly opened:

> In the literature of surgery there is little to be found on resection of the lung. . . . The majority of surgeons appear to have been content with palliation. . . . To refuse to operate upon a wretched [lung] patient, otherwise incurable, merely because the [operative] statistics may be unfavorable, seems hardly fair; one of the functions of our profession is the prolongation of life.[21]

Contrasted with intra-abdominal operations, procedures inside the chest were not as straightforward; air pressure, a crucial physiological difficulty, had to be overcome. The lungs consist of spongy tissue that constricts and stretches during the act of breathing. Each lung is covered by a thin layer of tissue called the pleura, which also lines the interior of the chest cage: the pleura is akin in form and function to the abdomen's peritoneum. The space between the two layers of the pleura contains a small amount of fluid that protects the tissue by reducing the friction generated from rubbing as the lungs contract and relax. During inhalation, the expansion of the lungs increases the capacity of the thoracic cavity. This allows air to flow in and inflate the lungs. During exhalation, the thorax decreases in size. This increases the pressure in the chest and air from the lungs flows outward. The cycle of changing air pressure repeats with each breath. Because the air pressure in the pleural space is lower than outside atmospheric pressure, when the chest is opened and the vacuum is released outside air rushes in through the incision, which forces the lungs to collapse, and breathing becomes impossible. The deadly calamity of a collapsed lung during an open-chest operation had to be overcome if thoracic surgery was to advance.

In Breslau, Germany, a surgeon devised a unique way to alleviate the problem of collapsed lungs during an open-chest procedure. He had engineers construct a large, leakproof glass and iron chamber with an interior maintained at negative pressure. The patient's head and neck (and anesthetist) were situated outside the chamber while the chest, abdomen, and extremities lay inside where the surgeons and nurses worked surrounded by the negative pressure. Thus, the patient breathed air and received anesthetics at normal atmospheric pressure while the negative pressure in his or her pleural space was not affected and the lungs did not collapse when surgeons opened the chest. The negative pressure chamber was a technologic wonder and, according to a contemporary source, "created a sensation in the surgical world."[22] In quick succession, pressure chambers could be found in Berlin, Cologne, St. Petersburg, Vienna, and, shortly, New York City (at the German Hospital, presently Lenox Hill Hospital).

The pressure chambers worked reasonably well but were complex in form and unwieldy in function. Patients could not be moved and the heat and working conditions in the cramped chambers were oppressive. Their sturdy walls made communication between surgeon and anesthetist difficult, and hand signals had to be used. Even more problematic were the clicking valves, hissing air, and pumping cylinders that created a racket incompatible with normal hearing and speaking. Over time, the pressure chamber concept went out of fashion and the contraptions were sold as scrap metal. However, the pressure chamber idea was later reincarnated as the iron lung for patients with respiratory paralysis from polio and other neurological conditions.

To counter the obstacles with pressure chambers, surgeons and anesthetists experimented with delivering the anesthetic directly into the windpipe or trachea. This was accomplished by cutting a small hole through the skin on the front of the neck and dissecting down to the trachea—the procedure is termed a "tracheotomy." The windpipe was opened, a breathing tube was inserted, and the anesthetic could be directed by hand under positive pressure into the lungs. A tracheotomy was dangerous and impractical for routine use in surgical operations. It gave way to the less formidable technique of passing a tube through the mouth, navigating it by sense of touch between the vocal cords, and placing it into the windpipe. This feat, known as endotracheal intubation, required considerable deftness in a conscious and gagging patient. The placement of an endotracheal tube became easier with the invention of the electric light laryngoscope, a handheld instrument that allowed the anesthetist to directly view the opening between the vocal cords into the trachea. Coughing and gagging were reduced by spraying cocaine down the throat as a local anesthetic.

*　*　*

Positive-pressure endotracheal intubation kept the lungs inflated when the chest was opened; further refinement of intubation brought about modern thoracic surgery and a wide range of operations. Among the technical challenges was how to remove a lung in its entirety. The conundrum was solved in 1933 when Evarts A. Graham successfully performed the first excision of a lung as treatment for cancer. This operation is considered a masterpiece of American surgery and brought Graham worldwide recognition.

Similar to many knife bearers, Graham recognized at an early age that his life's calling was surgery. In 1902, during his sophomore year at Princeton, he told a roommate, "Following medical school and internship [I] have three objectives—to do major surgery, to engage in research work, and to have a clinic of younger men who would be interested in studying and developing ideas."[23] Graham's father was a professor of surgery in Chicago and encouraged his son to attend Rush Medical College and then complete training as a surgeon while also pursuing graduate work in pathology and chemistry. When America entered World War I, Graham received a captain's commission in the Army Medical Corps. His combined laboratory and surgical experience led to an assignment to study the treatment of empyema (i.e., pus in the pleural space) in soldiers, a frequent complication of the influenza pandemic of 1918.

Prior to World War I, there was no effective treatment for empyema. Surgical drainage of the pus and aspiration with a needle and syringe were tried but with limited success. Instead, Graham proposed a conservative three-step treatment plan: avoidance of an open thoracic procedure and danger of a collapsed lung until the acute phase of the infection had passed and scar tissue formed; sterilization of the empyema site with antiseptic drugs and fluids; and careful attention to the nutritional status of the patient. Equally important, Graham provided a clearer explanation of the air pressure relationships within the chest; his straightforward clarification had a direct bearing on the future growth of thoracic surgery.

Graham's budding reputation led to his joining the faculty of the Washington University School of Medicine in St. Louis as its first full-time salaried professor of surgery. With his continued interest in surgical disorders of the lungs, Graham emerged as the most influential person in the growing field of thoracic surgery. In April 1933, he was consulted for treatment of a lung abscess in a long-standing smoker. Graham jolted the individual with his opinion: this was no pulmonary pustule; it was an aggressive cancer and the man's only chance of survival was removal of the diseased portion of the lung.

The distraught patient went home to discuss the findings with his family and friends. In a few days, he returned, ready to undergo the operation, and mentioned to Graham that he had some teeth filled prior to the procedure. The surgeon laughed: "I like an optimistic patient." The patient responded, "Yes, but I ought to tell you that I also bought a cemetery lot." A friend, who accompanied the patient, was a gynecologist and Graham invited him to sit in the upstairs gallery of the operating room and observe the operation. When the surgical exploration revealed the tumor to be more extensive than originally believed, Graham glanced up: "I'm not going to be able to remove the cancer without removing the whole lung," he said through the layers of his cloth mask. "What do you think about it?" The gynecologist answered, "Has it ever been done before?" Throughout Graham's career, he was known for his pugnaciousness and refusal to tread lightly to avoid an argument. As the patient's friend was about to see, this confrontational attitude made the surgeon a formidable opponent. "No," replied Graham, "but I've done it in animals. . . . I think I'll go ahead."[24] He did. Three hours later, surgical history was made.

Despite the virtuosity of Graham's achievement, he was not considered a technically adept surgeon. When Graham, known for his enthusiasm for laboratory research involving animals, first arrived in St. Louis, he was labeled by critics as only a "mouse surgeon."[25] Decades later, a visiting professor of surgery was blunter: "I judged [Graham] as rather heavy-handed and lacking in practical flair. . . . I thought how remarkable it was that such a great surgeon who had made such very great contributions to surgery could be such an indifferent practical performer."[26] Graham's defense of his technical skills was straightforward:

> The frontier of surgery is capable of indefinite expansion if we think of a surgeon as one who is interested in something more than just cutting and sewing.[27]

At the time of the historic operation, Graham, like his patient, was a heavy cigarette smoker. As evidence accumulated about the relationship between lung cancer and cigarette smoking—Graham was among the investigators—he ceased smoking in 1951. Graham was concerned enough about data that showed a time lag could occur between the end of smoking and appearance of cancer that he surmised, "I shouldn't be surprised if I died of lung cancer."[28] Six years later, Graham, unable to shake off the symptoms of flu, was diagnosed with a widely spread cancer of the lung. He was soon dead. In a poignant irony, one of the last visitors to Graham's bedside was his grateful patient. Twenty-three years after his historic lung removal, the gentleman was still smoking; his cemetery plot remained unoccupied for several more years.

*   *   *

In April 1939, *Time* magazine covered a seventieth-birthday party for a surgeon said to have "almost singlehanded" assured that an "operation for brain tumor is no more dangerous than a stomach operation." Despite this bit of hyperbole, Harvey Cushing, whom the reporter also described as "living for medicine,"[29] was not only among the leading voices in the creation of modern neurosurgery; he also had an eclectic personality that dominated much of American surgery. Resolute, standoffish, and taciturn Cushing's clinical accomplishments are legendary, ranging from the earliest safe excision of cancers of the brain to invention of the electric cautery for coagulating and cutting tissue. At a time when the printed word was the primary source for the communication of viewpoints within society—movies and radio were gaining in popularity but had not yet replaced journals, magazines, and newspapers—Cushing's achievements in the literary world were equally impressive.

Thirteen years prior to his birthday party, Cushing received the Pulitzer Prize for a two-volume biography of William Osler, one of the founding professors of The Johns Hopkins Hospital and celebrated as the Father of Modern Medicine. Cushing remains the only surgeon to be awarded the coveted honor. Several years later, an editorial in the *New York Times* further extolled Cushing's writing abilities: "The author's sense of atmosphere and form, the restraint and delicacy of his literary art, will stir professional writers to envy or humility."[30]

This encomium was followed by a request from the editor of the highbrow *Atlantic Monthly* (presently *The Atlantic*) to publish a set of articles based on the private diaries that Cushing kept during his service in World War I. In turn, Cushing fashioned the series into a full-length best seller, *From a Surgeon's Journal*. Cushing's acclaim as a literary wunderkind was underscored when a book reviewer implored that if *From a Surgeon's Journal* could be read by as "many millions of the post-war generation as there were of the preceding generation who served in the war, the likelihood of there ever being another such suicidal conflict would be greatly lessened if not entirely removed from the earth."[31]

Cushing's literary skills brought him respect, but it was his clinical skills that endeared him to the public as the genius brain surgeon. Operations on the brain, even more than abdominal or chest procedures, presented formidable problems. There was the existential puzzle of how the brain worked beyond an appreciation that it was an important control of the self; what areas of the brain regulated what areas of human behavior was guesswork. Secondly, there was the physical puzzle of how to operate on an organ with the consistency of tofu that was crisscrossed by a myriad of blood vessels more convoluted and fragile than anywhere else in the body.

For thousands of years, knife bearers feared to operate on the brain with the exception of trephination of the skull (strictly speaking, opening the cranium is not actual brain surgery). This apprehension lessened during the closing decades of the nineteenth century when advances in neuroanatomy and neurophysiology led to the localization of brain function and the pinpointing of malignant tumors. Cushing, more than other neurosurgeons, appreciated the importance of laboratory research for surgeons-to-be and established the first neurosurgical training program that combined investigative work, operative experience, and surgical experimentation. He explained:

> I personally feel that for the development of surgical technique no place is comparable to the experimental laboratory, and I feel that every young surgeon should begin to acquire his operative training in a series of operations on the lower animals . . . it has the advantage of giving them a sufficient laboratory experience to enable them subsequently to pursue to the only place where they are likely to be solved some of the many problems which arise.[32]

* * *

In the fall of 1896, Cushing, a recent graduate of Yale College and Harvard Medical School, arrived at The Johns Hopkins Hospital to train with its fastidious professor of surgery William Halsted. "A prior short visit," recalled Cushing, "was enough to show an outsider [me] something of the spirit which permeated the early group of workers there."[33] Cushing's organizational abilities and surgical skills were outstanding and, by the following spring, it was apparent that Halsted favored his new protégé over the other residents and would name him as his first assistant. "I need hardly to tell you that I am in hearty sympathy with your efforts to correct some of our many bad habits," Halsted wrote to Cushing. "We have never had a man on the staff who understood the management of his assistants [like you]."[34] Chief resident surgeon was a coveted position and entitled Cushing to oversee the hospital's surgical department.* Imbued with Halsted's operative dictum of deliberate, gentle, and slow dissections, Cushing performed a majority of the major operations—he took the first X-ray picture in the history of Johns Hopkins—and by the end of his training showed a special interest in neurosurgical cases.

Cushing's relationship with Halsted was cordial but distant. "I saw relatively little of Halsted during my three years as chief resident," explained Cushing, "less and less as he perhaps began to feel that I might be trusted with the bulk of the routine work."[35] Instead, the young surgeon enjoyed a close relationship with Osler, the hospital's professor of medicine and director of America's first formal residency training program for physicians. The two men were the veritable opposites who attracted each other. Distinct from Cushing's brusque intensity, Osler was a good-natured extrovert, who was equally praised for his clinical acumen and his efforts as a bibliophile, historian, and gourmand. Their lifelong friendship had a profound effect on Cushing's maturation as a physician and culminated with his writing Osler's biography.

In June 1900, after forty-four months under Halsted's and Osler's tutelage, Cushing departed for a year of neurophysiological laboratory work in Europe. In late summer of 1901, he returned to Baltimore, joined the surgical staff at Johns Hopkins, and was soon practicing neurosurgery on a full-time basis. Cushing emphasized a painstakingly slow and meticulous style of dissection in removing tumors of the brain. He devised tiny clips of silver wire to compress bleeding points and used electrical stimuli to study various areas of the brain. In 1910, Cushing reported on sixty-four cases of brain tumor removal, a quarter of whom had complete restoration of normal bodily function. His results were far superior to any of his contemporaries with markedly improved survival rates for patients undergoing difficult brain operations.

---

* In late September 1897, within days of Cushing assuming his responsibilities as Halsted's chief assistant, he began to experience abdominal discomfort. After much deliberation by Halsted, Osler, and members of the medical and surgical staff, it was decided to perform an exploratory operation. Halsted and another senior surgeon found an "infected" appendix with its tip lying deep in the pelvis. Cushing suffered a superficial wound infection but, by mid-November, was back to full-time duties.

Two years later, Cushing authored the first of what would be eight books on neurosurgical topics. Clear and forthright, *The Pituitary Body and Its Disorders* brought Cushing international prominence and led to his being named professor of surgery at Harvard and first surgeon-in-chief to the Peter Bent Brigham Hospital (presently Brigham and Women's Hospital). There Cushing organized a surgical training program with an emphasis on neurosurgery:

> Neurological surgery is fascinating, and will long continue an important and profitable field for intensive cultivation, partly because it has been largely unworked from an operative standpoint, partly because it deals with one of the two most important systems of the body—nervous and circulatory. It is gratifying to see that a number of young men are fitting themselves to specialize in it, with a preparation which makes envious one who has wriggled into the subject and, like the proverbial squid, has left little but a trail of ink behind him.[36]

* * *

Cushing's initial work in Boston included a three-month stint with the Ambulance Américaine in France. This was a philanthropically sponsored hospital in Paris that provided care to soldiers prior to America's formal entry into World War I. Cushing's management of the hospital's surgical unit opened his eyes not only to the shortcomings of military medical care throughout Europe but also to the incomprehensible scope of the conflict. Furthermore, the establishment of the hospital by wealthy Americans and its staffing by American doctors brought the need for military medical preparedness to the public's attention while serving as a model for the wartime training of surgical personnel.

Once Cushing returned to the United States in mid-1915, he decided that a fully functioning army field hospital had to be set up proactively for the sake of the country's military medical preparedness. His goal was to bring military life to the forefront of people's consciousness and prepare them for America's possible entry into the war. Cushing's idea was to construct an army hospital on the Boston Common, a proposal that never came to fruition. In May 1917, he ended his crusade when he was mobilized and sent overseas to France to manage a Harvard-sponsored base hospital as America entered the war.

Many horrific surgical stories came out of World War I, but one that involved Cushing, Osler, Osler's son, Edward Revere, and George Crile is among the saddest. On his mother's side, Revere, the Oslers' only child who survived infancy, was the great-great-grandson of famed American patriot Paul Revere. Revere spent his adolescence in England, where his father was professor of medicine at Oxford—the older Osler had left Johns Hopkins in 1905 to assume the new position. At the outbreak of war, nineteen-year-old Revere enlisted in the British military service and received an appointment as lieutenant in the Royal Artillery Force. In an afternoon in late August 1917, Revere was on the front lines in northern Belgium when he was struck by a German shell. He was carried by stretcher to a dressing station and, four hours later, arrived by ambulance at a field hospital in Dozinghem.

As fate would have it, several of his father's surgical friends were on duty nearby. Cushing, who was consulting at a neighboring field facility, rushed over in a motor ambulance through pouring rain. He found his mentor's son in shock and drifting in and out of consciousness. In Cushing's words, "It could not have been much worse . . . one [wound] traversing through the upper abdomen, another penetrating the chest just above the heart, two others in the thigh."[37] Several hours later, Crile, who was stationed in Rémy, France, arrived with a transfusion apparatus and immediately began to replace the blood that had been lost. As midnight approached, a surgical operation began. Large rents were found in the colon with feces spilled throughout the abdomen as well as blood in the chest and a collapsed lung. Revere's condition never stabilized and, just before sunrise, Cushing wrote in his diary that "this world lost this fine boy, as it does many others every day."[38]

The young Osler was buried in an alder branch–lined grave, dug by members of the British government–recruited Chinese Labour Corps, and wrapped in an army blanket covered by a weather-worn Union Jack. His grave is located in what became the Dozinghem Military Cemetery. Revere's renowned father never recovered psychologically from the loss. He caught influenza in the great pandemic and died. On Osler's bedside table was found a slip of paper on which he had written: "The Harbour almost reached after a splendid voyage with such companions all the way and my boy awaiting me."[39]

*   *   *

When Cushing returned to Boston at the end of the war, his understanding of neurosurgery was greatly broadened by his overseas experience. He brought the ultra-refinements of preoperative preparation and operative techniques into neurosurgery to such a degree that many of his brain procedures now required five or even six hours. Distinguished surgeons, from all over the world, visited to watch him operate. Cushing enjoyed the limelight along with the public's growing adulation. In the spring of 1930, the admiration reached a new level when his middle daughter married the oldest son of the governor of New York, Franklin Roosevelt. "Betsey's wedding day. Temp. 90° +/−," Cushing wrote to a friend:

> The town is full of Delanos, Roosevelts and motorcycle policemen and detectives. Our front yard looks like a circus and I feel like Mr. Ringling—the wedding ringling. I have reserved a special tent for myself . . . 10 cts. extra—peanuts and lemonade and camels (cigarettes).[40]

There was a telling admission in this letter. Cushing smoked incessantly and the circulation in his legs (and later his heart) was failing secondary to his heavy use of tobacco. The discomfort and unsteadiness were so severe that Cushing had to be intermittently hospitalized. Despite his ill health, Cushing rarely altered his daily schedule and, in mid-1931, performed his two thousandth operation on tumors of the brain, surrounded by moving picture cameras and still photographers to record the occasion. The next year he identified a previously unrecognized condition caused by an excess growth or tumor of the pituitary. The pituitary gland, located at the base of the brain, behind the nose, is often called the master gland because it controls the production of hormones in several other glands, including the adrenals, ovaries, thyroid, and testicles. In what is eponymously referred to as Cushing's disease, the pituitary releases too much of a hormone that, in turn, overstimulates the adrenal glands and affects their control of blood pressure and the body's water balance.

According to guidelines that Cushing established at the time of his appointment to Harvard, it was mandatory for him to retire at age sixty-three. No longer able to operate and with his health in decline—Cushing's circulatory difficulties worsened and he began to suffer from a stomach ulcer—he moved to Yale as professor of neurology. He continued to write and spent more time cataloging his collection of rare medical and surgical books. Cushing had a particular interest in Vesalius—a pastime begun under Osler's influence—and was working on a catalogue of publications by and about the famed anatomist.

One evening in the fall of 1939, Cushing was doing research on the planned bibliography when he lifted a heavy volume by Vesalius and was seized with severe pain in his chest. Three days later, Cushing died. An autopsy showed that the main blood vessels to his heart as well as those going to his legs were blocked by fatty deposits, a finding commensurate with his substantial use of cigarettes. The cremated remains of Cushing, arguably the most honored American surgeon of his generation, were taken to Lake View Cemetery in Cleveland to rest beside his parents and other members of his family.

*   *   *

Through the centuries, the practice of surgery has been largely defined by its tools and working with one's hands. Advances in surgical instrumentation and surgical technique paralleled one another. From the crude implements of ancient Greeks and Romans, through the hand-crafted instruments of the sixteenth century, to the complex surgical appliances developed in the eighteenth century, new and improved apparatuses led to better surgical results. During the closing years of the nineteenth century, growth in science brought possibilities into surgical practice not necessarily related to instrumentation and/or technique. Barely a half century later, progress in surgery was so pronounced that every organ and area of the body had been explored and few mysteries remained.

The essence of surgery—the invasion of people's bodies for cure—had become an accepted part of life. Indeed, surgery, with its ethos of sweeping action and continuous refinement, defined much of America's medical culture. The surgical profession was a juggernaut of clinical triumphs backed by the ability to diagnose diseases at earlier stages and supported by effective pre- and postoperative treatment that enabled patients to survive complex operations.

At the same time, surgery was undergoing a maturation process of organization, professionalization, and specialization that represented a reaction to emerging economic, political, and social forces. This transformation brought the men and women who performed surgical operations together in formalized, well-structured associations that served as powerful voices to affect policies, promote skills, and restrict competition. Paradoxically, it was in the United States, which had been much slower than European countries to recognize surgeons as a distinct group of clinicians separate from physicians, that the drive toward organization and specialization was centered.

The process of professionalization generated a fundamental change in the way surgeons viewed themselves and their interactions with a society distinguished by its rapid industrialization and growing prosperity. Automobiles ruled the highways, tractors reigned over the farmland, and planes mastered the skies. Speed meant everything and nothing was faster than the new electric industry and its mass radio audience and instant information. Suddenly advertising and news were immediate, which advanced the Americanization of immigrant communities and brought about new social structures including a well-defined middle class. Reflecting this affluence, by the late 1920s the United States achieved a position of paramountcy in total world industrial production never before attained by any other nation: 35 percent of the whole, compared with England's 11 percent, Germany's 10 percent, and France's 5 percent. As Americans grew richer so did their surgeons, especially those who became surgical specialists.

15.

PROFESSIONALIZATION

Surgery does the ideal thing—it separates the patient from his disease. It puts the patient back to bed and the disease in a bottle.

Logan Clendening, *Modern Methods of Treatment*, 1924

But after all, when all is said and done, the king of all topics is operations.

Irvin S. Cobb, *Speaking of Operations*, 1915

In 1927, Will Rogers, the American humorist, was at the end of a fund-raising campaign for victims of a disastrous Mississippi River flood when he developed severe abdominal pain. Rogers was diagnosed with gallstones, which were remedied by removal of his gallbladder. Reports of the operation were front-page news, including details of a persistent postoperative fever and other minor setbacks, as well as celebrity gossip concerning the hundreds of get-well telegrams Rogers received from such diverse personalities as President Calvin Coolidge, Ty Cobb, W. C. Fields, Ring Lardner, and Flo Ziegfeld. Two years later, a fully recovered Rogers used his comedic wit and turned the tale of his operation and convalescence into a best-selling book, *Ether and Me or "Just Relax."* The slim volume was an immediate success, fueled by sales in hospital gift shops. It went through eighteen printings, the last one in 1943, eight years after Rogers's tragic death in a plane crash. Among the various aspects of surgery that Rogers poked fun at, the notion of specialization was a major target:

This is a day of specializing, especially with the doctors. Say, for instance, there is something the matter with your right eye. You go to a doctor and he tells you, "I am sorry, but I am a left-eye doctor; I make a specialty of left eyes." Take the throat business for instance. A doctor that doctors on the upper part of your throat he doesn't even know where the lower part goes to. And the highest priced one of all of them is another bird that just tells you which doctor to go to. He can't cure even corns or open a boil himself. He is a Diagnostician, but he's nothing but a traffic cop, to direct ailing people.[1]

Rogers's pique was not without precedent. The clinical, financial, and social implications of specialization for surgeons had been a concern since the mid-nineteenth century. In 1861, Julius Homberger, a newly arrived immigrant from Germany, began to advertise his skills as an ophthalmologist, the first surgeon in the country to market his specialty. He had studied with several of Europe's leading eye doctors and his claims, although dubbed by critics as a "peculiar method of procuring practice,"[2] appeared credible. The following year, Homberger published the *American Journal of Ophthalmology*, the earliest periodical to be devoted solely to a surgical specialty in the United States, and was named ophthalmic surgeon to the Brooklyn Medical and Surgical Institute and the New York Eastern Dispensary.

While local practitioners resented how Homberger peddled his skills, he was quick to point out that the men he worked with in Berlin and Paris had long marketed their expertise in magazines and newspapers. Homberger saw no reason that he should not be allowed to promote what he considered specialized services and superior talents. He was adamant that what was acceptable in Europe should be acceptable in America and, either way, specialists would soon become a majority of United States' practitioners.

Homberger's major adversary was the recently established AMA, its state affiliates, and their Code of Ethics:

It is derogatory to the dignity of the profession, to resort to public advertisements or private cards or handbills, inviting the attention of individuals affected with particular diseases . . . or to publish cases and operations in the daily prints, or suffer such publications to be made, or to invite laymen to be present at operations, or to adduce certificates of skill and success. . . . These . . . practices . . . are highly reprehensible. Equally derogatory to professional character is it, for a physician to hold a patent for any surgical instrument.[3]

In 1865, he was censured by the Medical Society of the State of New York when its members passed a resolution, without mentioning him by name, that condemned medical advertising.

An aggrieved Homberger continued to advertise while renouncing his membership in the AMA and the state society: "I will follow my own views on questions ethical in procuring the extensive practice to which I have a right to consider myself entitled."[4] The war of words carried on for several years and an increasingly badgered and ostracized Homberger finally abandoned his practice, ceased publishing the *American Journal of Ophthalmology*, and resettled in French-speaking New Orleans, where he joined the staff of Touro Infirmary. In 1869, he issued a bitter attack against the AMA, a twenty-page bizarrely titled pamphlet, *Batpaxomyomaxia*, in which he reiterated the reasons why surgeons should be permitted to market themselves. Shortly after the broadside was published, Homberger suffered a mental breakdown and was confined to the Louisiana Retreat insane asylum. Nothing further was heard from or about him.

Homberger can be easily dismissed as an insignificant, rebellious, and troubled individual, but it was his spoken and written words and the actions taken against him that brought the question of surgical specialization in America to the fore. Prior to Homberger's activities, the notion of professionalization for surgeons along with its main components—organization and specialization—posed few conflicts since virtually every knife bearer was also a general practitioner.* "In the United States any attempt to separate the practice of [medicine from surgery] is altogether

---

* Professionalization is an economic and social process by which a craft, trade, or occupation transforms itself into a "profession," a disciplined group of individuals who adhere to an established set of ethical standards. At its core, a profession is intended to be an indicator of expertise and trust. The group positions itself as possessing special knowledge and skills in a recognized body of learning, derived from education, research, and training at an advanced level, and is regarded by the public as such. Professions enjoy prestige, privilege, status, and socioeconomic power, and their members comprise a class of individuals set apart from the common man. A professional agrees to abide by a code of conduct marked by altruism, competence, integrity, and accountability to those served and to society. The milestones that mark an occupation's maturation into a bona fide profession include establishment of specialty education, organization of specialty societies, publishing of specialty journals, and setting self-regulated standards for licensure and training.

futile," explained a doctor, "the most distinguished surgeons having been, and yet being . . . the most accomplished physicians of their respective localities."[5] Matters changed during the 1880s and 1890s following the wide employment of anesthesia and antisepsis and the return of thousands of Americans who had studied in specialized surgical clinics in Europe. Surgery was now safer and the number of surgical operations increased, such that specialization was increasingly viewed as a financially rewarding, practical, and worthwhile endeavor.

Despite the growing enthusiasm for surgical specialization, in early-twentieth-century America, use of the word "surgeon" connoted a wide range of professional identities. At the top of the pyramid was a small group of surgical elites, represented by East Coast professors of surgery from the leading urban medical schools. These men belonged to exclusive national surgical societies, dominated debates at meetings, performed research, wrote textbooks, and educated and trained others. A second and somewhat larger category consisted of individuals with a primary interest in surgery who taught in second-tier medical schools, maintained private surgical clinics, and staffed nonteaching hospitals. They were members of state and local surgical societies, wrote mostly for local journals, and rarely did research. The first and second groups were limited in number since it was difficult during these years to make a living as a full-time surgeon. A third group of individuals claimed to be "surgeons" but, unlike the first two groups, did not restrict the bulk of their practice to surgery. These were general practitioners with a local reputation as surgical consultants for other general practitioners who did not operate. The third group overlapped with a fourth group, the large mass of general practitioners who performed only an occasional operation. The latter two groups completed the majority of surgical procedures in the United States during the first half of the twentieth century.

The inevitable consequence of professionalization for surgeons was that clinical relationships between specialists and generalists turned rancorous. "Specialism has become an avenue of escape for hard labor," cautioned a general practitioner in the Midwest, "a harbor for a one-cell brain."[6] Less damning and more pragmatic was the founder of the AMA: "[Specialists and generalists] have become, in a great degree, separated into distinct and independent organizations. . . . So much so, indeed, it has become quite common to hear the interest of the general practitioner and the wants of the specialist spoken of as essentially distinct."[7]

The assessment was correct; surgical specialists, with their additional education and training, entrepreneurial spirit, and sophisticated gadgetry, not only earned more money but also were powerbrokers within American health care. Surgeons managed most of the newly opened hospitals, were repeatedly elected as presidents of the AMA, and established their own elite specialty organizations—American Ophthalmological Society (1864), American Otological Society (1868), American Gynecological Society (1876), American Laryngological Association (1878), American Surgical Association (1880), American Association of Genitourinary Surgeons (1886), and American Orthopaedic Association (1887).

Generalists argued that specialty societies fragmented Medicine and reduced the effectiveness of the AMA. They also feared that competition from surgical specialists would cut into their livelihood and whittle away their responsibilities. Although there was truth in their opinion, specialty organizations served as vital lynchpins in the process of professionalization for surgeons. They provided forums where the nation's knife bearers gathered under the auspices of duly constituted and legally recognized associations to discuss the pressing clinical and socioeconomic issues of the day, the "body politic" of surgery. "The only question which can arise relates to the manner in which the specialist shall proceed," cautioned a prominent general practitioner:

> Whether any or no attention shall be paid to the feelings and wishes of the profession; whether an individual shall pursue that course which is generally considered gentlemanly and honorable, or assume an ideal superiority over his brethren, and thus temporarily obtain a meretricious reputation and an undeserved reward.[8]

For decades, members of the AMA debated whether a specialist should be required to serve time as a generalist before having the right to advertise his or her specialty. While doctors dillydallied in their discussions, specialism flourished, propelled by the meteoric rise of surgical science and the burgeoning financial and political strength of surgeons.

*   *   *

Surgical specialists were initially found in the large cities of the Northeast, but they rapidly fanned out across the nation as their influence and clinical activities increased. "Every cross-road village has its ophthalmologist, aurist or gynecologist," observed a journalist at Fort Scott, Kansas, "not mentioning the gentlemen who in a minor way make the rectum, urethra, throat, nose, pharynx, etc. their particular field of onslaught."[9] The spread of specialists was facilitated by the explosive growth of railroads, whose steam-powered carriages bridged the physical miles between rural and urban America. The advance of railroads and the wide distribution of specialists brought about the now-forgotten field of "railway surgery," the nation's earliest large surgical specialty.

In 1869, the tracks of the Union Pacific Railroad and the Central Pacific Railroad were joined at a point called Promontory in the Utah Territory. A golden spike was driven as a symbol of the completion of the first chain of railroads to span the North American continent. A dozen years later, the linking in New Mexico of the Santa Fe Railroad from the east and the Southern Pacific Railroad from the west marked the completion of a second transcontinental rail route. Americans reveled in their expanding railroad network along with the glamour and excitement of moving at breakneck speeds. But railroads, that era's metaphor for progress, had a sinister side. The Interstate Commerce Commission reported that at the turn of the century 1 of every 28 railroad employees was injured and 1 in 399 died on the job. "That much danger to life and limb is incurred by those who are thus engaged in this special vocation is self-evident," wrote one expert. "Even in localities where the strictest supervision and management are employed to avoid danger, the number of accidents is painfully large."[10]

Not only were railroad employees injured, but railway calamities affected thousands of passengers also. There was the widely reported 1887 Great Chatsworth train crash in Illinois that resulted in over eighty fatalities and three hundred injuries when a trestle collapsed and twenty wooden passenger coaches plunged 150 feet into a ravine. Equally horrendous was the 1888 Mud Run collision in the mountains of Pennsylvania. A host of conventioneers were returning from a meeting of the Catholic Total Abstinence Union when two trains plowed into each other, causing sixty-six deaths. These new kinds of domestic mass-casualty accidents, as opposed to war injuries, required innovative surgical techniques and treatments as well as inventive methods of first response.

Out of this necessity arose railway surgery, which quickly developed into a bona fide specialty with its own journals, textbooks, and local, state, and national societies. Railway doctors were usually small-town general practitioner/surgeons, often retained by railroad companies, who offered a full spectrum of medical and surgical care, from treating injured travelers to advising officials on employee workplace safety. In 1888 the National Association of Railway Surgeons was established, and within several years it had over fifteen hundred dues-paying members. Whether the Association's annual meeting was in Detroit, Houston, or Kansas City, it was one of the largest conventions in the country. Manufacturing and pharmaceutical companies were usually on-site to promote their products—at the meeting in Chicago in 1897, representatives from Eli Lilly, Johnson & Johnson, McKesson & Robbins, Parke-Davis, the Pasteur Vaccine Company, and Searle & Hereth were present. "The associations of railway doctors are wholly scientific, in their objects, and you might say philanthropic," asserted one railway surgeon, "and only seek to improve themselves by coming together and discussing the various methods of taking care of the maimed and injured victims of accidents."[11]

The Association lobbied for railroads to maintain medical and surgical departments and build private hospitals under the authority of a company's chief physician/surgeon. By 1896, thirteen railroads managed twenty-five hospitals that treated over 165,000 patients annually. Several of the larger hospitals were state-of-the-art facilities and became celebrated as training centers for interns and residents. In these financially flush hospitals, managers could be cutting-edge in their ability to care for patients. "In all ways the policy of the management is broad-gauge and liberal," wrote a reporter describing the availability of surgical specialists, horse-drawn ambulances, and a twenty-eight-hundred-volume library at the Missouri Pacific Hospital in St. Louis. "No effort is made to economize in any matter wherein the welfare of a patient is concerned."[12]

Hospital administrators provided novel outpatient services through specially equipped "emergency department" railroad cars. These relief cars reached the far-flung outposts of any railway system and foreshowed the United States Army's famed M(obile) A(rmy) S(urgical) H(ospital) units. They had full-service operating and recovery rooms and hot water from the locomotive's boiler to sterilize bandages and instruments. "The patient has more chances of recovery," wrote a railway surgeon describing the emergency car, "and he himself, as well as the surgeons and officials of the road, rests content with the knowledge that every effort has been made for the best possible results."[13]

Despite the rapid ascent of railway surgery as a specialty, it ultimately failed to gain traction within mainstream Medicine and suffered a precipitous decline. This occurred because the majority of the nation's physicians, especially those in large urban areas, opposed the contract practice of railway surgeons. The fear was that corporate capitalism would dominate American Medicine and strip doctors of their clinical and financial independence. Thus, railway surgeons and virtually any doctor who worked for railroads and/or other businesses were regarded with suspicion and shunned by their non-company-employed peers. By 1920, the Association was moribund and its journal, *The Railway Surgeon*, dropped the word "Surgeon" from its title.

Notwithstanding the demise of the specialty, ex-railway doctors had learned a great deal and, over time, many of these general practitioner/surgeons turned their interests toward the full-time practice of surgery. "Specialism is a necessary phenomenon of progress, and cannot be ignored," claimed a longtime railway surgeon. "Nay, I would go farther and would say that it should be fostered and encouraged, for in this direction, only is healthy growth to be obtained."[14]

* * *

The rise of science, technology, and specialization shifted surgical care away from people's homes and toward hospitals, institutions that only several decades before were considered nothing but stopgap measures on the final journey to the cemetery. A boom in building—the number of new hospitals far outpaced the percentage rise in population—accelerated this change, providing centers for surgeons' expensive services as well as costly bacteriological and chemical tests and elaborate microscopic and X-ray studies. Architects and urban planners designed the new facilities to be organizationally original, physically impressive, and scientifically sound while leaders within American surgery called for surgeons to assume managerial control of the hospitals and their staffs. It was contended that the ultimate power of accreditation, licensing, policy, and standardization needed to be in the hands of those who made greatest use of a facility. "The hospital is essentially part of the armamentarium of medicine," argued a scalpel wielder from Chicago. "The independence and honorable position of medicine rests on the full control of its tools. If we wish to escape the thralldom of commercialism, if we wish to avoid the fate of the tool-less wage worker, we must control the hospital."[15]

The mounting costs of technologies and treatments forced hospitals' administrators to turn to surgical patients as a key source of income. In return, since surgeons referred the majority of paying patients to hospitals, governing boards expanded the number of management and trustee positions for knife bearers, especially those with high-volume practices. As their ranks swelled, surgeons became the dominant voice in hospital administration, which heightened the public's perception of their clinical authority and economic and social status. With surgery increasingly inpatient oriented, surgeons, who wanted to be viewed as scientifically responsible and socially respectable, were obligated to join the staff of a hospital. The transformation was so complete that, by the mid-1930s, most individuals practicing surgery had some form of hospital admitting privileges.

There was also no gainsaying the obvious; surgical outcomes were better evaluated in medical institutions than in the far-flung offices of individual practitioners. The more that surgeons congregated and worked in hospitals, the easier it was to study and standardize their practice routines. One consequence was that in the opening decades of the twentieth century reform-minded doctors, nurses, and administrators—this was the height of Progressivism,* when activists worked to improve public facilities—began to ask fundamental questions of surgeons: How long did it take for a hospitalized patient to be diagnosed? What operation was performed? Did the patient recover? If not, was the surgeon or the hospital to blame? Progressives looked to transform hospital care through a scientific approach to management and treatment. They demanded answers that correlated hospital outcomes with surgeon performance, and especially how scientific and technologic advances were incorporated into the care of a patient.

"Efficiency" became a key word, a simple metric for interest groups to determine if surgeons and hospitals were providing optimal care. Efficiency experts touted the conviction that a well-organized hospital and surgical staff would offer excellence in surgical procedures and pre- and postoperative care. For instance, the era's most renowned efficiency expert, Frank Gilbreth, used time and motion studies to show how an operating room nurse could be more efficient in passing instruments to a surgeon—he is also remembered for the book written by two of his children about him, *Cheaper by the Dozen*. Progressives wanted hospitals to

---

* Progressivism is a political philosophy that reached its peak in the opening decades of the twentieth century. It was a response to what was viewed as undesirable changes brought by the modernization of American society, exemplified by uncontrolled growth of large corporations and rampant corruption in politics. Progressives believed that advancements in economics, science, social organization, and technology were vital to the improvement of the human condition and social reforms needed to be integrated into the everyday life of Americans.

impose discipline on their staffs, especially with regard to the scrutiny of surgical outcomes. One result was that audits, statistics, and success-or-failure data came into use for the first time.

* * *

A major void still faced American surgeons in their drive toward professional status. The various elite specialty societies with limited memberships were not capable of serving as a national lobbying front, nor were the regional surgical societies—the Southern Surgical Association (1887), the Western Surgical Association (1891), the New England Surgical Society (1916), and the Pacific Coast Surgical Association (1925)—with their geographic-related concerns. At the same time, a change was occurring in medical school and postgraduate surgical education. The didactic and rote method of learning was being supplemented with practical demonstrations. Large classrooms of students served by one lecturer, who would drone on for hours were separated into smaller groups taught at the bedside and in the clinical laboratory. Surgeons in practice sought out technical masters by visiting them and observing their clinical prowess. "Show me" was suddenly more convincing than "tell me."

It was demand for a "show-me" attitude that led one thousand blue- and scarlet-robed surgeons to march into the Gold Room of Chicago's Congress Hotel in November 1913. Leading the procession was Franklin Martin, a dynamic, plain-speaking surgical gynecologist who had been long involved in the politics of American Medicine. The surgeons were to be sworn in as members of the newly chartered ACS. Martin, the founder, contended that an organized group of surgeons with sophisticated technical skills could easily demonstrate to the public the limits of a general practitioner's surgical abilities. "Patients with intelligent judgment in other matters, were cheerfully hopping up on operating tables and allowing a medical school graduate with one year of training in an internship to peer and search aimlessly within their abdominal and other body cavities,"[16] complained a member of the ACS. For Martin and his followers, such surgical recklessness had to stop. They saw the ACS as the appropriate instrument to allow them to attain organizational and political dominance over the general practitioner who did little more than dabble in surgery.

Martin understood the immensity of the turf war and the need for professional jurisdiction. "A renaissance of surgery was dawning," he explained. "The wilderness with its jungle was being explored, and this most perplexing of problems had to be solved."[17] Martin—his biographer described his bearing as severe and "Indian-erect"[18]—was neither an academic nor a renowned elite surgeon, but his personal narrative as a general physician who had restricted his practice to surgical gynecology, combined with his involvement in grassroots medical politics, made him an ideal spokesman for those who wanted to be considered specialists in surgery. In this capacity, Martin championed endeavors both to prohibit nonspecialists from performing surgeries and to circumscribe the role of the general practitioner.

Martin first became a national surgical powerbroker in 1905, at forty-eight years of age, when he founded one of the earliest journals devoted to the surgeon as specialist. "I was convinced," wrote Martin, "that the profession needed a practical journal for practical surgeons, edited by active surgeons instead of *littérateurs* only remotely connected with clinical work."[19] *Surgery, Gynecology & Obstetrics* (renamed the *Journal of the American College of Surgeons* in 1994) succeeded immediately and afforded Martin a direct line of communication with thousands of surgeons.

Martin exploited this opportunity, sharply demarcating the boundaries between general practitioners who rarely performed surgery, self-professed surgeons who continued to treat nonsurgical patients, and legitimate full-time surgical specialists. He pushed and prodded his peers to understand that simply reading *Surgery, Gynecology & Obstetrics* was not sufficient by itself. Surgeons and surgeons-to-be had to see master surgeons perform operations to truly understand technical complexities. For Martin, "show me" became a surgical imperative:

> The phenomenal acceptance of *Surgery, Gynecology & Obstetrics* was conclusive proof that the profession preferred to receive information directly from practicing surgeons rather than from non-practicing editors who acted merely as interpreters. And it was far better to have a practicing surgeon demonstrate his work than to have him tell about it.[20]

In 1910, Martin placed announcements in his new journal for a clinical meeting to be held in Chicago where physicians, as long as they had the slightest interest in surgery, could visit the operating rooms of the city's great surgeons. "It was an innovation," claimed Martin, "that the academic orators and medical politicians watched with amusement that they did not conceal, but it stirred in the minds of practical surgeons a hope."[21] He expected two hundred attendees. One thousand and three hundred doctors showed. The registration booths were underserved and the operating rooms were overcrowded. The attendees urged perpetuation of the clinical meeting through some type of organization that would ensure a yearly opportunity to observe the work of master surgeons in different cities.

With much fanfare, the Clinical Congress of Surgeons of North America was established. A second Clinical Congress convened in Philadelphia the following year with over fifteen hundred attendees. Several hundred watched a hernia repair on John Coombs, pitcher for the Philadelphia Athletics and hero of the 1910 World Series. Newspapers hailed the operation with banner headlines ("Baseball Player Undergoes Treatment at University Hospital") and provided the Congress widespread publicity ("Over 1,000 Delegates Attend Surgical Clinics").[22]

At a third Clinical Congress in New York City in 1912, over twenty-six hundred doctors registered and hundreds more attended without paying. Swarming crowds brought chaos to the live surgical sessions. Martin's Congress had turned into a logistical nightmare. His attempt to provide hands-on surgical education to Medicine's rank and file, to democratize surgical education, and to upgrade the operative skills of physicians had succeeded beyond his expectations. However, political and practical dilemmas became apparent. Many attendees were not interested in restricting their practices to surgery. Instead, they registered to learn surgical techniques in order to augment their general practice and increase income. Moreover, these men declared themselves well-educated and -trained surgeons based simply on the imprimatur of attending a Clinical Congress. Similar to American doctors who studied in German specialty clinics and received "diplomas" for their work abroad, general practitioners hung their certificates of attendance on the walls of their office to impress patients that they were "surgical specialists."

Once Martin realized that his Clinical Congress functioned as merely another pathway to part-time surgical specialization, he searched for ways to limit admission. "There must be a change; there must be a change," he preached. "I formulated my program. It involved a new organization, through which definite qualifications for membership would be established."[23] Martin proposed an organization, the ACS—loosely modeled on the Royal College of Surgeons of England—that would establish minimum requirements for a doctor to be allowed to perform surgical operations. The ACS would award those who qualified the title of Fellow of the American College of Surgeons (FACS) and disseminate their names to hospitals and the public as qualified specialists in surgery.

Martin's attempt to distinguish surgeons from general practitioners enjoyed wide support, including backing from several state medical societies. "If it holds itself aloof and free from medical politics and politicians, it is destined to become the most potent factor in directing and establishing the standards and requirements for all who desire to devote their life to surgery,"[24] wrote an official from Michigan. But there were also those who challenged Martin's idea. "Do you have in mind the establishment of a glorified surgical union, along labor union lines?"[25] asked one foe. Another general practitioner suggested calling Martin's organization the American Surgical Society so that the "mystic letters" after his name would spell "quite nicely, ASS."[26]

Neither the relentless ad hominems nor concerns about personal safety—fisticuffs broke out and threats were hurled at meetings—dissuaded Martin. When the thousand soon-to-be fellows of the ACS assembled in Chicago on that chilly autumn morning in 1913, they established benchmarks that changed the course of surgery in America. For the first time, capable surgical specialists were identified for the American public. The ACS emphasized the specialist's professional authority and clinical competence over general practitioners by standardizing the very idea of a surgeon. From that day on, no one could deny the notion of specialization in surgery.

The establishment of the ACS set an exceptional precedent: the profession of surgery, rather than federal or state governments, would determine who could be called a specialist in surgery. Surgeons began to police themselves and, in so doing, introduced a hierarchy into everyday surgical practice that left generalists with unsettled professional prospects. Animosities were inevitable by placing general practitioners on the defensive and for good reason. Surgical specialists were on top of the clinical and socioeconomic ladder; by the end of 1915, almost thirty-three hundred surgeons had been admitted to the ACS.

*　　*　　*

Two years after its founding, the ACS was forced to consider a stronger role in the movement to reform America's surgeons and hospitals. The reason was a classic catch-22 situation. Although the ACS was busily endorsing doctors as capable surgeons and hospital administrators used the information to weed out incompetents,

Martin and his supporters realized that they could not properly evaluate the competency of knife bearers independent of detailed information about the hospitals where they practiced. "We found evidence that much surgical work was being done in hospitals that lacked many facilities essential in the scientific care of the patient," recounted Martin. "Cases were unsystematically recorded and the professional work was generally without supervision."[27]

The ACS was denying over half of its applicants and the excluded physicians were upset. Under pressure from those who were rebuffed, hospital administrators asked the ACS to furnish examples of acceptable operative records, define standards for laboratories, and outline staff requirements. In turn, leaders of the ACS issued guidelines, known as the "Minimum Standard," and created a national commission on hospital standardization. The program clarified the manner in which a hospital should organize its medical staff and explained that positions must be restricted to individuals "competent in their respective fields and worthy in character and in matters of professional ethics."[28]

Doctors were instructed about how to behave and collaborate with one another and staff meetings were to be scheduled monthly to review their clinical outcomes. The program expected that physicians would maintain accurate and detailed records of all patients and that the case histories would be accessible to outside inspectors on a moment's notice. Lastly, hospitals had to provide laboratory facilities ("chemical, bacteriological, serological, histological, radiographic and fluoroscopic services")[29] under trained supervisors.

The ACS's hospital evaluations started in mid-1918 and the strategy worked—magazines and newspapers touted the ACS's efforts. *Harper's* told of the "new control of surgeons" and how "their adoption of the Minimum Standard kills the old boarding-house hospital and makes the hospital itself responsible for everything that goes on within its walls."[30] An article in the widely read *World's Work* went further:

> With the ideals of the [surgical] profession visualized, and with practical plans made to insure their application, the country may confidently look forward to a new era that is already partly here; when the hospitals of America will be institutions for service, from which selfish interest and careless methods have been abolished, and to which the country may look for considerate and efficient treatment, confidently expecting and receiving the utmost that the [surgical] profession is capable of giving.[31]

By late 1922, as public support solidified, the ACS published a list of almost seven hundred approved hospitals of one hundred or more beds. Hospital administrators hung their new certificates of endorsement in front entranceways and announced their success in community newspapers. By the mid-1920s, the ACS had endorsed over 80 percent of the nation's largest hospitals and one-half of moderate-sized hospitals. Smaller hospitals continued to struggle with the criteria, but strong public condemnation led either to their compliance or to their closing.

*   *   *

The ACS's "Minimum Standards" helped regulate hospital care, but efforts were also underway to evaluate and certify surgical internships and residencies. Several medical colleges and state licensing boards had begun to require that graduates complete an internship or "fifth year" of hospital work to earn their MD degree. "The hospital internship is no longer for the privileged, but will soon be required of every graduate in medicine," explained an article in the *Journal of the American Medical Association*. "We must be willing to devote ourselves to the long years of patient, grinding tutelage, advancing slowly, under recognized masters, until we have laid broad and firm foundations."[32]

The process of approving hospitals for internships quickly became too burdensome for any individual medical school to handle. The AMA, which had grown uneasy toward the ACS and its status as a hospital regulator, seized the opportunity to counter its rival's influence. In 1920, the AMA introduced a competing hospital standardization program centered on the approval of internships and shortly published a list of 469 general hospitals with 2,960 "acceptable"[33] programs. Seven years later, the AMA expanded its involvement in evaluating postgraduate training when it authorized a list of approved residency programs in medical and surgical specialties. "The danger is not from an increasing specialization, but from those who pose as specialists without having secured the essential advanced training,"[34] explained a member of the AMA's Council on Medical Education and Hospitals. An AMA directory named 270 hospitals with 1,699 approved residencies, including anesthesia, dermatology, gynecology and obstetrics, medicine, neuropsychiatry, ophthalmology, otolaryngology, pathology, pediatrics, radiology, surgery, tuberculosis, and urology. Thus, the AMA formally declared its support for specialization, a key policy decision that had a profound impact on the future of the country's physicians and surgeons and the whole of American Medicine.

The AMA's efforts to upgrade hospitals, internships, and residencies complemented the ACS's Hospital Standardization Program. The two competing plans assisted hospitals to become responsible institutions from the clinical, educational, and organizational standpoints. The programs also provided information that allowed citizens to compare and contrast their local hospital with nearby institutions. "Certainly, the movement is in the right direction," applauded a member of the ACS board, "and out of it should come a generation of very much better trained men than the last generation furnished."[35]

*　*　*

The surgeons who founded the ACS wanted to distinguish themselves from general practitioners and to raise the level of performance of individuals who performed surgical operations to the highest standards. Despite these intentions, the organization initially set membership guidelines relatively low in its haste to expand enrollment—by the mid-1920s there were over seven thousand Fellows of the ACS, the majority of whom had not taken any form of an examination or undergone a personal interview. In view of these "low" qualifications, there was concern that membership was increasing at too alarming a rate. Critics, mostly academic and full-time surgeons, demanded a more thorough accounting of an applicant's character, intellect, and training. "There is about as much distinction in being a member of the American College of Surgeons as in belonging to the mob in Grand Central Station, New York City," complained one surgeon. Another added: "As compared with the analogous organization in Great Britain, the American College of Surgeons has about the relative standards of a 5 and 10 cent store as compared with any first-class department store."[36] In essence, those in the ACS who were well-trained full-time surgeons threw down a gauntlet to the organization's self-taught and part-time surgeons with regard to their credentials.

Initially, little action was taken, possibly due to a lack of unanimity of opinion but more likely because control of the ACS remained entrenched in the hands of Martin and his aging supporters, especially George Crile and the Mayo brothers. In the early 1930s, a faction of surgeons decided that the status quo was no longer tolerable. They were mostly young and well-trained surgical educators from the large cities, individuals who would ultimately advance American surgery through the middle decades of the twentieth century. For now, they were idealists with a steadfast opposition to surgical mediocrity who sought a national organization composed only of full-time, well-trained surgeons.

Evarts Graham, a man who minced few words, led this breakaway group. He was well known for his recent successful removal of a lung for cancer. He was aloof, determined, and patrician in comportment, and it was no surprise that he served as the main instigator for the dissidents. "The deftness of the operator, the number of operations performed and even the income of the surgeon is often chosen as criteria upon which to measure the greatness of the surgeon," explained Graham. "These are the false standards which lead to unwise operating, too much operating and the commercialism of the profession."[37]

Graham and his surgical insiders knew that if the profession did not move to better regulate specialists in surgery, the state governments would eventually step in to fill this role, a situation that few scalpel wielders wanted. There was lay pressure as well. Patients, increasingly dependent on surgeons for their health care, could not determine who was truly qualified—licensure from a state government only established a minimal floor for education, and training and membership in medical societies revealed little about competency. The public needed reassurance from the surgical profession that their caregivers had the imprimatur of a respected authority.

At a series of acrimonious meetings, Graham and his supporters told the leaders of the ACS about their plans to organize a society that would certify surgeons as being properly educated and trained and in a full-time surgical practice. The ACS, said the insurgents, had allowed "fingers to replace brains" while "handicraft outruns science."[38] Graham's group threatened to turn the ACS's annual meeting into a "surgical circus"[39] unless its leaders cooperated in the founding of an independent board for certification. Representatives of the College, who feared a collapse of their organization, grudgingly agreed to cooperate.

Graham's appeal for a new certifying body was patterned after several existing models. He recognized that the integrity of any profession was largely dependent on the control it exercises over the competence of its members. Therefore, the certification of expertise, whether through government mandate or voluntary compliance, was of crucial importance. In America, the first surgical specialty to attempt to rein in practitioners by certification of their competency was ophthalmology. Unlike other "specialists" in surgery, ophthalmologists had an organized presence that dated back to the Civil War—they were the first group of knife bearers to establish a specialty organization, the American Ophthalmological Society (1864). Despite the Society's existence, ophthalmologists were beset with competitive and political difficulties.

By the turn of the century, non–medically schooled optometrists were making claims, through extensive advertising campaigns, of greater competency in prescribing eyeglasses and treating various ailments than their medical-schooled peers. Full-time and part-time ophthalmologists were restrained from advertising their services by the ethical codes of the medical profession—Julius Homberger is the exemplar. As a result, ophthalmologists could do little to effectively counter the boasts of their optometric competitors. Just as problematic was the growing number of general practitioners who, after attending an ACS Clinical Congress or other postgraduate courses, trumpeted their investiture as specialty "ophthalmologists" capable of treating diseases of the eye.

Full-time ophthalmologists were outraged at what they considered the usurping of their hard-earned professional skills. Especially troubling was the obvious fact that there were no established criteria with which to distinguish well-qualified ophthalmologists from lesser-trained general practitioner/ophthalmologists or even optometrists. To resolve the situation, the idea of a self-regulating professional examining board, sponsored by the leading ophthalmological organizations, was proposed as a means to certify competency. In 1916, uniform regulations and standards were established that included educational and training requirements as well as oral and written examinations. Thus, the American Board of Ophthalmic Examinations (later renamed the American Board of Ophthalmology) was formally incorporated—the first instance of what the American public began to know and value as "board certification." Several years later, a National Board of Examiners in Otolaryngology (currently the American Board of Otolaryngology—Head and Neck Surgery) was organized, followed shortly by the American Board of Obstetrics and Gynecology.

Other surgical specialties attempted to create their own certifying boards, but the absence of a central body to coordinate the growing number of efforts prevented an orderly approach. To remedy this lack of leadership, an Advisory Board for Medical Specialties (later renamed the American Board of Medical Specialties)* that

---

* Presently, the American Board of Medical Specialties sets guidelines for board certification in its twenty-four constituent specialty boards (date of founding): Ophthalmology (1916), Otolaryngology (1924), Obstetrics and Gynecology (1927), Dermatology (1932), Pediatrics (1933), Colon and Rectal Surgery (1934), Orthopedic Surgery (1934), Psychiatry and Neurology (1934), Radiology (1934), Urol-

represented an independent coalition of the three existing surgical specialty boards, some seventy medical schools, state licensing committees, and numerous hospitals was formed in 1933. Once the new organization issued a set of standards for certification, a number of specialty boards were established in rapid succession, including the American Board of Surgery (ABS) in 1937.

The founding of the ABS was a crucial step in upgrading surgical education and training in America. Though Graham and his followers denied any intent to impel board certification as a requirement for membership on hospital staffs, it was not long before board-certified surgeons were receiving preferential treatment. In World War II, board-certified knife bearers obtained higher military rank and assumed more responsibility than their colleagues without certification. In civilian life, the public came to regard board certification as an indicator of clinical competency, while hospitals began to limit surgical privileges to only board-certified individuals.

Despite Graham's expectations that the ABS could formulate a certification procedure that covered the whole of surgery, its actual power was truncated. He tried to broker ties between the ABS and the established surgical specialty boards of ophthalmology, otolaryngology, obstetrics and gynecology, and orthopedic surgery. As convincing as Graham could be, it was to no avail. The leaders of the previously organized surgical boards pointed to the economic and educational rewards their certifications represented as reason enough to remain independent of Graham's board. In fact, the ABS should more accurately be titled the American Board of "General" Surgery, because it largely represents the needs of the general surgeon contrasted with the wishes of the orthopedist, otolaryngologist, neurosurgeon, plastic surgeon, urologist, et cetera.

*   *   *

---

ogy (1934), Internal Medicine (1935), Pathology (1936), Surgery (1937), Neurological Surgery (1940), Anesthesiology (1941), Plastic Surgery (1941), Physical Medicine and Rehabilitation (1947), Preventive Medicine (1948), Thoracic Surgery (1948), Family Medicine (1969), Allergy and Immunology (1971), Nuclear Medicine (1971), Emergency Medicine (1976), and Medical Genetics and Genomics (1980). Most of the specialty boards have areas of subspecialty certification. For instance, the American Board of Orthopaedic Surgery awards certificates in orthopedic surgery but also offers two subspecialty certifications, Surgery of the Hand and Sports Medicine. Similarly, the American Board of Urology awards board certificates in urology and offers subspecialty certification in pediatric urology and female pelvic medicine and reconstructive surgery.

On June 30, 1982, I completed seven years of general surgical residency during which I also attended classes at the Johns Hopkins School of Hygiene and Public Health and received a doctorate in public health. It was a time of celebration for my family (Beth and I were the parents of a four-and-one-half-year-old daughter and a one-and-a-half-year-old son); I was to join a general surgical practice in central New Jersey. The endless work of a surgical residency was over, but one crucial element remained: I had to become certified by the ABS—my ultimate standing in the practice I joined and my admitting privileges at the local hospital were contingent on being board-certified.

Certification by the ABS is a two-step process that requires successful completion of an eight-hour multiple-choice Qualifying Examination followed, a year later, by an oral Certifying Examination of three thirty-minute sessions conducted by six examiners. Fortunately, I passed the Qualifying Examination in November 1982 and, one year later, sat for the Certifying Examination. Shortly, I received a letter with an opening sentence: "The American Board of Surgery is pleased to inform you that you have successfully completed the Certifying Examination and are now a Diplomate of the American Board of Surgery."

Two memories stand out during my process of board certification. The first was driving home with the worst headache I had ever experienced from the overwhelming stress associated with taking the Qualifying Examination. The second involved my interest in surgical history. At the conclusion of the final session of the Certifying Examination, one of the poker-faced examiners asked a simple question: "Dr. Rutkow, can you tell me who discovered heparin and when?" Heparin is a blood thinner that prevents the formation of blood clots. Although I had already written a number of journal articles on surgical history,[40] I doubt that the surgeon knew of my interest. I looked at the examiner, smiled, and answered, "Yes, it was Jay McLean, a second-year medical student at Johns Hopkins in 1916." A surprised look came over the surgeon's face. "No one has ever been able to answer that question. How and why do you know about McLean?" I simply stated, "I studied at Johns Hopkins and have an interest in surgical history." The examiner's impassive expression returned: "Dr. Rutkow, thank you and good luck with your career."

* * *

From 1910 to 1940, the development of surgery in America gathered tremendous momentum. A consolidation of professional power, marked by an interplay between internal organizational issues, external political/socioeconomic concerns, and startling clinical advances, predominated events. Efforts to devise new operations called for greater reliance on experimental surgery and laboratory investigations. A scientific basis for surgical therapies—consisting of empirical data, collected and analyzed according to nationally and internationally accepted standards and set apart from individual assumptions—demonstrated the validity of surgery to the public. Longstanding quarrels with poorly trained and under-educated "surgeons" were settled. Knife bearers lobbied for stronger medical licensing laws, established board certification programs, and turned the management of hospitals into safeguards of support. In short, surgeons shaped their profession so that its sovereignty was sustained while the division of scalpel wielders into various specialty areas was strengthened.

The many vast changes placed new responsibilities on surgeons. They had no choice but to allay society's fear of the surgical unknown by making certain that surgery was viewed as an accepted part of Medicine's present and future. This was not an easy task, because the aftermath of surgical operations, especially discomfort and worry, was often of more concern to patients than the knowledge that an operation could eradicate devastating disease processes. Thus, the most consequential achievement by surgeons during the first part of the twentieth century was ensuring the acceptability of surgery as a legitimate scientific and social endeavor backed by a confident and well-organized profession.

Despite any uncertainties about surgery's future, two things were clear: Americans were now the key players on the world's surgical stage and specialization, with its organizational complexities and technologic wizardries, was about to produce spectacular clinical triumphs upon spectacular clinical triumphs.

PART V

TRIUMPHS

16.
THE BLOOD OF WAR

America, it has been said, was a land of practical men. . . . It was there-
fore a land of surgeons. The same ingenuity in mechanical contrivance
which was proving so beneficial in industry was exhibited also in the
operating room.

Lloyd G. Stevenson, *Yale Journal of Biology and Medicine*, 1960

In surgery all operations are recorded as successful if the patient can be
got out of the hospital or nursing home alive, though the subsequent his-
tory of the case may be such as would make an honest surgeon vow never
to recommend or perform the operation again.

George Bernard Shaw, *The Doctor's Dilemma*, 1906

In 1946, following the end of World War II, Frank Slaughter, a thirty-eight-year-old surgeon who doubled as a best-selling historical novelist—he would author fifty-six books with worldwide sales of 60 million copies—wrote *The New Science of Surgery*, a work that introduced readers to recent advances in surgical research and technologies. His message was simple: "Without the skill of the surgeon's fingers, there would be no surgery, no lives saved. But without science there would be no way for that skill to operate."[1] Slaughter, who is largely overlooked in present-day surgery, was part of a notable literary tradition: the surgeon as writer. He, more than any other American scalpel wielder in the mid-twentieth century, established a pathway for contemporary surgeon/authors exemplified by William Nolen, Sherwin Nuland, and Richard Selzer.

Slaughter, who attended The Johns Hopkins University School of Medicine, completed four years in surgical training at the Jefferson Hospital, Roanoke, Virginia, followed by twelve months as a resident in thoracic surgery at Herman Kiefer Hospital in Detroit, Michigan. He was board-certified in surgery and thoracic surgery and a Fellow of the American College of Surgeons. Whether telling the story of the surgeon/anatomist Andreas Vesalius in *Divine Mistress* or describing the medical and surgical training of Luke the Evangelist in *The Road to Bithynia*, many of Slaughter's books contained surgically related story lines based on real events backed by exhaustive research. He became so successful in the early stage of his writing career that at the completion of Slaughter's wartime service as an army surgeon he closed his surgical practice in Jacksonville, Florida, and devoted himself to literary pursuits. Year after year, Slaughter produced one or two novels, writing several thousand words a week.

The New Science of Surgery was one of only three nonfiction books that Slaughter wrote. A reviewer described it as "highly readable . . . extremely entertaining . . . concise and authoritative"[2] The work's premise examined the close cooperation between surgeons and researchers in the basic sciences of biology, chemistry, physics, and physiology, along with engineering. For example, Slaughter detailed the development of sulfonamide drugs, the first broadly effective antibacterials to be used systemically, and how their availability paved the way for the antibiotic revolution in Medicine. In World War I, the death rate from bacterial pneumonia was 18 percent; in World War II, following the use of sulfonamides, it fell to under 1 percent.

Slaughter also described the discovery, in 1928, of the first bacteria-killing antibiotic, penicillin, and explained that, initially, researchers could not produce adequate quantities for routine use in clinical practice. Even as late as 1940, America's doctors only had enough penicillin to treat ten patients at a time. To relieve this shortage during wartime, the federal government initiated a coordinated effort into the mass production of the drug, forging a relationship between scientists in academia, government-funded laboratories, and the chemical, distilling, and pharmaceutical industries. The various groups worked together to perfect the necessary fermentation techniques and increased penicillin production exponentially. "The development of penicillin afforded a striking illustration of the effectiveness of a well-financed, coordinated approach to surgical research," claimed a participant. "No private, uncoordinated procedure could have secured comparable results in anything like the same time."[3]

By 1944, sufficient amounts of penicillin had been stockpiled and newspaper articles and radio broadcasts lauded cases in which army surgeons used penicillin to radically improve clinical outcomes. "Penicillin saves flier on first use in Rumania [*sic*]," ran one headline in the *New York Times*. The reporter told a dramatic story of how the airman was "blown from his [Liberator] plane but managed to get his parachute open." He suffered fractured hips and injuries of the arms and legs and peasants from the village of Ploesti carried him to a small hospital. American personnel operated, but the flier went into surgical shock. In a desperate gambit, the surgeons had penicillin flown in from Italy. "He is now on his way to a full recovery," extolled the journalist.[4]

*   *   *

The impact of World War II on surgery was enduring and profound. For the first time in the history of American warfare, deaths from military action exceeded those from diseases and causes not related to hostilities. Various factors contributed to this circumstance: better organization of the U.S. Army Medical Department and its personnel; recognition that early surgery was paramount in the resuscitation effort; improvements in the management of surgical shock, including the wide availability of blood and plasma for transfusions; use of sulfa drugs and penicillin; rapid evacuation of the wounded by handheld stretchers, ambulances, and airplanes; presence of surgical nurses to assist at operations and provide pre- and postoperative care with an emphasis on cleanliness; establishment of specialized treatment centers for the seriously wounded; and the organization of Portable Surgical Hospitals (they were forerunners to the famed Mobile Army Surgical Hospitals of the Korean War) plus the presence of large hospital ships, both born of necessity in the hostile jungles and island-hopping campaigns of the Pacific combat theater.

Despite improvements in surgical care, the lethality of the tissue destruction caused by artillery-shell fragments and large-caliber bullets, and the general force of the bigger munitions employed in World War II is impossible to overstate. Nothing seen in civilian surgery had ever remotely approached the extent of the trauma to the human body encountered in this war. Ranging from America's tank-mounted "Calliope" Rocket Launcher T34, which fired a barrage of deadly shells from sixty separate launch tubes to Germany's "Bouncing Betty" S-mine with its explosive charge of 360 steel balls that tore an individual to pieces to the various flamethrowers and the horrendous burns they inflicted, the injuries were devastating. Even when a soldier was not directly hit, the concussive force of these large weapons could shred intestines into ribbons while solid organs like the kidney, liver, and spleen exploded.

The demand for surgery was overwhelming and could only be met by a well-coordinated organization able to conduct operations efficiently and promptly under widely varying settings. In addition, the surgical infrastructure had to be mobile, so it could move with the battle; otherwise its effectiveness was lost. At the same time, surgeons had to have the capability of treating soldiers on the front lines who were slightly wounded and could be promptly returned to duty as well as those who were seriously injured and required immediate treatment, which precluded further evacuation. "The record which has been made in this war by American surgeons in their treatment of the wounded is enviable," claimed an eyewitness:

> This saving of life has been achieved primarily by the skill of American surgeons and their ability to develop rapidly the concepts which were necessary for the intelligent management of the wounded. Few if any of the surgeons had ever experienced the flow of gross trauma which faced them when the battle was on and casualties began to pour in . . . their intellectual flexibility, their ingenuity at improvisation, and their constant attention to detail in the care of the wounded provided a great tribute to the system of medical education which developed their surgeons. Their record was not equaled by that made by any other nation.[5]

The initial care of a wounded soldier was provided by medical corpsmen, or medics. On the front line, the distressed cry of "Medic!" brought them on the run. Medics were not trained doctors, let alone surgeons, but they rendered sophisticated first aid: control of gross hemorrhage, dressing of wounds, initiation of sulfonamide and/or penicillin therapy, management of pain with injections of morphine, and splinting of fractures. Bill Mauldin, the Pulitzer Prize–winning editorial cartoonist, celebrated for his popular depictions of bedraggled and weary infantrymen, called the medical corpsman the "private soldier's family doctor."[6] The medic's dangerous responsibility was readily evident; in the European theater alone, more than two thousand medical corpsmen were killed in action and five were awarded the Medal of Honor.

Once medics completed their treatments, stretcher-bearers carried the patient to a battalion aid post, generally located one half mile behind the front line of combat, where definitive resuscitation began. The junior medical officers who staffed battalion aid posts tried to ensure that the wounded soldier remained stable for further evacuation. Therapies included additional control of bleeding, placement of tourniquets, intravenous administration of plasma, closure of open chest wounds to prevent collapse of a lung, and injections of tetanus toxoid. From the battalion aid post, the wounded were transported farther back to a collecting post and then driven approximately five miles to the rearmost point in the active combat zone, the clearing station. It was there that the formal triage of patients occurred. The diagnosing and sorting were of such importance that only experienced medical officers were given the responsibility.

Adjacent to the clearing station was a tented surgical complex, the field hospital, equipped to support a variety of surgical operations. A soldier who needed care at the field hospital usually had life-threatening injuries to the abdomen, chest, or head and neck and further evacuation jeopardized any chance of survival. Surgical conditions in a field hospital were not ideal. The surgical staff was small in number and the surgeons were not the most experienced. Furthermore, field hospitals were usually near artillery positions. Incessant bombarding made it difficult for the recently operated-on soldier to obtain rest, and during periods of intense military action pre- and postoperative care was less than optimal.

From the field hospital, a soldier was taken to an evacuation hospital, located twelve to fifteen miles behind the lines. These facilities were fully equipped and staffed with surgeons who were proficient in managing the most devastating of wounds. The evacuation hospitals served as the backbone of the army medical service and handled the majority of the wounded in the active combat area; it was there that the bulk of lifesaving surgery occurred.

A wounded soldier could remain in an evacuation hospital for two weeks but, once stable, was transferred to a general hospital. These facilities were typically grouped as a hospital center where specialty surgical care (i.e., hand surgery, head and neck operations, neurosurgery, plastic and reconstructive surgery, and thoracic surgery) was available. By segregating casualties, surgeons gained confidence with new and complex procedures that would have taken years to evaluate and master in a civilian practice. Moreover, the relatively unsupervised and urgent nature of combat surgery encouraged technical innovation, allowing surgeons at general hospitals to attempt novel operations. During the early years of the war, the hospital centers were located in Great Britain and Ireland, but their locations changed as military successes were achieved. By the closing months of the hostilities, the final portion of the evacuation plan for a wounded soldier involved air and sea travel to a general hospital center as near to their home as possible.

* * *

The organization of the evacuation system and the manner in which the wounded soldier was resuscitated were among the critical aspects of surgical care that most distinguished this war from those before. In World War I, the pulse rate and the presence of nausea, sweating, and vomiting were seen as evidence of surgical shock. However, research conducted between the wars showed that these indicators were far from accurate. At the start of World War II, blood pressure, degree of thirst, and the soldier's mental status—none of which had received much attention in World War I—were found more useful in evaluating the extent of shock. Still, the diagnosis of surgical shock remained confusing and needed clarification. In response, shock wards and shock teams were organized (similar in function to those of World War I) and casualties, believed to be in shock, were admitted to these facilities, regardless of whether they required a surgical operation. The legacy of the World War II shock ward is seen in the modern surgical intensive care unit with its staff of critical care specialists. In fact, the American Board of Surgery presently offers subspecialty certification in Surgical Critical Care.

As with evacuation and resuscitation, if overall surgical care was to be successful, then the framework of clinical activities had to be fairly standardized. The uniformity of surgical treatments afforded efficiency and safety and many of these principles became cornerstones in the care of civilian patients. Despite concerns about surgeons and their possible opposition to the strict regimentation of clinical activities, treatment of the sick and wounded was detailed in a myriad of directives and written manuals. These advisories provided in-depth instructions on how army surgeons should treat the wounded soldier, from the battlefield to the rearmost hospital. Notwithstanding the guidelines, individual initiative was permitted such that the skill of the experienced surgeon was encouraged and the less experienced surgeon was provided with supervised training.

To discuss the various clinical advances in surgery, from orthopedic procedures that preserved limbs to the treatment of burns with skin grafts or the skilled repair of injured arteries, is to ignore what was perhaps the most important clinical distinction between World War II and its predecessors. In the Civil War and World War I, American surgery leapt forward, largely due to the unparalleled experience that battlefield surgeons gained in a short period of time. World War II also provided the nation's knife bearers with intensive practical experience, but the hostilities commenced at a time when American Medicine was in ascendance, an era when the federal government had newfound faith in the surgical profession and actively partnered with its practitioners to further its development.

Importantly, the federal government's activities dampened the long-running tussle between generalists and specialists. The military's decision to award higher ranks to surgeons with advanced levels of training and specialized knowledge, especially board certification, provided doctors with an incentive to specialize that trumped ongoing debates within American Medicine concerning the prudence of specialization. Indeed, it was the reservoir of specialists formed in the late 1920s and through the 1930s that made possible the competent medical and surgical care given in World War II. The military became so dependent on the expertise of board-certified specialists that as the war wound down, the surgeon general of the army instituted a point system for the discharge of doctors skewed toward the retention of specialists. "New Army Separations Board, Setting Score," explained a newspaper caption, "Aims to Keep the Scarce Specialist."[7]

Although military authorities did not explicitly support the process of board certification, they de facto recognized the importance of the education and training necessary to obtain such an imprimatur. By rewarding surgeons who were board-certified with pay and rank, the military effectively catalyzed medical and surgical specialization in postwar America, thus ensuring that specialty boards and the notion of specialization became mainstays of the health care delivery system. Tens of thousands of returning physicians responded by vesting their professional futures in specialty training.

*   *   *

With the start of World War II, the federal government began to devote financial resources to scientific research on such a grand scale that it created a fertile environment for surgical innovation. Among these investigations, surgeons were at the forefront of studies regarding the preservation and use of blood and its main constituent, plasma.* The government of Great Britain acknowledged this expertise when it reached out to America's medical community for assistance in providing blood for emergency transfusions after Nazi Germany initiated its siege of England. The British Ministry of Health estimated that if the German Luftwaffe's aerial bombardment escalated, six hundred thousand people could be killed and twice that many injured.

In mid-June 1940, a group of high-ranking physicians, who concentrated on blood research, met in New York City to discuss how to supply the embattled British with the needed blood. The attendees included the Nobel Prize–winning French surgeon, Alexis Carrel, various administrators of biological and pharmaceutical firms, and other experts representing the army, navy, Rockefeller Institute, and federal government's National Research Council. The British request appeared straightforward but was logistically challenging and pushed the boundaries of America's capabilities. To organize a nationwide blood collection effort—one significantly larger than any before and that preserved the blood for several weeks while awaiting shipment overseas—would be a massive undertaking.

It was only twenty-five years earlier that an American physician first determined how to preserve blood for transfusions. The use of a powerful anticoagulant allowed the blood to be maintained in a liquid nonclotted form, which slowed its decomposition and made it available for transfusions for up to a week. In World War I, a United States Army medical officer took advantage of this discovery and set up a rudimentary blood storage facility near the front lines. He completed fewer than two dozen transfusions, but his ice-cooled refrigeration unit, with its supply of anticoagulated blood, was one of the world's earliest blood depositories. Several years later, American researchers identified the A, B, O, and Rhesus (Rh) blood compatibility groups, discoveries that dramatically decreased the threat of fatal blood mismatches.

As blood transfusions became safe, in 1937 a physician at Chicago's Cook County Hospital established a laboratory that stocked donated blood. He coined

---

* Plasma is the liquid component of blood and makes up 55 percent of its total volume (the remaining 45 percent consists of red blood cells, white blood cells, and platelets, all of which are suspended in the plasma). Plasma is over 90 percent water and contains vital proteins, such as albumin and gamma globulin, along with hormones, salts, and vitamins. Plasma serves four major functions: maintaining blood pressure; supplying critical proteins for blood clotting and immunity; transporting electrolytes, such as potassium and sodium; and preserving a proper pH balance in the body.

the phrase "blood bank," explaining that the term "is not a mere metaphor. . . . Just as one cannot draw money from a bank unless one has deposited some, so the blood preservation department cannot supply blood unless as much comes in as goes out."[8] Blood banks, with their ready availability of blood for transfusions, gradually spread across the nation and led to the development of broad-based donor programs.

Around the same time, a privately managed nonprofit blood service in New York, the Blood Transfusion Betterment Association, was organized. Despite its quaint name, the organization was as modern as any feature of American Medicine. For the first time, it brought blood researchers together to study the science of blood transfusion as well as to stimulate physician education and training in an emerging specialty, hematology. The Betterment Association also provided the administrative and scientific know-how to match hospitalized patients in need of blood with donors, who were on call twenty-four hours a day and paid according to the amount of blood they gave. In a nod to its philanthropic bent, the Association also raised funds to provide transfusion services to the indigent or, as they were labeled, "impecunious patients."[9]

Much of the blood research in the years leading up to World War II focused on how to extend the shelf life of stored blood beyond the seven-day barrier. Investigators looked to blood plasma as a possible solution. To obtain blood plasma, medical technicians first separate freshly drawn blood so that the blood cells settle to the bottom. They then pour off the liquid plasma. Although blood plasma cannot substitute for a transfusion of whole blood, it can temporarily sustain a victim's blood pressure during transportation to a hospital or, in the case of combat, initially resuscitate casualties on the battlefield.

At the New York meeting, those in attendance were told that researchers had recently determined how to safely preserve blood plasma in a refrigerator for almost two months, eight times longer than what was possible with whole blood. Although researchers still considered the use of blood plasma experimental, the meeting's participants could not ignore its lengthy shelf life and potential usefulness. They decided to organize a "Blood Plasma for Great Britain Project"—colloquially known as the "Blood for Britain" plan—which would provide blood plasma to the English and other allies in amounts never before attempted. There was also an ulterior motive for the Americans; they acted out of concern for their country's national defense program and its capability to supply whole blood and plasma to the armed forces.

The administrators of the Blood for Britain project moved quickly to coordinate the collection and delivery efforts. The presence of the Blood Transfusion Betterment Association, particularly its managerial capabilities to procure and service large numbers of donors, led the organizers of the Blood for Britain project to locate their program in New York City. Within several weeks, the Blood for Britain managers hired a staff of twenty-two secretaries as well as numerous clerks and telephone operators. Engineers designed a refrigeration truck to carry blood away from the various hospitals where it was donated. The American Red Cross coordinated the public call for volunteer donors, while the Blood Transfusion Betterment Association supervised the actual collection of the blood and the technical separation of the plasma. "Plans Are Laid to Get Blood for British," declared a bold-faced headline in the *New York Times* in mid-August 1940, "Red Cross and Unit Here to Supply Plasma Solution."[10]

Alongside these technical preparations, the Blood for Britain administrators worked assiduously to garner public support. Radio announcements ran around the clock. Volunteers distributed descriptive pamphlets. Publicity posters appeared on buses and subways. Reports in newspapers touted the project with touching stories: "19 Members of Family Donate Blood to Britain" was the lead for one article.[11] By Labor Day, program staff had registered over one thousand volunteers, and one month later the number climbed to five thousand. Eager donors, acting in support of their across-the-Atlantic ally, filled collection centers at Hospital for Joint Diseases, Lenox Hill Hospital, Long Island College Hospital, Memorial Hospital, Mount Sinai Hospital, the New York Hospital, New York Post-Graduate Hospital, and The Presbyterian Hospital. "It apparently had a very strong popular appeal," wrote one of the project's managers, "judging by the immediate enthusiastic response from every stratum of society."[12]

Despite Blood for Britain's success in attracting volunteer donors, the program soon encountered technical problems with regard to the preparation of plasma on such a large scale. "When we began this work, we were led to believe that it would be relatively simple," bemoaned the project's director. "We received the impression that preparing plasma would not be much more difficult than mixing a cocktail, but we soon learned, much to our distress, that such was not the case."[13]

The handling of mass amounts of plasma for shipment abroad simply differed from the preparation of small quantities for immediate use in nearby hospitals. There were vigorous debates on how to store plasma (liquid or dried form), the size and shape of the collecting bottles (cylindrical, dumbbell, or square straight-sided), and how to withdraw the volunteer's blood (vacuum versus suction versus simple venous pressure). There were also discussions about the criteria for donors, including age range, presence of high blood pressure, and quality of the blood itself as determined by a red blood cell count. The first batch of liquid plasma the American team sent to England had a milky appearance. British authorities raised the question of bacterial contamination and rejected it. Mounting difficulties forced the project's organizers to take what they termed a "radical step."[14] A full-time, salaried surgeon was hired to answer scientific questions, formulate a standardized collection technique, solve shipping dilemmas, and better coordinate the cooperating hospitals.

* * *

When executives of the Blood for Britain project appointed Charles Drew as their campaign's supervisor, they were told there were few things the thirty-six-year-old could not master. Broad-shouldered, handsome, and tall, he carried himself with an obvious air of authority. "He commanded respect by his presence," recalled Drew's older sister. "He stood very straight, a big powerful man."[15] Drew was a highly ambitious, well-organized, multitalented individual, starting with his academic and athletic success at Washington's Dunbar High School and continuing through his studies at Amherst College and medical school at McGill University, where he graduated as salutatorian.

The Blood for Britain executives, however, wanted Drew as much for his medical and surgical background as for his personal strengths. Drew represented the new breed of American surgeon, one whose clinical expertise rested on in-depth education and training combined with proficiency in leading-edge scientific research. He spent two years following medical school as a resident in internal medicine at Montreal General Hospital. This was followed by a three-year surgical residency at Freedmen's Hospital, which was associated with the Howard University School of Medicine in Washington, DC. In 1938, Drew was awarded a two-year fellowship to complete his surgical training at Columbia University and The Presbyterian Hospital in New York City. "For years I have done little but work, plan and dream of making myself a good doctor, an able surgeon," he soon wrote to his wife. "I have known the cost of such desires and have been quite willing to do without many of the things that one usually regards as natural."[16]

There was little argument that Drew possessed stellar personal and professional qualifications, but his appointment at Columbia was also a key cultural and social milestone in American surgical history. Drew was African-American and had reached the zenith of the American surgical establishment at a time when racial segregation was rampant in Medicine and racist attitudes affected large segments of the profession of surgery. No black surgeon had trained at Presbyterian or at other prestigious surgical residencies and, similar to white-administered hospitals of the era, no black surgeon had been offered staff privileges at Presbyterian or at other famed hospitals. Drew, however, was resolute in wanting to complete his surgical training at one of the finest residency programs in the United States. "He was intense," said a friend, "always sticking to anything that needed to be done and not sparing his own energy."[17]

The erudite and soft-spoken Drew made many friends at Columbia, most notably the influential chairman of the department of surgery; he would provide the crucial backing that Drew needed to be deemed eligible to take the examination of the American Board of Surgery for certification as a general surgeon. In addition to Drew's clinical training, the chairman assigned him to work with a team of researchers involved in studies relating to blood banking and transfusion. "There are some grand people here," Drew wrote to his mother, "it's good to feel the impact of new ideas and the surge of creative activity."[18] After several months, an always-competitive Drew realized that the results of his research could be turned into a doctoral thesis on banked blood that would fulfill the requirements for him to obtain a second doctoral degree, a doctor of science in medicine (M.D.Sc.). Drew believed that having an additional doctorate would help distinguish himself from other surgeons, black and white.

Drew's training for his eventual stewardship of the Blood for Britain program began in early 1939 when, in conjunction with his research, he established Presbyterian's first blood bank. "[As a researcher], Drew was naturally great," wrote his research mentor:

> A keen intelligence coupled with a retentive memory in a disciplined body . . . [and] a personality altogether charming flavored by mirth and wit, stamped him as my most brilliant pupil. His flair for organization with his attention to detail; a physician who insisted on adequate controls in his experiments. These were the hallmarks of a budding scientist.[19]

Drew used this storage facility as the primary source material for his doctoral dissertation, an imposing, two-hundred-plus-page compilation of facts and figures about blood banking. The thesis and a half-dozen published papers, some of which were sponsored by the Blood Transfusion Betterment Association, established the young surgeon as one of the nation's most knowledgeable authorities on blood banking and blood preservation. "Intelligently employed during the first week of storage," Drew assured the public and the profession, "[banked blood] need be neither dangerous nor disappointing."[20]

When Drew took control of the Blood for Britain project, he set about remedying the problems that had plagued the early batches of plasma. "The job here is big, hard and important," he explained to his mother. "Mistakes will have international sequelae and must not be made."[21] Drew introduced stricter manufacturing criteria, including a rigid two-week-long bacterial culture quarantine, random checks to monitor for continued sterility, and routine tests of blood samples for syphilis. He improved and standardized the blood collection technique at the participating hospitals and instructed donors not to fast in the morning in order to lessen the chance of their having low blood sugar and fainting at the afternoon's bloodletting. Drew also revised record keeping and insisted that donors receive decorative cards from the Red Cross to note their blood group and provide recognition for their volunteer efforts.

Six weeks after Drew assumed charge, the cooperating hospitals were handling over two hundred donors daily and the Blood for Britain project had shipped 1,575 pints of plasma to England, which tested sterile upon arrival. In addition, Drew's program technicians were processing another 3,000 pints of collected blood and were holding 1,700 pints of plasma for a final quarantine check before release for overseas shipment. "Since Drew, who is an excellent organizer, has been in charge," wrote one of the project's trustees, "our major troubles have vanished."[22]

The Blood for Britain project, the world's first successful mass donor procurement program, provided the British with the blood that the country desperately needed. However, the program, which had been conceived as a short-term venture, continued for less than a year and officially ended in mid-January 1941. By that time, the British were self-sufficient regarding their own volunteer blood donor programs. In addition, the German army's overhyped land invasion of England never materialized and the British Royal Air Force had thwarted the Luftwaffe's campaign to gain air superiority in the Battle of Britain.

Drew prepared a final report on the Blood for Britain program that detailed its popular appeal. His account described the 14,556 total donations and how they represented the first effort in the United States to collect large amounts of blood from voluntary civilian donors for wartime use. Drew not only summarized the results of the Blood for Britain project, but he also gathered the latest research studies and clinical updates from both sides of the Atlantic. By all accounts, Drew was now an internationally acclaimed leader in blood studies as he shifted his interests toward America's wartime needs, blood supplies and the use of dried blood plasma.

*   *   *

The liquid form of plasma had been the mainstay of the Blood for Britain project for several reasons. The urgency of England's appeal favored using liquid plasma, which could be obtained speedier than dried plasma. Liquid plasma was also less expensive to manufacture than the dried type, which required specialized equipment. In addition, medical researchers at the time considered the use of dried plasma experimental when contrasted with their growing experience with the liquid form. However, over the early course of World War II, Drew and other scientists learned how to store dried plasma safely for months at a time, far longer than liquid plasma. This dried plasma could be reconstituted into a liquid form with sterile water and be easily transfused under battlefield conditions.

With the Blood for Britain project coming to an end, Drew conceived a plan for the mass production of dried plasma. He sent letters to leading blood researchers and commercial and pharmaceutical laboratories around the country to gather information about their dried-plasma research and to press for further investigations. Drew submitted his ideas to the American Red Cross, including a suggestion that the organization initiate a three-month pilot program for manufacturing dried plasma on a massive scale. Moreover, he proposed plans for a cloth packet, containing two easily opened tin cans—one containing dried plasma and another holding sterile water for reconstitution—to be available for emergency transfusions on the battlefield.

In early January 1941, as the nation's war footing intensified, the surgeons general of the army and the navy, noting the success of the Blood for Britain program, solicited the Red Cross to create a national blood donor program:

The national emergency requires that every necessary step be taken as soon as possible to provide the best medical service for the expanded armed forces. Even though the need for proper blood substitutes may not be immediate, there seems every reason to take steps now which shall provide in any contingency for an adequate supply of these substances for use in individuals suffering from hemorrhage, shock, and burns.[23]

It would be an immense undertaking, and Red Cross officials considered an experimental pilot project a necessary first step. They looked to Drew to be its medical director. Less than a month later, he was formally appointed administrator of the first American Red Cross Blood Bank and assistant manager of blood procurement for the federally sponsored National Research Council. The Council replaced the Blood Transfusion Betterment Association as the organization responsible for the technical side of the program, including the maintenance of standards.

Drew was soon sitting in a Red Cross ambulance with a crew of nurses as they hauled a trailer left over from the defunct Blood for Britain project thirty-five miles to an elementary school that served as a blood procurement center in Farmingdale, Long Island. Shortly, the Red Cross began to place mobile blood collection units (aka bloodmobiles) at department stores, government offices, industrial plants, and public schools and universities. Drew's New York–based pilot program and the technical information it gathered was pivotal for the Red Cross's soon-to-start nationwide effort to collect blood and provide the armed forces with millions of parcels of dried plasma. By the end of the hostilities, the Blood Donor Service of the American Red Cross collected and processed over 13 million blood donations gathered from across the United States.

Despite the success of Drew's pilot program, his tenure with the Red Cross was a short-lived two months; his resignation coincided with the start of one of the uglier instances of institutionalized racism in American Medicine. Drew never fully articulated the reasons he left the managerial post. Two weeks before he gave notice, he cryptically wrote to his wife: "There are some things that I will leave unfinished here which I naturally would like to finish, but I feel that the moment is propitious for pulling out."[24] Drew had recently completed the final stage of the American Board of Surgery's certification process and may have simply wanted to pursue professional goals other than those related to blood banking. Or, perhaps, it was the

Red Cross's failure to offer him the managerial position for the about-to-commence nationwide blood program that was based on his pilot program.

It remains unknown how much race factored into either the Red Cross's or Drew's decision. However, when the federal government sponsored publication of a book on the details of the Red Cross's National Blood Program, no mention was made of Drew and his New York pilot program. Admittedly, Drew left the national blood-banking scene a half year before America entered the war and the National Blood Program was not the massive organization it later became. Given that the author of the government volume explained the role of virtually every doctor who played a part in the project other than Drew, whether some degree of institutional racism factored into his resignation should be considered.

What is known is that a few months after the start of the National Blood Program the Red Cross, under pressure from the military and in an act of blatant prejudice, moved to exclude black donors. Not until several years later did the Red Cross begin to accept blood from black Americans, albeit rigidly segregating the blood supply. The black press drew sharp notice to the racist overtones of the policy and looked to Drew among others for answers. He acknowledged that under the Blood for Britain program blood was accepted and mixed from all donors, despite official claims to the contrary. "I feel that the recent ruling of the United States Army and Navy regarding the refusal of colored blood donors is an indefensible one from any point of view," declared Drew:

> As you know, there is no scientific basis for the separation of the bloods of different races except on the basis of the individual blood types or groups.[25]

Protests grew. Newspapers across the country ran front-page stories with bold-faced headlines such as "Red Cross Bans Negro Blood!"[26] and "Red Cross Rejects Negro Blood Donors."[27] In Chicago, twenty-eight-year-old Gwendolyn Brooks, five years away from becoming the first African-American to be awarded a Pulitzer Prize, wrote a poem for the literary magazine *Common Ground*:

> In a Southern city a white man said,
> Indeed, I'd rather be dead.
> Indeed, I'd rather be shot in the head

Or ridden to waste on the back of a flood
Than saved by the drop of a black man's blood.[28]

On the opposite side of the political divide, a segregationist congressman from Mississippi labeled Drew and his fellow critics as "crackpots, Communists, and parlor pinks," who were attempting to "mongrelize this Nation." He inveighed on the floor of the House against the prospect of pumping "Negro blood into the veins of our wounded white men on the various fronts." The demagogic politician implied that Drew and other African-American doctors were unpatriotic, endeavoring to destroy the blood donor service and damage the war effort. "They had better remember," he warned, "that there is still a Congress of the United States, and that Congress represents the American people and that the American people through their Congress are not going to permit such outrages against our wounded boys . . . or against our men, women, and children who are injured in local disasters."[29] The Red Cross's segregation policy on blood donations continued through the Second World War and did not end until 1950.

*　　*　　*

Drew largely ignored the continuance of perverse claims and race-baiting around blood collection. Instead, he turned his attention to other medical and surgical matters. Drew's major interest had always been surgery, but his involvement with blood banks left little time for the operating room or his favorite role, educating and training surgeons. As one of the most well-known of the nation's board-certified African-American surgeons, Drew considered it his personal mission to create a tradition in surgery for black knife bearers. Thus, part of his decision to resign from the Red Cross involved his return to Washington, DC, as chairman of the department of surgery at Howard University Medical School and chief surgeon at Freedmen's Hospital.

Drew's academic life was focused on his teaching responsibilities. "The boys whom we are now helping to train," he wrote a friend, "I believe, in time will constitute my greatest contribution to medicine."[30] During the 1940s, over half of the black American surgeons who received board certification studied under his direct supervision. Drew's skills as a surgical educator were officially recognized when he became the first African-American surgeon selected to serve as an examiner on the American Board of Surgery.

As busy as Drew was, his teaching responsibilities did not distract from his commitment to the fight for racial justice within the whole of American Medicine. He waged what has been described as a "rather bitter battle"[31] with the ACS as well as the AMA over their unwritten policies that barred black surgeons from membership. At the turn of the century—when initially faced with little likelihood of obtaining membership in the AMA, its state societies, or their well-known Sections on Surgery—African-American physicians joined together to form the National Medical Association (NMA) with its own surgical section.

During the 1940s, Drew served as chairman of the NMA's surgical section. Under the auspices of the NMA, surgical clinics were inaugurated at "Negro" hospitals that offered section members the opportunity to develop their decision-making abilities as well as technical skills under the direct supervision of prominent African-American surgeons. The NMA's surgical clinics preceded the Clinical Congress of Surgeons of North America (i.e., the forerunner to the ACS) by half a decade and were the earliest examples of formally organized "hands-on/show-me" surgical education in the nation.

The surgical clinic sites were in predominantly African-American communities in the East, Midwest, and South; hotel reservations in the face of "Jim Crow" barriers made the events logistical nightmares. Among the facilities, including the St. Joseph and Presbyterian Hospitals in Lexington, Kentucky, Lincoln Hospital in Durham, North Carolina, and Wheatley-Provident Hospital in Kansas City, Missouri, those held at the John A. Andrew Memorial Hospital in Tuskegee, Alabama, proved extremely popular and provided the most intensive course in surgery for practicing African-American surgeons through the first six decades of the twentieth century.

Drew never became a member of the AMA or a fellow of the ACS; not until 1968 did the AMA amend its founding documents to forbid racial discrimination at its local, state, and national levels. With regard to the ACS, in 1945 he applied for membership, but his application was denied. Drew was not surprised by the rejection. That year, other African-American surgeons were similarly rebuffed. "It will be very deleterious with [*sic*] the College to give any particular recognition to these men," explained one of the leaders of the ACS:

Recognition by the College is different from certification by a Board. The College fellowships work closely into the social relationship. It wouldn't be safe for the College to get mixed up in this subject. I don't think it would be a good thing.[32]

Instead, several months later Drew became a fellow of the International College of Surgeons (ICS), a rival organization that had been established by individuals who had been turned down by the ACS.

When the ACS was first founded, its leaders faced accusations of gender, racial, and religious bias. For example, Arthur Dean Bevan, who served as director of general surgery in the surgical division of the surgeon general's office in World War I, was a founder of the ACS, president of the AMA, and longtime chairman of its influential Council on Medical Education and Hospitals. A colleague described him as a "man with a driving personality; a forceful character . . . [with] disdain for personal criticism."[33] Bevan was also an outspoken anti-Semite and racist who pushed an anti-immigrant policy for the nation. In 1926, he specifically urged that action be taken against the large number of Jewish applicants to medical school, who were supposedly "over-crowding the profession":

> The physician must cultivate and acquire the judicial attitude, the judicial quality of mind, in order that he may decide properly the important questions that confront him. Above all, the physician must be a man of character. He must in his life and professional work accept a high code of ethics which controls all his actions. He must always and at all times be governed by the [AMA's] code of ethics and practice the Golden Rule. He must not commercialize his profession . . . there is one phase of this problem which must be studied carefully . . . the great number of Jewish applicants. . . . In the present over-crowded condition, no group [that is, Jews] should be permitted to enter medicine in such numbers as to crowd out of medicine the members of other groups who desire to enter.

Bevan went so far as to assure his listeners that "leaders of Jewish thought and culture . . . are making a determined effort through Jewish publications and societies to lower the great number of Jewish students who are overcrowding into medicine." Bevan's depiction of such an "effort" as representative of mainstream Jewish organizations was speculative at best.[34] What was not theoretical was the whispered belief, held by members of the Jewish medical community at large, that prior to the 1960s anti-Semitism was particularly rife in general surgery. Although Jews held responsible positions in various surgical specialties like otolaryngology, ophthalmology, and urology, no general surgeon of acknowledged Jewish heritage would assume presidency of the ACS until 1960.

Bevan's "zero-growth" suggestion was never explicitly adopted, but little doubt exists that elements of his attitude and others with the same thinking insinuated themselves into mid-twentieth-century American surgery and the makeup of organizations like the ACS. Bevan was correct that there were objectionable numbers of poorly educated individuals practicing Medicine in America, but just as serious was the grave injustice he and others championed that forced many worthwhile persons to be excluded from the surgical establishment due to their gender, race, and/or religion.

Drew believed bigotry permeated the leadership of the ACS and that the organization had become largely social in nature with less interest in academic or professional achievements. By 1950, this opinion had changed when he saw that conditions for qualified black surgeons to become Fellows had improved. Drew again began the process of applying for admission. As time passed and individuals with similar views to Bevan died, the ACS became a more egalitarian organization, and presently it is less restricted by questions of gender, race, and religion.

In 1944, the National Association for the Advancement of Colored People awarded Drew its Spingarn Medal for his work in blood plasma research. The *New York Times* described this as the "highest achievement of a Negro."[35] The award's prestige further increased Drew's public profile and he used this heightened status to advocate against all forms of racial injustice. He marched in labor parades, gave speeches at public rallies, and participated in lesser-known efforts, including attempts to end a policy of racial segregation in Washington's private hospitals. Five years later, at a meeting of the Association for the Study of Negro Life and History, Drew summarized his view about black scientists and surgeons:

> While one must grant at once that extraordinary talent, great intellectual strength and unusual opportunity are necessary to break out of this prison of the Negro problem, we believe that the Negro in the field of physical sciences has not only opened a small passageway

to the outside world, but is carving a road in many untrod areas, along which later generations will find it more easy to travel. The breaching of these walls and the laying of this road has not been, and is not easy.... But there is a team ship which extends far beyond the realms of physical science; this team must include all of us who are interested in achieving goals higher than those of merely great scientific or technological achievement. There must always be the continuing struggle to make the increasing knowledge of the world bear some fruit in increased understanding and in the production of human happiness.[36]

Sadly, Drew spent only a few years in the surgical and public limelight. In the early hours of April 1, 1950, he was driving to a medical conference in North Carolina with three colleagues when he fell asleep at the wheel. The car flipped over at more than 70 miles per hour and Drew suffered massive damage to his head and chest. Though he received prompt medical attention, his injuries were too severe for doctors to save his life.

Certain publications speciously reported that Drew, the nation's pioneer blood researcher, had died from blood loss after physicians at a racially segregated hospital refused to treat him. In truth, the white surgeons who cared for Drew were well aware of his professional reputation and worked diligently to prevent his death, including a blood transfusion. The racially charged allegations concerning Drew's death likely originated from frustrations with the widespread southern policy of hospital segregation and the denial of medical services that caused the deaths of countless black accident victims in that era.

Over time, the circumstances of Drew's death evolved into an emotional urban legend that persists today. The myth of the extraordinarily talented black surgeon, who saved countless lives through his pioneering medical research on blood and was himself refused blood due to his race when he most needed it, still resonates in the American racial narrative. In death, Drew continues to be venerated: in addition to the many schools and medical facilities named after him, including the Charles R. Drew University of Medicine and Science in Los Angeles, in 1976 the National Park Service designated the Charles Richard Drew House in Arlington, Virginia, where Drew lived with his parents from the age of fifteen years until his marriage in 1939, as a National Historic Landmark. In 1981, the United States Postal Service issued a stamp in its Great American Series to honor his memory, and in 2010, the United States Navy launched the USNS *Charles Drew*, a Lewis and Clark class dry cargo ship.

* * *

The explosion of atomic devices over Hiroshima and Nagasaki ended World War II. For surgeons, the detonations showed how a concatenation of basic and applied sciences could yield technologic breakthroughs never before thought possible. New directions were about to appear that brought surgical therapies far beyond the simple manual craft of just a few decades before. From a logistical and therapeutic standpoint, America's surgeons had embraced the mantle of world surgical leadership. Everything was in place, from the acceptance of surgery as a true science, through the blossoming of specialization, to the establishment of strict guidelines regarding surgical education and training. The postwar era would showcase American surgical ingenuity and its immensity while setting the stage for changes in the socioeconomic structure of surgery.

17.

THE CENTER OF THINGS

Of all the ailments which may blow out life's little candle,
heart disease is the chief.

William Boyd, *Pathology for Surgeons*, 1925

The surgeons of the future will not tolerate the divorce of the hand
from the brain, and the surgery of the future will not again be merely
a handicraft. . . . In the surgery of the future, the individualist will be
left by the roadside, for after all surgery is part of that broader field of
experimental pathology to which all the medical sciences belong.

Isidor S. Ravdin, *Annals of Surgery*, 1948

The years of economic expansion following World War II had a dramatic impact on the scale of surgery in America. During the 1950s and 1960s, the number of individuals in the health care workforce increased from 1.2 to 3.9 million. The nation's expenditures on Medicine grew from $13 billion to $72 billion (approximately $530 billion in 2022). In 1963, Congress passed the Health Professions Educational Assistance Act, which for the first time provided unrestricted federal funds for the construction, equipping, and renovation of America's medical schools. In 1950, 7,042 individuals matriculated in first-year classes. By 1975, 14,763 freshmen students were beginning their medical education. With graduation rates approaching 100 percent, the American public anticipated a steep rise in the aggregate of the nation's surgeons. It was as if health care had suddenly become big business with the delivery of medical and surgical treatments comprising the country's largest growth industry.

Society afforded surgical science unprecedented recognition as a prized national asset. Many surgeons, who were baptized during the war with the performance of technically complex surgical operations, became leaders in the construction and improvement of hospitals, multispecialty clinics, and surgical facilities in their hometowns. Hospitals—once considered a depressing final stop before the funeral home—became gleaming citadels of health care with astonishing surgical equipment, flashing lights, stainless steel, tempered glass, and wide corridors. These facilities contained the most recent scientific and technologic advancements while the complexes' presence and size embodied the strength of the socioeconomic boom.

Patients welcomed new surgical treatments once thought possible only as science fiction. Large city and community hospitals established surgical residency programs, finding it relatively easy to attract residents. In 1940, the vast majority of physicians in active clinical practice (77 percent) classified themselves as either general practitioners or part-time specialists. Ten years later, the 23 percent of doctors reporting themselves as full-time specialists had increased to 37 percent. By 1960, the number had grown to 55 percent, and a decade and a half later it was nearly 80 percent of American physicians. The trend toward specialization was so profound that the possible extinction of the old-fashioned general practitioner seemed inevitable.

This change in demographics was especially dramatic for the surgical specialties. In 1930, only 10 percent of American Medical professionals considered themselves full-time practitioners of either general surgery or one of the other surgical specialties. Thirty years later the proportion had risen to 26 percent, and by 1975 slightly more than one-third of doctors were full-time practitioners of surgery—this represented over one hundred thousand individuals. In 1970, of the forty-seven thousand total residency positions offered, seventeen thousand were in surgery. The emergence of surgical programs as the most sought after of residencies reflected the growing economic and social clout of the nation's knife bearers. Surgeons commanded the highest salaries (in 1975, the average heart surgeon was earning $200,000 to $300,000 per year) and the public was increasingly enamored with the drama and secrets of the operating room.

Progress in Medicine became part of the nation's cultural and social fabric as the media helped shape American expectations about surgery and its practitioners. In 1929, Lloyd C. Douglas's best-selling novel *Magnificent Obsession*—later adapted as a radio play, released as a film in 1935 starring Irene Dunne and Robert Taylor, and remade in 1954 starring Jane Wyman and Rock Hudson—revealed a main character whose life's tale involved redemption as he became a neurosurgeon. Five years after *Magnificent Obsession* was published, *Men in White*, a play about surgeons in a large city hospital, was awarded the 1934 Pulitzer Prize for Drama; it was soon adapted into a namesake film starring Myrna Loy and Clark Gable. In 1959, the mystery movie *Suddenly, Last Summer*, based on a play by Tennessee Williams and starring Katharine Hepburn, Elizabeth Taylor, and Montgomery Clift, told the story of a brain surgeon who is offered a million dollars for his clinic if he performs a lobotomy on a troubled young woman.

Beginning in the mid-1950s, television brought surgery to the fore of national consciousness. *Medic* aired in 1954 and was the first doctor drama to focus attention on different types of surgical procedures. In November 1960, Rod Serling's series *The Twilight Zone* contained a chilling episode, "Eye of the Beholder," in which a dictatorial state compelled its citizens to undergo plastic surgical procedures to achieve an acceptable facial appearance. Serling exploited the growing number of cosmetic surgical procedures as the lens through which the American public considered questions of personal attractiveness. The following year, tens of millions of Americans tuned into evening prime time as Ben Casey, an idealistic chief resident in neurosurgery, or Dr. Kildare, an intern on his way to becoming a surgeon, worked in fictional large metropolitan institutions, while learning the fundamentals of their profession. From 1969 to 1973, *The Bold Ones: The New Doctors* focused on the life of a successful neurosurgeon, played by E. G. Marshall, who enlisted two young surgeons to help manage his exclusive private clinic. In addition to the evening prime-time shows, there were several daytime soap operas set in hospitals. *General Hospital* premiered on April 1, 1963, and remains one of the longest-running TV shows in America. On the same day, *The Doctors*, a rival medical-themed soap opera, also debuted and would have over five thousand episodes produced. The mainstream programs portrayed surgeons as heroes of American Medicine while the story lines confirmed the links between modern science and sophisticated surgery. Patients were shown as active and knowledgeable consumers who searched for the best surgical service for their money. Viewers grew conversant with ERs, ethical dilemmas, operating theaters, surgical intensive care units, and startlingly new forms of surgical therapy.

Television further piqued the public's fascination with live broadcasts of surgical operations. These programs offered compelling visual images distinct from those created by televised melodramas, thereby promoting in real time the notion of America's scientific superiority and surgical authority. In June 1952, surgeons in Chicago performed the first operation televised live coast-to-coast to a potential audience of 30 million Americans. "Major Operation to Save a Life Put on Network TV for First Time," read the next morning's front-page headline in the *New York Times.*[1] While the entire procedure (excision of a portion of the stomach and duodenum to treat a bleeding ulcer) lasted over three hours, the public saw an eight-minute excerpt.

Viewers observed anesthesiologists, nurses, and surgeons dressed in white caps, gowns, and masks. They watched the deftness of a surgeon's gloved fingers and were privy to the admonishments of his assistants: "Don't jiggle the instruments, boys; keep them steady."[2] The sights of gleaming metal retractors holding back blood vessels and other tissues as well as the sterile cloth drying pads (increasingly saturated with blood) were particularly vivid. In truth, only those with a knowledge of abdominal anatomy and surgery had an inkling of the technical aspects of what transpired, but the live broadcast was a defining moment in the history of surgery in America. The *Times* reporter said the event "proved fascinating"[3] and a critic for the weekly entertainment publication *Variety* termed it a "blue ribbon winner." "This TV venture into the heretofore hush-hush world of [surgery]," wrote the reviewer, "literally oozed with human drama and human interest . . . the slicing . . . the surgery was, of course, the topper."[4]

The media coverage of surgery became particularly intense following President Dwight Eisenhower's operation for intestinal obstruction. It was a risky situation, involving thorny surgical decisions made difficult by the fact that the president had suffered a severe heart attack only nine months previously. The president endured crampy abdominal pains for over twenty-four hours when X-rays revealed an unrelenting obstruction of his small intestine secondary to regional enteritis (aka Crohn's disease). In the early morning of June 9, 1956, a team of surgeons conducted an exploratory operation that resulted in a bypass of the diseased section of bowel.

What made this event so unique was that a sitting president underwent an abdominal operation for the first time in the annals of American surgery. The entire saga and safe outcome were dramatically reported by the press corps. "Doctors Say President Can Run," blared the banner headline in the *New York Times*, "Condition 'Most Satisfactory'; Hospital Stay Is Put at 15 Days."[5] In the midst of all the tumult, the chief surgeon reigned supreme as he held a postoperative news conference and stood at a blackboard with a sketched outline of the intestinal tract and diagrams of the procedure. "At the end, as at the start," wrote a reporter in a compliment to the world of surgery at large, "[the surgeon] appeared to be the coolest and perhaps the calmest person in the room, which had been heated to oven-like temperatures by klieg lights and the presence of about seventy reporters and photographers."[6]

Less than a decade later, in October 1965, President Lyndon Johnson underwent an elective removal of his gallbladder and a kidney stone. The surgical procedure was considered so routine that the event barely caused a ripple in the daily life of the nation. "The President was helped to his feet to take a few steps in his hospital room a few hours after the operation," wrote a reporter. "Such exercise is common practice under modern surgical methods."[7] Several days following his operation, Johnson, in an act of surgical machismo, pulled up his polo shirt and sports jacket to proudly display a six-inch incision to a group of surprised news photographers. "What we had here, was two operations for the price of one," explained the president as he pointed to his abdomen. "[One surgeon] went in there and messed around a couple of hours, then he stood aside and let the other fellow in. There are footprints everywhere that hand went, and I can still feel them."[8]

With hundreds of magazines and newspapers carrying a picture of the President of the United States exhibiting his newly acquired scar, any lingering questions from the public concerning the relative risks and social acceptability of surgical operations were quelled. It also happened that Johnson needed every public relations victory he could muster to support his policies about the Vietnam War. The calculating display of his surgical wound had a subliminal message that he, too, was wounded by the war, understood pain, and was strong enough to survive. It was a moment when the outcome of a surgical operation became indivisible from the world of politics.

* * *

By 1950, the nation's surgeons had successfully operated on every bone, ligament, muscle, organ, and tissue of the human corpus but for the heart. This exception was disconcerting because more Americans were dying from heart disease than any other medical ailment—in 1940, it accounted for 27 percent of American deaths; by 1953, the figure had increased to 39 percent. Doctors desperately tried to resolve the situation and sought innovative techniques to treat cardiac conditions, but thoughts of surgery on the heart elicited deep-seated fears from the public and trepidation on the part of the profession. At the turn of the century, one of England's most renowned surgeons had synopsized the long-standing caution with words that echoed through much of the twentieth century: "Surgery of the heart has probably reached the limits set by Nature to all surgery: no new method, and no new discovery, can overcome the natural difficulties that attend an [operation] on the heart."[9]

Fascination with the heart goes far beyond clinical Medicine. From a perspective of art, culture, economics, literature, music, philosophy, and religion, the heart has represented the home of the soul, the seat of one's personal identity, even the cradle of the spirit of life itself. Imbued with goodness and described with noble sentiments, altruism, devoutness, empathy, and mercy among them, this muscular organ was also believed to contain more than humble emotions. For example, aptitude and insight are capacities over which the heart is said to compete with the brain. To memorize something perfectly, so that it can be performed, recited, or written without thinking, is to "learn by heart."

The explanation that credits the ability of the heart, instead of the brain, to remember things stretches back to the ancient Greeks, who believed the heart was the home of everyday emotions along with intelligence and memory. The Greeks also understood that the heart pulsed and bled when wounded. In referring to the death of a Trojan soldier who was injured in the chest, Homer wrote in the *Iliad*:

> He fell; the spear-point quivering in his heart,
> Which with convulsive throbbings shook the shaft.[10]

Hippocrates taught that trauma to the heart was usually fatal while his countryman Aristotle declared the heart was so essential to life it could never suffer a disease. Such thinking lasted for over two millennia, having been bolstered during the Renaissance when a renowned surgeon/anatomist concurred that if the heart was wounded it could never heal because it was always in motion and impossible to repair. The hands-off policy on the supposedly untouchable heart remained through the end of the nineteenth century.

Starting in the 1890s, a clearer understanding of injuries to the heart along with the occasional recovery—bolstered by the discoveries of anesthesia and antisepsis—emboldened surgeons. In 1891, a scalpel wielder at the St. Louis City Hospital operated on an individual who was stabbed in the chest with a knife that nicked his pericardium, the sac of tissue that supports and surrounds the heart and provides lubrication as the organ beats. In a surgical first, the surgeon successfully sutured the small laceration, but as he explained, "I had no precedent to guide me, no authority to uphold me, in attempting to sew up this wound over a heart that was beating at the rate of 140 per minute. . . . Medical literature seems to be particularly barren upon this particular form of injury."[11]

Less than two years later, Daniel Hale Williams, a founder of Provident Hospital in Chicago, the first hospital in the United States opened by African-Americans, completed a repair of a one-and-one-quarter-inch laceration of the pericardium. Williams incorrectly claimed that "this case is the first successful or unsuccessful case of suture of the pericardium that has ever been recorded."[12] He was unaware of the prior operation in St. Louis. However, because Williams's case was published in a respected "national" medical journal, contrasted with a "regional" periodical, he received considerable publicity and personal recognition. Shortly, he was named surgeon-in-chief at Freedmen's Hospital in Washington, DC, and, in 1895, the first vice-president of the newly organized NMA.

Williams, a graduate of the Chicago Medical College (presently the Northwestern University Feinberg School of Medicine), was a complex personality who crafted Freedmen's Hospital into an important source of training for African-American surgeons. In the late 1890s, he was audacious enough to open the operating theater at the hospital to the general public to demonstrate the technical skills of black surgeons. In 1913, when the ACS was founded, he was named a charter fellow, and he remained the only black member until the remonstrations of Charles Drew and others in the 1940s.

The milestone heart operations in Chicago and St. Louis should be considered in the surgical context of the time and the circumstances that made success unlikely. The patients were in pitiful conditions, had lost a large amount of blood, verged on shock, and were in poorly equipped hospitals. Blood transfusions were not available, endotracheal anesthesia had not been invented, and antisepsis was far from perfect. Still, Williams, sans cap, gloves, gown, and mask, emerged triumphant. "To this absence of infection," he wrote, "is probably attributed the successful progress and termination of the case."[13]

Other operations for wounds of the heart, including actual perforations of the organ's chambers, were attempted but with limited success. Even during World War I with the large number of cardiac injuries, surgeons shied away from operating on the body's center. Many soldiers had fragments of shrapnel left behind in their chests, some with splinters of metal lodged in their hearts. Even if a soldier might die without surgery, few surgeons were willing to take the risk.

In the 1920s, several intrepid surgeons in Boston began to blindly insert scalpels into beating hearts, trying to cut through calcified and scarred valves. The doctors attempted to open narrowed apertures and relieve patients of deadly shortness of breath from overtaxed hearts. The results of these early cases were grim: multiple attempts and only one short-term survivor. Though the consequences were serious and surgical failure generally meant death, surgeons continued to develop techniques to deal with hearts and their diseases. But in every instance, surgeons struggled with two ever-present and overwhelming physiological problems: large quantities of blood flowing through the operative area and the unremitting to-and-fro movement of a beating heart.

Surgeons tackled the problem of blood flow in the most dramatic of ways: they tied off all the blood vessels feeding the heart. This provided the scalpel wielder a window of three to four minutes to open the organ, complete whatever repair needed to be done, sew the tissues back together, and undo the tied vessels before the lack of blood permanently damaged the patient's brain. It was surgery ruled by a stopwatch: nerve-wracking and suitable for only a small number of patients (or surgeons for that matter). Surgeons worked to extend the available window of time but with limited success. They discovered that cooling a patient's body temperature down to about 85°—normal temperature is 98°—could provide several additional minutes. This reduction in temperature decreased the oxygen demands of the heart and brain and lessened the possibility of stroke. America's operating rooms soon contained anesthetized heart patients immersed in giant ice-filled bathtubs as surgeons went about their business at a more measured pace.

Notwithstanding the rare achievements, the clinical reality was that the various fields of surgery had grown largely based on the notion of extirpation. If an organ failed or an extremity was injured beyond salvage, then it was unceremoniously removed. However, the future of cardiac surgery was unlike that of the other surgical specialties; its progress required that forms of reparative treatment be available. Since the heart was little more than a sophisticated mechanical device with a muscle power source and one-way valves, its breakdowns and injuries needed repair—excision was not an option.

* * *

Dwight Harken could not understand why other surgeons refused to operate on injuries to the heart, especially when bullets and shrapnel were lodged inside. The issue became especially urgent following the Allies' D-day landing on the beaches of Normandy as planes and ships repatriated growing numbers of severely wounded soldiers back to England. In the rolling Cotswold Hills, the thirty-four-year-old Harken, a lieutenant colonel in the Medical Corps of the Army of the United States and head of the thoracic surgical team at the 160th General Army Hospital in Stowell Park, had petitioned his supervisors for permission to perform heart operations should the need arise. After weeks of refusal and mounting numbers of casualties, Harken received the go-ahead.

Few of his peers would argue that Harken was not ambitious, assertive, bold, and confident. With flaming red hair, matched by a hair-trigger temper, he shattered the surgical myth of the heart as an organ so intricate and vital that it was sacrosanct from surgical intervention. "We discovered," said Harken, "that the heart wasn't such a mysterious and untouchable thing after all."[14] He was born in Osceola, Iowa, where his father, the local general practitioner, visited his patients on horseback and conducted kitchen-table surgery. Harken went to Harvard College and Medical School and completed his surgical education and training at Bellevue Hospital in New York City. He pursued further studies in London, where he worked with several renowned thoracic surgeons and devised surgical approaches to treat heart infections.

At the 160th General Army Hospital, Harken became known for removing bullets and shrapnel from the hearts of over 130 wounded soldiers without a single fatality. Admittedly, for Harken and his patients, they now had science and technology on their side. Penicillin was available, endotracheal anesthesia had improved, transfusions of plasma and whole blood were accessible, antisepsis was of better quality, and X-rays, including the use of newly invented moving X-ray images (aka fluoroscopy), were present. Day after day and night after night, Harken studied where the bullets and shrapnel were located and how to safely reach them. Thoracic cavities were opened, torrents of blood escaped, heart lacerations were closed, and lungs reflated, all before blood pressure dropped and the patient died. Harken repeated this procedure over and over, each time presenting the recovered soldier with the removed bullets and metal fragments.

Harken's feats required audacity mixed with composure and courage. News of the remarkable outcomes spread and celebrities visited Harken to bask in his success. Generals, politicians, royalty, and even the legendary Glenn Miller and his band dropped in. Reporters referred to Harken as the "generalissimo" and composed striking headlines: "13 GI's Still Alive With 'Fatal' Hurts: U.S. Corps in England has 100% Record in Saving Hopeless Heart-Wound Cases."[15] Harken accomplished more than simply removing pieces of inanimate metal. He demonstrated that it was possible to cut into the "untouchable" beating heart without the patient dying. "Unquestionably, the surgical experience of this war will broaden our knowledge of this field," wrote Harken, "and point out important technical aids in the surgical management of individual cases."[16]

Building on his war-related experiences, Harken returned to Boston and was named chief of thoracic surgery at the Peter Bent Brigham Hospital. By the late 1940s, Harken moved beyond the retrieval of foreign bodies and established surgical protocols to operate on cardiac valves. He extended his surgical reach by rigging his index finger with a small knife to operate on patients suffering from mitral stenosis. This disease affects the mitral valve, which controls the flow of blood between the two chambers on the left side of the heart. Mitral valve disease is commonly the result of rheumatic fever, an inflammatory condition that develops when strep throat or scarlet fever is not properly treated with antibiotics. Once the flaps of the mitral valve stiffen or even fuse together, the opening between the left atrium and ventricle is narrowed and blood flow to the body is reduced. Sufferers from mitral stenosis experience a myriad of problems associated with a weakened heart, including fatigue, an irregular heartbeat, poor circulation, shortness of breath, and a premature death.

Having shown that surgery on the heart was possible and safe, Harken's technique was exquisitely simple. An incision was made between the ribs, a small opening was created in the wall of the heart, a finger with an attached tiny knife was inserted, and the valve was freed. No surgeon could visualize the area he or she was operating on; everything was conducted by touch and pressure. Not only were surgeons blindly groping around inside the heart; they also still worked against a ticking clock—four minutes to be precise.

Heart surgeons could make diagnoses and temporarily ease symptoms, but they could not permanently solve cardiac defects without some method to stop a beating heart and allow themselves sufficient time to repair the organ's problem. To attempt anything more ambitious, surgeons needed to see what they were doing and, above all, they needed more time. The solution to the dilemma of a beating heart became the cardiac surgeon's holy grail.

*　　*　　*

John Heysham Gibbon Jr.—his friends called him Jack—came from a long line of physicians, stretching from his father, a professor of surgery at Jefferson Medical College in Philadelphia (presently the Sidney Kimmel Medical College—Thomas Jefferson University), to his great-great-grandfather, a general practitioner with a medical degree from the University of Edinburgh. Gibbon was an intellectual, an independent thinker who considered self-reliance among the most important of character traits. Some colleagues found him self-centered— he was notoriously moody, shy, and stubborn—and labeled him a self-absorbed egoist. Gibbon also displayed an innate persistence that was evident as a youngster. He could sit for hours playing chess with his father or reading by himself and barely move when his mother served a meal. These peculiarities provided Gibbon the demeanor necessary to spend a lifetime attempting to construct an artificial heart-lung machine.

As a sixteen-year-old Gibbon matriculated at Princeton University, and four years later he entered Jefferson, from which he graduated in 1927. Gibbon completed an internship at Pennsylvania Hospital followed by a fellowship in surgery at Harvard's Massachusetts General Hospital. In Boston, a clinical event occurred that proved crucial to his future calling. Gibbon was assigned to care for a female patient who had suffered major heart and lung damage following the removal of her gallbladder. Her surgeons were stymied because they were unable to safely operate on her rapidly beating heart. One night, when Gibbon was recording her blood pressure, pulse, and respiratory rate, she worsened and died.

This incident and watching the patient struggle for life troubled Gibbon. He imagined that surgeons could have saved the patient if they had a device to relieve the work of the heart during an operation. "The thought naturally occurred to me," recalled Gibbon, "that the patient's life might be saved if some of the blue blood in her veins could be continuously withdrawn into an extracorporeal [outside] blood circuit, exposed to an atmosphere of oxygen, and then returned to the patient by way of a systemic artery."[17] It was an ingenious idea that would allow a surgeon time to cut into a heart emptied of blood. Thus, the scalpel wielder could see what needed to be accomplished, instead of depending on touch. The concept of performing cardiac surgery in a bloodless field was a magnificent proposal. It seemed simple enough: all that was needed was a system of pumps, a method to oxygenate the blood, and a supply of blood adequate to maintain flow at the necessary rate. Gibbon's idea was also absolutely preposterous given the state of science and Medicine in 1931.

A brief review of how the heart functions will clarify what Gibbon's machine needed to accomplish. The heart is actually two distinct muscular organs, each lying on opposite sides of a shared wall or septum. Both sides have an upper chamber, or atrium, that receives blood, and a lower chamber, or ventricle, that pumps it out. The two separate pumps work in a coordinated fashion that produces the well-known *lub-dub lub-dub* sounds of a normal heartbeat. The right side of the heart receives "used" blood from the body and then propels it to the lungs, which remove carbon dioxide and replenish oxygen. From the lungs, the rejuvenated blood heads for the heart's left side, where it is gathered and then pushed out to nourish the body's tissues. Because the heart's left side has to work much harder to accomplish its mission, the pressure within its chambers is markedly higher than that of those on the opposite side. Whatever apparatus Gibbon devised, it needed to temporarily replace this entire process mechanically.

He began his quest to engineer his fantastical device independently—his wife was his research assistant and muse—and with no outside financial support. "The Federal Government," he later remarked, "was not then pouring out hundreds of millions of dollars to doctors to perform research. . . . I bought an air pump in a second-hand shop down in East Boston for a few dollars."[18] Gibbon made his initial valves out of solid rubber corks and built the circuitry for blood flow from rubber and glass tubing pushed together (plastic was unavailable). When he believed his rudimentary prototype functioned properly, Gibbon started to perform research trials on animals. He and his wife walked the city streets at night with bait and nets hunting for stray alley cats. By 1940, Gibbon had refined his makeshift device into an apparatus that could bypass the heart and lungs of a cat for twenty-five minutes, with no ill effects and no damage to the animal's nervous system.

World War II interrupted Gibbon's research and clinical studies. As a reserve officer in the Medical Corps, he was among the earliest of surgeons to enter active service. Gibbon shipped out in January 1942 and the following year was made chief of surgery at a military hospital in New Caledonia, the French-controlled, Pacific archipelago located near the about-to-be-famous Guadalcanal battlefield. He was stationed there for three years until a back injury brought about reassignment to a military hospital in Illinois. Following Gibbon's discharge in 1946, he became a professor of surgery at his alma mater in Philadelphia (ten years later, he was named chief of surgery), where he resumed research on a heart-lung machine. After numerous failed attempts at resolving how to adequately oxygenate the large amounts of blood that would necessarily flow outside the body, Gibbon decided he needed "some good engineering advice."[19]

A student at the medical school, who previously worked with engineers associated with the International Business Machines Corporation (IBM), put Gibbon in contact with their director of research. In turn, the director introduced Gibbon to Thomas J. Watson Sr., one of the country's leading industrialists, who was the company's president. Watson immediately supported Gibbon's endeavor and concluded their initial meeting at IBM's headquarters in New York City with, "You name the place and time and I will have engineers there to discuss the matter with you."[20] Subsequently, IBM not only provided Gibbon engineering assistance but also assumed a large part of the cost of constructing the heart-lung apparatus.

Though Watson ardently supported the effort to develop an artificial replacement for the human heart and lungs, he strongly opposed medical research using animals and refused to provide funds for animal experimentation. This proved a conundrum to Gibbon, who lacked sufficient resources to pay for animal-based clinical trials. Then, in 1949, Gibbon received a grant from the federal government for almost $30,000, nearly all of it for animal research.

With the assistance of Watson's engineers and the federal money, Gibbon improved his device, making it more automatic and versatile. He experimented with metal screens, perforated steel plates, and plastic and wire mesh to enhance the transfer of oxygen to blood. The new machine was larger than previous ones, had more elaborate control designs, and was filled with a myriad of blood pumps, electrical motors and switches, electromagnets, revolving cylinders, and water baths. Gibbon enclosed the baby-grand-sized works in an air-conditioned and temperature-regulated metal and glass container.

The entire contraption resembled a Rube Goldberg–like invention. The machine caused bleeding problems, damaged blood cells, and was still not putting enough fresh oxygen into the red blood cells that flowed through a mechanical bypass, but his colleagues praised it and the media started to pay attention. In late September 1949, *Time* informed its readers how Gibbon's mechanical device had taken over the heart and lung functions of dogs for up to forty-six minutes. The reporter remarked that Gibbon's colleagues believed his work on a mechanical heart would "open 'the last field of surgery."[21] "Come on, Jack," his friends encouraged him, knowing of the two decades of time invested in his invention. "When are you going to stop working on dogs and start working on man?"[22]

Less than four years later and after further animal experimentation, Gibbon concluded that his heart-lung machine was safe for humans. Around this time, Cecilia Bavolek, a college freshman with a worsening heart murmur, was admitted to Jefferson's hospital. Doctors diagnosed her condition as an anomalous hole in the shared wall between her heart's two upper chambers. Each minute, several pints of the oxygenated blood returning from her lungs to her heart's left atrium leaked back through the hole and into the right atrium (due to the pressure gradient between the atria) instead of being normally distributed throughout her body. Bavolek's heart was working tirelessly in an effort to compensate for its own endless cycle of inefficiency. She had been hospitalized multiple times in the prior six months for severe shortness of breath, fatigue, and palpitations—symptoms of congestive heart failure. It was just a matter of months before the eighteen-year-old would succumb to a heart attack.

Gibbon explained the situation to Bavolek and her mother. He told them of his research on a heart-lung machine and how this apparatus could be the key to Bavolek leading a normal life. They agreed that experimental surgery with the heart-lung machine was the only medical option. On the morning of May 6, 1953, Gibbon and three assistant surgeons laid bare Bavolek's heart. They opened the large veins carrying blood to her heart's right side and slipped in plastic tubes that drained Bavolek's life source away to the heart-lung machine. Inside the device, one pump drew in the blood and a second speeded it through the oxygenation chamber. Electronic controls maintained Bavolek's vital functions, from the blood's flow rate to the oxygen added and carbon dioxide taken away. A third pump sent the refreshed blood back into an artery above the left side of Bavolek's heart where it was distributed to her body.

Operations on the heart had always been a bloody affair, but when Gibbon lifted up Bavolek's heart and opened it with a scalpel he had a view unlike anyone before. He scrutinized a living but bloodless heart and plainly saw its internal architecture, including the abnormal half-dollar-sized opening between the atria. He stitched the hole shut. "It went very quickly and easily," explained Gibbon in his operative note, "giving a secure closure."[23] The operation lasted forty-five minutes. For twenty-six minutes, Gibbon's machine served as Bavolek's heart and lungs. She awoke without difficulty and showed no signs of brain damage or harm to any of her vital structures. Bavolek was home within two weeks and enjoyed a healthy life thereafter. Thus, for the first time in history, man's ingenuity had successfully substituted for the heart and lungs given him by nature.

The first successful open-heart operation in the world involving a heart-lung machine was a momentous surgical triumph and stands as one of the landmarks of American surgical achievements. The self-effacing and intensely private Gibbon insisted that the operation receive no publicity and refused to pose for a photograph with his device. The world had other ideas. Newspapers and magazines carried every last detail of the procedure, running headlines like: "Heart's Job Done by New Apparatus; Surgeons Close Hole in Empty Organ While Circulation Is Maintained Mechanically."[24] *Time* termed it a "historic operation . . . nothing has been dearer to the surgeon's heart."[25] A newspaper editor wrote: "Surgical history was made the other day in Philadelphia. The accomplishment indicates what we may expect in the future."[26] Gibbon subsequently received numerous awards including the nation's highest honor in Medicine, the Lasker Award, in 1968, and was nominated three times but never won the Nobel Prize.

Gibbon's later years were spent in early retirement at his farm in rural Pennsylvania. His invention of the heart-lung machine made difficult operations, such as valve replacement, easier and led to the development of new procedures, including heart bypass for blocked coronary arteries. "I suppose," reminisced Gibbon, "that I had opened some kind of Pandora's box."[27] Gibbon's tinge of remorse/sarcasm had some responsibility in what was an ironic end to his life. In the early 1970s, he developed signs of cardiac difficulties: a heart attack followed by symptoms of angina. Gibbon knew what treatment was needed: an X-ray of his coronary arteries probably followed by a bypass operation using a heart-lung machine. He was stubborn regarding any form of surgical therapy and, in 1973, died of a massive heart attack while playing tennis.

Gibbon's development of the heart-lung apparatus is a high point in the surgical family of remarkable achievements. His invention meant that heart surgery, a vision in 1950, became practical by 1955 and routine by 1960. In turn, there were few American surgeons as well known as the pioneers of open-heart surgery. Their surnames, Cooley, DeBakey, Gibbon, and Harken, became part of everyday household conversations. Cardiac surgeons were courted by the media and their faces were found on the front pages of the nation's magazines and newspapers.

In 1957, *Time* ran a lengthy cover story titled "Surgery's New Frontier." In the article, the reporter described how the innovators in heart surgery pushed "far beyond what was considered possible only five years ago . . . nothing is impossible in surgery."[28] The triumphs of cardiac surgery were soon seen by millions of TV viewers. Within a year, a special called *Heart Surgery* was broadcast from the New York University Bellevue Hospital, where a three-year-old child underwent correction of a congenital anomaly. A reviewer called this first live transmission of a heart operation along with the use of a heart-lung machine one of "epic proportions in the history of tv . . . this was the scalpel and lancet at their true best."[29] Six weeks later, a live open-heart operation was televised to an estimated 1.25 million viewers in the San Francisco area. There was an unprecedented level of public attention and the TV station was inundated with almost sixty thousand sympathetic queries about the condition of the eight-year-old patient. The congressman from the district even introduced a resolution into the *Congressional Record* praising the broadcast: "Whereas the local and national press did bring this program to the attention of the bay area, the State, and the Nation: Be it therefore *Resolved*, That the Open Heart Surgery program represented the optimum use of the television medium for the public interest, information, and education."[30]

*   *   *

The field of cardiac surgery, with its death-defying operations and uncompromising refinement, served as an exemplar for much of surgical culture in the late twentieth century. The dangers of slicing open a person's body to remedy a deadly heart disorder, offset by the rewards of operative successes, dramatically showcased surgery's promise. No area of cardiovascular disease validated this potential as did the surgical treatment of diseased coronary arteries. The operation's signature scar was visible on those who wore bathing suits, open shirts, or low-necked outfits; it stretched the length of their breastbones.

Among the various procedures performed by cardiac surgeons, coronary artery bypass surgery stands supreme in its ubiquity. Formally known as coronary artery bypass graft (CABG, pronounced "cabbage") surgery, and colloquially heart bypass or bypass surgery, the operation restored blood flow to a narrowed or obstructed coronary artery. The coronary arteries are the arterial blood vessels that wrap around the heart and provide a continuous supply of oxygenated blood to its muscle. Narrowing or obstruction of the arteries is caused by a process known as atherosclerosis or arteriosclerosis. This occurs when plaques (aka atheromas) build up over time in the walls of the arteries. These plaques or atheromas consist of microscopic pieces of cellular debris, including calcium, cholesterol, and fibrous tissue, which create an area of inflammation on a blood vessel's inner wall. As an atheroma matures, it turns craggy and rigid and seeks out the company of neighboring atheromas. The result is a network of crusty, unyielding atheromatous plaques that line and constrict the inner contours of an artery, similar to the rust and mineral deposits that clog old water pipes. It is a degenerative condition, and the collective process of atheroma development, plaque formation, plaque coalescence, and artery deterioration is called atherosclerosis.

Atherosclerosis has many catalysts: cigarette smoking, diabetes, a fast-food diet, high blood pressure, lack of exercise, and obesity. When these elements combine with further circumstances, including advanced age, maleness, and a genetic predisposition, atherosclerosis quickly becomes an efficient killing machine. The tissue that surrounds the narrowed blood vessel gasps for life-preserving oxygen in a condition known as ischemia. Ischemic attacks are harbingers of impending medical disasters and serve as one of the body's most dependable early-warning systems.

When the affected arteriosclerotic artery supplies the heart, the ischemic attack is termed "angina" and is accompanied by chest pain, shortness of breath, and sweating. In a catastrophic scenario, the cardiac tissue dies and the victim suffers a myocardial infarction, or heart attack, which can be fatal. For almost a century, atherosclerotic heart disease has been the nation's most proficient medical killer. Over 650,000 Americans die of the condition yearly, and 20 million individuals live with a history of heart attack or symptoms of angina. Not only is atherosclerosis the leading cause of death in the United States, but its treatment consumes the largest expenditure of any single class of diseases—almost $400 billion annually.

One way to treat blocked or narrowed arteries is to bypass or graft the blocked portion of the coronary artery with a piece of a healthy blood vessel from elsewhere in the body. Blood vessels/grafts used for the bypass procedure are commonly sections of a vein taken from a patient's leg or an artery in his or her chest. The plumbing involved and the rerouting of blood vessels is quite simple. Heart surgeons attach one end of the graft above the blockage and the other end below the blockage. Oxygenated blood bypasses the blockage by circulating through the new graft to reach the heart muscle. The blocked vessel itself is not tied off or removed.

The ability to surgically restore blood flow to diseased coronary arteries, supported by the development of coronary catherization, was a long-awaited solution for patients with ischemic heart disease. In 1929, Werner Forssmann, a German medical student, inserted a plastic catheter into a vein in his arm, safely threaded it to the right side of his heart, and had an X-ray taken. This feat of self-experimentation and the beginning of cardiac catherization brought Forssmann—he went on to become a urologic surgeon—the 1956 Nobel Prize in Physiology or Medicine. Continued advances in coronary artery catherization led to its present-day use as both a diagnostic tool (i.e., taking X-rays of radio-opaque dye injected through a catheter to search for diseased coronary arteries is called coronary angiography) and a therapeutic device (i.e., placement of a stent through a catheter to open up a blocked or narrowed coronary artery is termed "percutaneous coronary intervention [PCI]").

In the late 1960s, prior to the development of PCI, the option of surgical revascularization of diseased coronary arteries was quickly adopted. The annual number of CABG procedures in America increased rapidly, to almost 40,000 in 1974, and exceeded 110,000 by 1979. In 1986, a report on the sizeable and sustained increase in cardiovascular operations pointed out that "these changes have occurred entirely because of coronary artery bypasses."[31] By the mid-1980s, more than a million Americans had undergone a heart bypass operation. The growth continued through the 1990s with CABG operations becoming routine and ranking among the country's most frequent surgical operations, topping out at almost 350,000 per year.

No other surgical procedure had undergone such an astronomical percentage rise—the closest comparisons were cataract extractions and hip replacements—and, in sheer volume, rivaled the number of celebrated and long-established surgical operations like appendectomy and tonsillectomy. This is astonishing given the rapidity of the CABG's utilization, underscored by the serious risks and sophisticated technology involved in its performance. Indeed, hospitals and heart surgeons prospered as the explosion of investment in cardiac bypass technology created a multi-billion-dollar industry built around this single operation. By the mid-1990s, virtually every medium-to large-sized city in the nation claimed one, if not two or three, costly open-heart surgery center(s) as coronary artery bypass surgery became the single biggest money-maker in American Medicine. Likewise, the relative safety of cardiac bypass surgery helped it to spread rapidly throughout the wealthier countries of the world.

Starting in the 1980s, when cardiac stenting via PCI developed, initially for the treatment of acute heart attacks and soon for coronary artery disease, its usage also grew exponentially. Further technical improvements in PCI, including the place-ment of increasingly sophisticated stents, along with a wide range of up-to-the-minute medical therapies, allowed a broader variety of diseases of the heart to be treated percutaneously. By the turn of the millennium and an apparent saturation of the market for surgical treatment of ischemic heart disease, the utilization of CABG procedures declined and steadied in the 150,000 range per year. As a result, CABG operations became reserved for and remain the gold standard for patients with com-plex and multi-vessel arteriosclerotic lesions of their coronary arteries.

*   *   *

In little more than fifty years, along a pathway littered with cast-off operations, dead patients, and rejected theories, the United States transformed itself from a backwater surgical province to the unrivaled global leader in heart surgery. Cardiac surgeons grew bolder with each passing decade and stood apart from their surgical colleagues as almost every heart operation was a matter of life or death. This urgency is the most striking thing about the story of heart surgery in America. A surgical specialty rooted in a history of operative complications and dying patients becoming firmly established as an essential tool for helping people live long and healthy lives by as-suring the safety of its risky procedures is a remarkable achievement.

As the barriers to open-heart operations lessened, another complex field of surgery captured the attention of the country's knife bearers and researchers. The conquest of this new frontier and the difficulty of obtaining its objective required physicians and surgeons of varied specialties to work together, a clinical approach that would define American medicine in the closing decades of the twentieth century. Like open-heart surgery, the transplantation of organs started out as a near-hopeless field. Technical limitations simply appeared too great and operative achievements too few. Once patients were diagnosed with problems related to the failure of a specific organ, they were effectively given a death sentence, but that was about to dramatically change.

18.

OUT WITH THE OLD

Be not slow to visit the sick: for that shall make thee to be beloved. Whatso-
ever thou takest in hand, remember the end, and thou shalt never do amiss.

Ecclesiasticus 7:35

The human body is the only machine for which there are no spare parts.

Hermann M. Biggs, radio talk on WGY, Schenectady, New York, 1922

Few performance spaces are as striking as Stockholm's Concert Hall with its black main ceiling, golden coffer balcony ceiling, and choir loft framed by a sixty-one-hundred-pipe organ—the largest tube measures thirty-six feet in length. Built in 1926, the Hall is home to the Royal Stockholm Philharmonic Orchestra and is where the awarding ceremonies for the Nobel Prize are held. To walk through the lobby with its life-sized statues of the four Muses—Erato, Euterpe, Polyhymnia, and Terpsichore, the inspirational goddesses of the arts, literature, and science—and enter an auditorium set up for the Nobel Prize award presentation, resplendent with decorative flowers and elaborate textiles, and see the royal family and dignitaries seated on the podium is at once daunting and inspiring.

Since 1901, the Nobel Prizes have been presented to the Laureates at ceremonies on December 10, the anniversary of the death of Alfred Nobel, the industrialist who established the awards. Presentation speeches extoll the winners, after which the King of Sweden hands each of them a diploma and medal. In 1990, the awarding of the Nobel Prize in Physiology or Medicine was especially important because for the first and only time an American surgeon was honored for an operative surgical feat.* The prize committee's announcement was straightforward:

> Joseph E. Murray discovered how rejection following organ transplantation in man could be mastered . . . [and] successfully transplanted a kidney . . . for the first time. He pioneered transplantation of kidneys obtained from deceased persons and could show that patients with terminal renal insufficiency could be cured. The field was then open for transplantation of other organs such as liver, pancreas and heart. . . . Murray's discovery is crucial for those tens of thousands of severely ill patients who either can be cured or be given a decent life when other treatment methods are without success.[1]

Murray's award was a singular honor that highlighted the public's growing interest in and the scientific community's research on immunology. Doctors understand much about the body's immune system, but seventy-five years ago its functions as well as the know-how to transplant an organ were wrapped in mystery. For a transplant to be successful, two formidable barriers needed to be breached: the body's immunologic defenses required analysis and understanding, and the skills necessary to perform the operation had to be worked out. The foremost technical obstacle was devising a technique that allowed blood vessels to be successfully sutured together. Blood vessels are circular in diameter, easily damaged, and can feel and look like wet, slippery spaghetti. Surgeons could not transplant organs without the ability to attach blood vessels, but knife bearers lacked the necessary know-how to fashion such connections.

---

* In 1966, Charles B. Huggins, a Canadian-born American-educated surgeon, who specialized in the treatment of prostate cancer, received the Nobel Prize for Physiology or Medicine for his discovery that hormones could be used to control the spread of some cancers. Huggins graduated from Harvard Medical School, completed a residency in general surgery at the University of Michigan, and, in 1924, joined the surgical faculty at the University of Chicago. At the latter institution, he was asked by the chairman of surgery to manage the growing number of urologic cases related to diseases of the prostate. Without a background in surgical research or training in urology, Huggins grudgingly accepted the offer, bought a standard textbook of urology, and committed portions of it to memory within a month's time. Fifteen years later, he had established a method to measure the effect of hormone changes on how the prostate functioned and realized that removal of the testicles to stop the production of testosterone or the administration of estrogen led to a decrease in size of the gland. Huggins remained at the University of Chicago for the rest of his academic career.

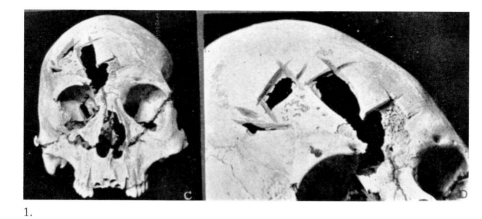

1.

Above: A Neolithic skull showing multiple crude cross-hatchings used to remove a section of bone. Whether done for supernatural or trauma-related reasons, the successful opening of a skull by prehistoric man was an astonishing surgical feat.

Bottom Left: Galen was a renowned physician/surgeon of the Greco-Roman period, and second only to Hippocrates as the most important healer in antiquity. Galen's views would dominate European Medicine for the next fifteen centuries.

Bottom Right: Uneducated barber-surgeons found their calling within the monasteries of medieval Europe where monks hired them to care for their facial grooming. Over time, barber-surgeons began to assist the clerics in the medical and surgical care of patients.

2.

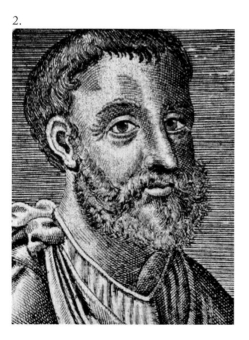

3.

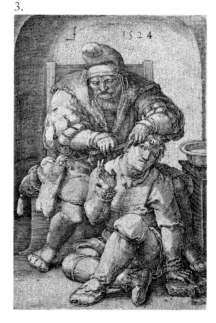

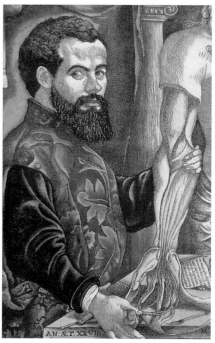

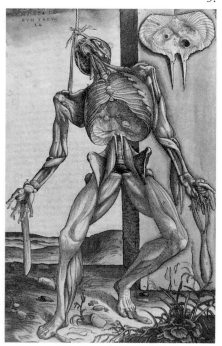

Top Left: Vesalius was a sixteenth-century physician/surgeon and widely recognized anatomist. His book, *De Humani Corporis Fabrica Libri Septem* (On the fabric of the human body), is considered one of the most important works in the history of Medicine and established the modern study of human anatomy.

Top Right: Among the reasons that Vesalius's *Fabrica* became so influential was its outstanding woodcuts. For the first time, illustrations were integrated with a written text that helped to clarify innumerable peculiarities and variations in structures encountered during the dissection of a human body.

6.

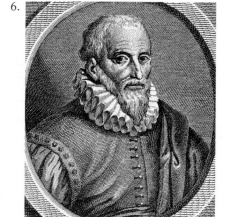

Right: Ambroise Paré's position in the history of surgery is of supreme importance. He severed the final link between the surgical thoughts and techniques of the ancients and the push toward the modern era.

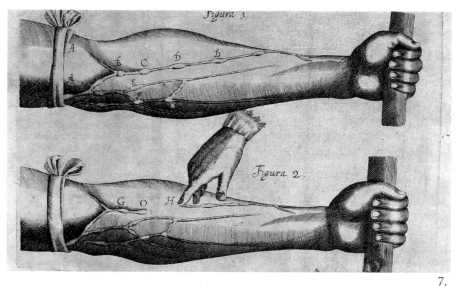

8.

7.

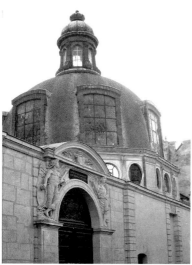

Above: William Harvey's *De Motu Cordis*, published in 1628, established that blood circulates throughout the body. He showed how the heart acts as a muscular pump and propels blood through the arteries such that its motion is continuous and circles back to the heart via the veins.

Left: The building at 5 rue de l'École de Médecine in Paris originally housed one of Europe's oldest surgical amphitheaters. Constructed in 1695, the structure was an unmistakable indication of the growth in prestige and prosperity of the French surgical community.

9.

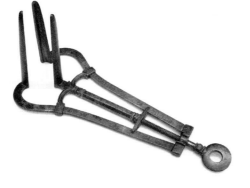

Left: In 1686, the surgical treatment of Louis XIV's anal fistula required construction of a handmade, three-pronged, metal retractor that allowed his surgeon to adequately view the king's anal canal. The success of the operation demonstrated the curative powers of a knife bearer's scalpel and brought about a key shift in how the public viewed the craft of surgery.

10.

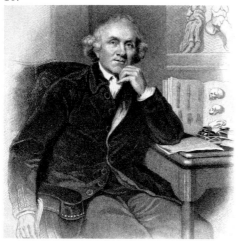

Left: John Hunter, a Scottish surgeon, is considered one of the most influential surgeon/scientists of all time. Through the breadth and depth of his research, surgery came to be regarded as a legitimate branch of Medicine firmly backed by studies in pathology and physiology.

Center: An operating amphitheater from the early nineteenth century located in the garret of St. Thomas's Church in London, on the original site of St. Thomas's Hospital. Note the uncomfortable appearing wooden operating table surrounded by a steeply banked standing-room-only area for observers.

Below: In March 1847, several months after the value of ether anesthesia had been established, daguerreotypes of surgical operations were taken at Massachusetts General Hospital. In this photo, John Collins Warren has his hands on the patient's leg and another surgeon readies an ether-soaked sponge by the patient's head.

11.

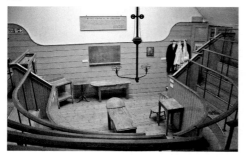

12.

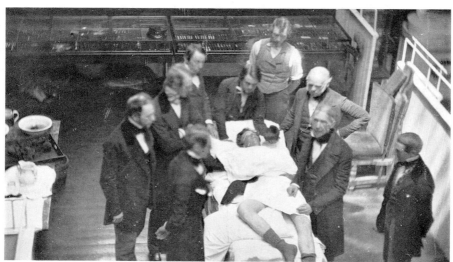

Right: In the long evolution of surgery, the contributions of a few individuals are preeminent. Joseph Lister joins the elite list because of his notable efforts to introduce systematic, scientifically based antisepsis in the treatment of wounds and the performance of surgical operations.

Center: Railway accidents in the nineteenth century were so common and catastrophic they brought about the long forgotten specialty of railway surgery. It was America's earliest large surgical specialty with its own journals, textbooks, and local, state, and national societies. However, railway surgery ultimately failed to gain recognition within mainstream Medicine and suffered a precipitous decline.

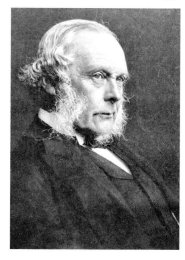

14.

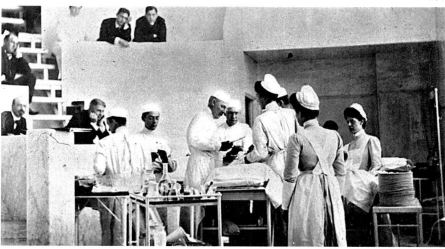

Below: William Halsted brought laboratory science into surgery. A brilliant innovator and awe-inspiring teacher, he, more than any other surgeon, created the foundation on which the school of modern American surgery rests.

15.

16.

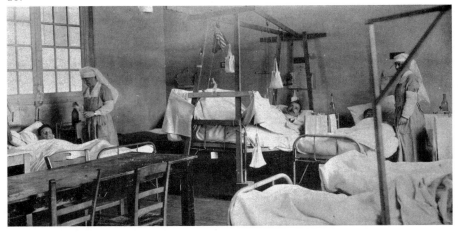

17.

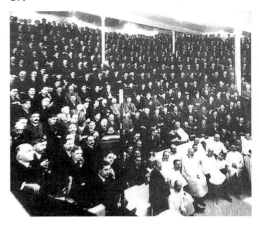

18.

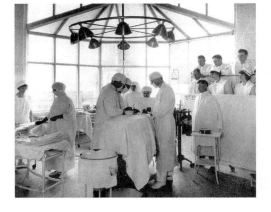

Above: For surgeons, war has always posed a moral dilemma: they gain greater clinical experience while surrounded by ever-mounting human suffering. World War I was no exception, a deadly conflict of attrition marked by trench warfare, unrelenting bombardment, and lethal new weapons that required the organization of sophisticated field hospitals to treat the severe casualties.

Left: At the turn of the twentieth century, the use of "wet clinics," where master surgeons demonstrated their operative techniques to a large audience of fellow knife bearers, became common. These presentations played an important role in improving the quality of America's surgeons and their operative skills.

Bottom Left: By the 1930s, dramatic changes occurred in the physical makeup of a surgical operating room. The viewing audience, in this case nurses, was plainly set apart from the patient as antiseptic and sterilization techniques now included surgeons, spectators, and support staff.

19.

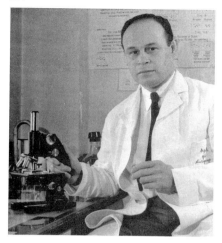

Left: Charles Drew was a celebrated African-American scientist and surgeon. His research in the area of blood banks and techniques for blood storage led to the large-scale use of blood transfusions during World War II.

Below: In 1965, President Lyndon B. Johnson's gallbladder surgery was extensively covered by the nation's press corps. The photo of the president showing off his scar was widely circulated and helped remove any lingering doubts about the social acceptability of surgery.

20.

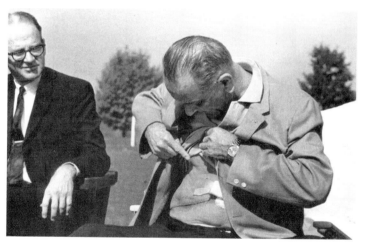

21.

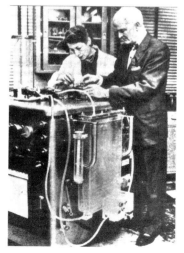

Left: Surgeons could not repair major cardiac defects without a way to stop the heart from beating while ensuring that the patient's blood was still oxygenated. John Gibbon, with the assistance of his wife, Mary, developed the heart-lung machine and their success meant that heart surgery, an elusive vision in 1950, became practical and routine by 1960.

22.

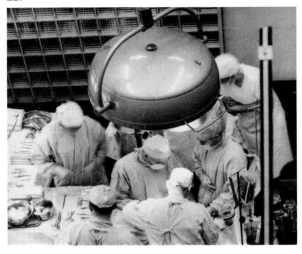

Left: In 1954, the world's first successful transplant of an organ, a kidney, changed surgery in profound ways. It broke a psychological, perhaps spiritual, barrier that viewed the human body as a sacrosanct object able to receive care but not designed to provide it. An individual's body could now provide a cure, along with drugs, minerals, and plants.

23.

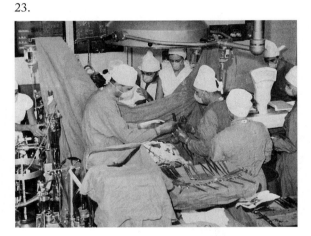

Right: The first successful heart transplant by Christiaan Barnard in South Africa in 1967 was one of the peaks of modern surgical triumphs. The operation rivaled the accomplishments of such contemporary fields as space exploration and cellular genetics.

24.

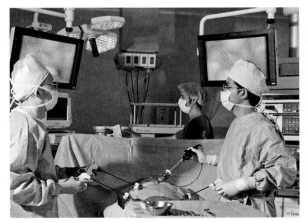

Left: In the late twentieth century, the rise of minimally invasive laparoscopic surgery combined with the advent of same-day surgery represented a dramatic change in the conduct of surgical operations. Gone were unsightly scars and multiple-week recoveries, replaced by wounds measured in inches and healing in days.

In the early years of the twentieth century, Alexis Carrel, a French surgeon working at New York City's Rockefeller Institute for Medical Research, developed a reliable method of securing blood vessels to one another. He was awarded the Nobel Prize in Physiology or Medicine in 1912 for this achievement. Carrel labeled his discovery the "triangulation method" of suture. He brought the ends of blood vessels together by placing three stitches equidistant around their edges. By pulling carefully on the sutures, he formed three straight lines. In this way, Carrel converted the circular vessels into a triangle at their ends. He then easily sutured along the straight lines between the sutures. Carrel made the difficult problem of joining the ends of flimsy blood vessels simple. Once this surgical skill was perfected, the field of transplant surgery opened up to greater experimentation as well as increasingly complex surgical challenges.

From a surgeon's perspective, the organ simplest to detach and reattach is the kidney; it only has three crucial points of connection with the body—the renal artery, the renal vein, and the ureter, which carries urine from the kidney to the bladder. In comparison, the anatomy of the liver or pancreas is more complex with multiple incoming and outgoing arteries and veins as well as difficult-to-manipulate secretory ducts. The heart and lungs cannot be removed without the use of elaborate temporary measures to sustain life during the transplant procedure, such as a heart-lung machine. Consequently, the thrust of early transplant research focused on the kidney.

These bean-shaped, fist-sized organs located near the middle of the back, just below the rib cage, are the body's primary filtration system. Every minute, one pint of blood travels to each kidney through its renal artery—the two kidneys receive 20 percent of the heart's output—and spreads through the organ's tiny filtering units, called nephrons. A healthy kidney contains more than 1 million of these, each with a glomerulus and a tubule, a collection of microscopic-sized capillaries. These tiny blood vessels are pockmarked with holes, like a sieve, and use a delicate chemical exchange to remove excess water and accumulated waste (known as urea) from blood. The refreshed blood then leaves the kidney via the renal vein and flows back to the lungs and heart. The waste, now in the form of urine, exits the kidney through the ureter. In addition to filtering the blood, the kidneys maintain the body's level of vital salts, especially sodium and potassium, thereby regulating blood pressure. They also control the production of red blood cells and vitamin D and constantly fine-tune the body's acid-base balance.

Problems mount when the kidneys stop working correctly (a person only needs one fully functioning kidney to remain healthy). Individuals in kidney failure grow lethargic. Their hands and feet may swell or feel numb. As unfiltered poisons congregate in the bloodstream, patients become comatose and eventually die. There is no way to repair damaged nephrons, surgical or otherwise. The only long-term solution is replacement with a healthy donor organ or lifelong dependence tethered to a dialysis machine.

At first, surgeons were uncertain what would be the most sensible way to attach a donor kidney. Early transplant researchers grappled with several questions that seem intuitive in hindsight: Where should a transplanted kidney be placed? Why not the abdomen or perhaps the thigh? What should be done with the ureter? Should the urine drain through a catheter to the outside or flow through the ureter to the bladder? The orthotopic or normal anatomical location for the kidney proved too difficult to maneuver about for transplantation. The answers to these questions did not become evident until the early 1950s, when Murray conducted a series of animal experiments that showed a donor kidney could be easily attached in relatively the same manner as the failed one but in the lower abdomen.

At its start, the field of transplant surgery blundered its way forward. One early operative success sounds more like a tale from a medieval alchemist's diary than a fascinating preface to future landmarks in surgical transplantation. In 1947, a woman was admitted to the Peter Bent Brigham Hospital in Boston with acute but recoverable kidney failure as the result of a botched illegal abortion. She had an infection in her uterus, which led to severe shock and the development of anuria (i.e., the total suppression of urine formation). Although her kidneys were otherwise sound, they needed a period of rest to recover from the trauma they had suffered. The doctors believed that this could be accomplished with a temporary donor kidney, a so-called bridge transplant. The donor organ was obtained from a deceased accident victim and attached to blood vessels in the patient's forearm. Surgeons then taped the now-external substitute kidney to her skin, covered it with a moist towel, and kept it warm with heat from a gooseneck lamp. The ureter, which normally connected to the bladder, drained her urine into a laboratory flask. As crude as the solution was, the donor kidney worked and, several days later, the patient's own kidneys recovered and functioned normally.

The "bridge transplant" performed admirably, but it could never be considered a long-term solution (and not simply because patients would have likely refused to walk around with kidneys hanging off their forearms). Microscopic examination of the donor kidney showed that the patient's body had begun to reject it at a cellular level after only forty-eight hours. A donor kidney or any organ perceived as foreign to an individual's immune system has little chance of survival. Doctors recognized this problem as the major hurdle in organ transplant, but they did not understand the underlying biochemical and physiological principles.

Only in the mid-1940s did medical researchers start to decode the nature of the immune reaction and the causes of organ rejection. The issue turned out to be a dilemma of human individuality. Each person's cells are biologically unique to that being and foreign to all others. The body's immune system instinctively attacks and rapidly deploys its defenses to eliminate unfamiliar tissues with an onslaught of killer white blood cells, hostile antibodies, and other antagonistic elements. This protection is mainly accomplished through the immune system's own distribution network, the lymphatic vessels, whose primary function is to transport lymph throughout the body, a fluid rich with foreign-body-and-infection-fighting white blood cells. The lymphatic vessels drain into lymph nodes, where the lymphatic fluid is cleared of debris. The hundreds of lymph nodes are located both deep inside the body and close to the surface, such as under the arm or in the groin. The spleen, thymus gland, and tonsils are also part of the lymphatic system. Researchers concluded that patients' chances for successful transplantations would increase exponentially if doctors could mute immune systems and make them tolerant to foreign tissue—a process labeled "acquired tolerance." But understanding the nature of a problem is not the same as having the solution. Immunosuppression and "acquired tolerance" proved to be incredibly complex research questions.

Nonetheless, in 1954, American surgeons performed the world's first successful long-term kidney transplant in advance of having answers to many immunologic issues, thus completing one of the greatest surgical achievements of the mid-twentieth century. This unlikely accomplishment was a testament to the cooperation, courage, and vision of two surgeons—one received the Nobel Prize while the other graced the cover of *Time*—and two patients, who were identical twins.

*   *   *

Francis Moore, the surgeon who oversaw this transformative surgical operation, was a man of grace and warmth, a master of repartee, and a giant of mid-twentieth-century American surgery with an unrivaled knowledge of biological science. According to one colleague, Moore's expertise would "intimidate anyone who disagreed with him or even appeared on the same platform."[2] A journalist, equally impressed, commented: "Men like Francis Moore . . . often seem to be peering even beyond the future."[3] In May 1963, *Time* magazine placed Moore's portrait on its cover, with six words: "IF THEY CAN OPERATE, YOU'RE LUCKY."[4]

Moore was well prepared to be a leader in America's advancement of surgery. He attended Harvard College, where he wrote both book and music and played the piano for the Hasty Pudding's 1934 theatrical show, *Hades! The Ladies*, which imagined the university as a coeducational institution. He then matriculated at Harvard Medical School, where his initial interest in internal medicine faltered because he found the discipline "Too much talk and theory; not enough action."[5] Instead, Moore shifted his focus to surgery, progressing over the course of a decade from intern to surgical resident to assistant in surgery at Massachusetts General Hospital. In 1948, at age thirty-four, he was appointed by Harvard Medical School administrators to lead the surgical department at the Peter Bent Brigham Hospital, the youngest surgical chairman in Harvard's history.

Physicians respected Moore for a wide range of medical achievements. He had a well-deserved reputation for solving difficult scientific puzzles, such as determining the body's normal amount of potassium, sodium, and water or quantifying the loss of fluids in a burn victim. Admirers claimed that his leadership of the Brigham's surgeons led to major breakthroughs in abdominal operations, heart surgery, and procedures on the blood vessels. "With their new machines and new skills," wrote one enthusiast, "surgeons [like Moore] know practically no limits to the range of patients they can help. Operations once regarded as foredoomed to failure and fatality . . . are now carried out on the youngest of babies or on the oldest and sickest of patients."[6] But Moore's influence went far beyond his research and clinical accomplishments. He encouraged the interplay between surgeons and physicians, believing that specialists from different fields needed to collaborate when faced with modern medical dilemmas. He argued that inter-specialty support would hasten Medicine's evolution. This approach is commonplace today, but in the 1940s it was a minority position.

When Moore assumed leadership of the Brigham's surgical department, a group of surgeons and physicians were already pursuing research into organ transplantation. "This was to become the most extensive area of clinical research in our department," Moore would later write, "and the largest entirely new field of medi-

cine and surgery in this century."[7] Murray joined this team in 1951, having graduated from Harvard Medical School and completed a general surgical residency at
the Brigham followed by a plastic surgery residency at the New York and Memorial
Hospitals and the Sloan Kettering Institute.

Murray's fascination with transplantation began during World War II when,
following his internship, he was inducted into the U.S. Army Medical Corps and
served in the plastic surgery unit at a military hospital in Valley Forge, Pennsylvania.
"We took care of thousands of casualties, many with severe burns," he told a reporter
for *Time*. "I was performing skin grafts and became interested in why skin wouldn't
graft permanently."[8] Many of Murray's patients were so badly burned that they did
not have enough of their own skin to use as a cover for the burnt areas. In these cases,
the surgeons took skin from another person to serve as a substitute. Inevitably, the patient's immune system mounted a defense against the foreign skin causing it to slough
off. At the time, the only solution, but wildly impractical, was to hope that the patient
had an identical twin with a similar immune system and harvest skin from him or her.

Murray's assignment within the Brigham group was to determine the technical
requirements for the performance of a kidney transplant. No one understood how
long a kidney could survive outside the body or the surgical techniques needed to
attach a donor kidney to the recipient's blood vessels and urinary system. Following several years of experimentation on dogs, he developed a procedure to place the
transplanted organ in the lower abdomen. Murray was a "builder," explained another
transplant surgeon:

> He began his plastic surgery career by building new faces and body
> parts for people who had been maimed physically and emotionally
> by war, accidents, and cancer. . . . He next turned to transplantation
> to rescue patients who could be healthy, were it not for the failure of
> a vital organ. In the long run, he built a stadium called the specialty
> of organ transplantation, began to populate it with high-minded
> people whom he trained, and welcomed with open arms those of us
> whom he did not even know.[9]

While Murray and his colleagues worked on the surgical side of the transplant
question, physicians at the Brigham were developing the country's first artificial kidney or dialysis apparatus. A European doctor had designed a prototype, but the Bos-

ton doctors improved it and made the device functionally reliable. For almost five years, the band of Brigham physicians worked in a coordinated fashion with their surgeon counterparts to perfect its mechanisms. Like Moore, they relied on interspecialty cooperation to tackle complex problems, what he referred to as "organized play for grownups."[10]

The dialysis machine had plenty of complicated issues to handle, from preventing the dialyzed blood from clotting or frothing to avoiding the development of bacteria. The finished apparatus looked precarious with its air traps, clot traps, Lucite hood, motors, switches, and thermometers along with a rotating stainless-steel drum and hot water bath. Despite its fantastically complicated and improvised appearance, the dialysis machine was an instant success. It mitigated several common kidney ailments, including acute but reversible kidney failure, and chronic kidney conditions, such as glomerulonephritis, an irreversible inflammation of the organ. In addition, the dialysis machine made procedures like the infamous Brigham "bridge transplant" obsolete. Its physician developer explained that the device represented an "integral part of a long-range program leading to the transplantation of kidneys for irreversible renal failure."[11]

* * *

In late October 1954, twenty-three-year-old Richard Herrick was at life's end. He was in the final phase of end-stage kidney failure with convulsions, headaches, out-of-control blood pressure, and psychotic behavior bordering on all-out madness. His only chance for survival was a kidney transplant—long-term dialysis was not an option—a surgical procedure that had never been successfully performed. The odds did not favor Richard, but two factors made his case surgically unique and proved lifesaving. First, he had been admitted to the Brigham Hospital, home of Moore, Murray, their surgical transplant team, and the newfangled kidney dialysis machine. Second, Richard had an identical twin.

Although doctors understood little of organ rejection and "acquired tolerance," they recognized one general exception to the rule of human individuality: identical twins. The different gestation processes of fraternal and identical twins show why this should be. More than 90 percent of twins are fraternal. At the time of their conception, two sperm fertilize two different eggs that become two distinct embryos nourished by separate placentas. Fraternal twins can look distinct from each other and be of opposite sexes. They generally have distinct chromosomal profiles as well as dissimilar immune systems. With identical twins, however, the moment of conception occurs when one sperm fertilizes one egg that then spontaneously divides into two embryos joined through a common placenta. Consequently, the individuals have nearly indistinguishable genetic makeups, including their immune systems. One identical twin's immune system will not consider tissue from his or her sibling to be foreign. Therefore, Richard would not reject a kidney donated from his brother Ronald.

Moore and Murray understood that Richard's identical-twin status made him an ideal candidate for a kidney transplant, but before addressing the possibility they needed to improve his critical condition and ensure the twin's immune compatibility. No patient could survive such invasive surgery like a kidney transplant while suffering from high blood pressure, persistent infections, and psychotic episodes, only to then face the deadly situation of possible graft rejection. The question of cleansing Richard's blood to stabilize his condition would not have been possible in any other hospital but the Brigham with its newly developed dialysis apparatus. The doctors decided to give Richard four hours of blood cleansing using the novel machine. The medical report concluded: "A good chemical response was obtained and 36 hours later the patient's sensorium had cleared and he was cooperative and able to take diet and medicaments by mouth."[12] In other words, the dialysis device accomplished everything that was asked of it, efficiently restoring Richard's mental and physical balance. He went home to recuperate while Moore and Murray contemplated a venture into the surgical unknown.

With Richard convalescing, it became easier to test the brothers to determine whether they were truly identical twins and immune compatible. The matching was completed through several ways including blood typing, fingerprinting, examining eye color, and even talking to the family doctor who delivered the brothers to see if they shared the same placenta. Over a dozen confirmatory assessments checked out, but one remained a mystery. Murray had grafted a small piece of skin from Ronald onto Richard. If the transplanted skin remained alive then surgeons knew that the twin brothers were truly identical. One month later, it was.

The Brigham's surgeons realized what an extraordinary opportunity it would be to perform the world's first organ transplant and save Richard's life, but they struggled with the magnitude of the procedure. The possibility of relocating a whole organ from one living being to another was among the most nerve-wracking operations ever deliberated. "Was it right and proper," asked Moore, "to sacrifice a normal kidney from a healthy person to rescue another who was ill?"[13] They discussed the issue with each other but ultimately decided to meet in mid-December for a final decision-making process with their team of anesthesiologists, immunologists, internists, nephrologists, pathologists, and surgeons plus clergy, lawyers, and psychiatrists. With this collective expertise, the interdisciplinary group was better positioned to consider the range of ethical and scientific concerns. Eventually, it was decided that the potential benefits outweighed the risks.

Besides convincing one another, the Brigham team also had to persuade Richard's brother Ronald. Part of the final preparations included meetings with him to explain the procedure and answer questions. They were asking him to do something no human being had ever done before: voluntarily allow doctors to remove an organ for the benefit of another person. Since Ronald only needed one healthy kidney, the short-term clinical risk was minimal, but the long-term effects were less certain. If his one remaining kidney somehow became diseased or injured, he did not have another identical brother to lend him a spare. Ronald was not dissuaded by what seemed remote concerns. The two brothers had, according to Moore, "an unusual emotional stake in each other's illness."[14]

Even with Ronald's consent, cultural and social concerns lingered. There was fear that the Boston doctors had unfairly pressured him or that he had felt coerced. Some suggested that using a live donor crossed an ethical threshold and that Ronald should bow out gracefully. But the world's first living organ donor did not find the situation morally unreasonable. "They left it up to me to decide," he later recalled. "I was the one who was going to do it; they weren't going to make the decision for me."[15] Ronald confirmed his resolve the night before the surgery. He was lying in a hospital bed, awaiting the morning's procedure, when his brother had a note passed to him that said: "Beat it, go home while you can." The guilt over Ronald's sacrifice had apparently grown too strong for Richard to handle. Ronald firmly responded: "I'm here and I'm staying here."[16]

* * *

The next morning, December 23, 1954, the two surgical procedures began at 8:15. Twin teams of surgeons operated on the brothers simultaneously to minimize the amount of time that Ronald's healthy donor kidney was disconnected from his body.

If the organ went without oxygenated blood for a prolonged period, its filtering mechanisms would deteriorate. At exactly 9:53, Murray, having prepared the site in Richard's pelvis where the transplant would be located, called for the donor kidney. Moore, who was waiting on the team handling Ronald, carefully walked down the hallway to Richard's operating room. At his waist, he carried a stainless-steel surgical basin swaddled in blue cloth that contained, in his words, "this sacred kidney."[17] Moore handed the organ to a nurse who passed it to Murray and his assistants. They examined the kidney under the shine of overhead lights and pronounced it completely normal. Moore stepped back from the table as Murray, knowing he had to reattach the donor kidney as quickly as possible using Carrel's triangulation method, joined the organ's artery and vein to Richard's blood vessels, then connected the ureter to his bladder.

Shortly after 11:00, Murray finished securing Ronald's kidney in Richard's lower abdomen, not far from the appendix. The kidney was without blood flow for an hour and twenty-two minutes. The tension in the operating room was obvious: quiet took over. "We watched—some with fingers crossed, some saying silent prayers," recalled Murray.[18] He undid the clamp on the blood vessels and blood started to flow. The dark red kidney turned pinkish red as it filled with oxygenated blood. A collective sigh of relief was heard. Within minutes, crystal-clear yellowish urine flowed through the ureter. Moore later remarked, "Although you may never have developed any affection for urine, if you or your patients are unable to make any, you come to appreciate it."[19] When the surgeons sutured Richard's abdomen closed, they had completed the world's first successful long-term kidney transplant.

The operation quickly became national news. The media publicized the accomplishment within days, before the Herrick brothers had even left the hospital. "Twin gains in operation, transplanted kidney working 'efficiently,'"[20] headlined the Associated Press account. A now-iconic photograph of Richard leaving the Brigham a month after the operation was widely distributed. It showed Ronald guiding his grinning brother in a wheelchair toward an ambulance to transport him home.

The medical profession took slightly longer to digest the seminal operation; the Brigham team did not submit the details of the Herrick operation to peers until early 1956. The article reaffirmed that American Medicine was moving in an increasingly interdisciplinary direction: the authors made certain that the physicians and surgeons of the Brigham Hospital were recognized jointly for their efforts. Their report also showed that cutting-edge research required enormous financial resources.

An accompanying list of acknowledgments included private foundations, like the John A. Hartford Foundation and the American Heart Association, as well as public sources, like the Office of the Surgeon General and the United States Public Health Service.

As for the Herrick brothers, they returned to their normal lives. Richard married one of his nurses from the hospital and raised a family. Unfortunately, the glomerulonephritis that destroyed his own kidneys returned to devastate the transplanted one as well as cause heart problems. He died from a heart attack in 1963. Ronald remained healthy for many years, but in 2010, at age seventy-nine, succumbed to complications following heart surgery. In 2012, Murray, having been the longtime chief of plastic surgery at the Brigham, died from complications of a stroke. Moore, a man who always cherished his personal independence and self-determination, became seriously debilitated with chronic heart failure in his mid-eighties. In 2001, at the age of eighty-eight, he took his own life.

* * *

While the Herrick operation was a clinical triumph of the highest order, it provided few answers to fundamental questions about organ rejection. Since the brothers shared the same genetic structure, the kidney transplant circumvented the issue of immunologic intolerance altogether. Moore, Murray, and the teams of physicians and surgeons still had to resolve the underlying immunologic problem of tissue rejection. Their most promising early research in tissue rejection involved the suppression of lymphocytes.

Lymphocytes are a type of white blood cell that both produce antibodies and attack bacteria and viruses. They are fearsome defenders and come in two main forms: B and T, a detail of cell biology that was not understood in the 1950s. The former produce antibodies that attach to the surface of foreign invaders. These antibodies will either disable the intruders or mark them for annihilation. T cells come in two different varieties, helpers and killers. Helper T cells assist their B cell brethren to manufacture antibodies. The killer T cells are vicious and destroy any cell identified by B cells as alien. The Brigham doctors knew that lymphocytes were produced in the bone marrow and were among the most important cellular elements of an immune reaction. They also knew that the bone marrow is extremely sensitive to radiation.

Consequently, Brigham doctors first tried to solve the dilemma of immune compatibility with X-rays. They exposed test patients to full-body X-rays, hoping to create an environment where a transplanted organ could survive. Problematically, irradiation also tended to lower immune defenses so efficiently that a patient could not respond to even a simple infection, like the common cold, and might die of the most commonplace of illnesses. In the late 1950s, of the various patients who received whole-body X-rays and a kidney transplant at the Brigham Hospital, only one survived. It was a transplant performed by Murray between two fraternal twins. Despite the overall dismal results, the Nobel Prize Committee cited this operation as a significant "first" in the effort to achieve immunosuppression.[21] Moore later commented that the technique's clinical failure gave a new twist to an old cliché: instead of "the operation was a success but the patient died," he quipped, "the graft lived but the patient died."[22]

The use of whole-body X-ray in transplant surgery was a shotgun blast, but surgeons needed the precision of a rifle shot. In the early 1960s, they found their weapon of choice. Chemists had recently synthesized drugs that achieved immunosuppression safely: 6-mercaptopurine and its close relatives, azathioprine and cyclosporine. These new "wonder drugs" had the potential to treat a host of medical dilemmas, including autoimmune diseases, cancers, and organ rejection. Unlike X-ray therapy, which the Brigham doctors administered in one irreversible blast, immunosuppressive drugs could be prescribed in small amounts on a daily basis. Physicians could decrease or suspend dosage levels if a patient's immunologic defenses deteriorated too swiftly. The immunosuppressive drugs revolutionized the field of transplant surgery by providing doctors the control and precision that they had lacked with whole-body irradiation.

The Brigham's surgeons rapidly transitioned away from the X-ray technique of immunosuppression and prepared protocols for a kidney transplant using the new drug-based technology. By mid-1963, Murray and his assistants had performed over a half-dozen successful transplants from a nontwin donor based on drug-induced immunosuppression. One of the successful procedures included a kidney from a cadaver donor and was cited by the Nobel Committee as the third key operation in the history of transplant surgery performed by Murray.[23]

The Brigham's accomplishments provided the model that most subsequent organ transplants followed. The use of the immunosuppressive drugs allowed host patients to safely tolerate kidneys from unrelated donors. The era of identical twins as the only individuals who could undergo a successful kidney transplant was officially over. The techniques that Moore and Murray developed spread to other academic medical centers, and kidney transplants became part of the fabric of American and international Medicine. "We were no longer unique,"[24] explained Moore.

The world's first successful kidney transplant changed Medicine in profound ways. It helped break a psychological, perhaps spiritual, barrier that viewed the human body as a sacred object able to receive medical care but not designed to provide it. The Brigham team's transplant research showed that an individual's body could serve as part of the universe of curatives, along with plants, minerals, and synthesized compounds. The research and application of this new concept in medical care—that one person's healthy body could cure another's sickness or that a patient's own tissue could be modified to serve as a source of healing—was a wellspring that helped fuel subsequent accomplishments in transplant surgery.

*   *   *

Once kidney transplants based on immunosuppressive drug therapy were shown to be feasible, a door opened to other organs, especially the most prized of all, the heart. However, unlike the kidney, transplanting the human heart posed problems apart from rejection. At its core, the heart is a complex muscle, and without oxygen it fails within minutes, making it impractical to store. Following its removal, the heart must be transplanted with rapidity. Despite this difficulty and the familiar affairs associated with one's heart, the growing incidence of heart disease meant that a breakthrough in cardiac transplantation would have enormous value in treating the health of the American public. However, it was not until the heart-lung machine was developed that human cardiac transplantation became a possibility. Thus, in the mid-1950s, studies that led to the first human patient receiving a human donor heart began in earnest. And like the "arm kidney" operation with the organ hanging from the patient's forearm, the first attempt at a human heart transplant had an unexpected twist.

In January 1964, an elderly man with severe coronary artery arteriosclerosis was admitted to the University of Mississippi Medical Center. There, surgeons had already completed over two hundred animal heart transplants and were organizationally and technically prepared to carry out a human heart transplant. With their patient's heart rapidly failing, he was placed on a heart-lung machine and prepared for the first transplant between humans. The donor was to be a young man on a respirator who was dying from irreversible brain damage. But when the elderly patient's heart ceased altogether, the donor's heart was still beating. At the time, medical protocols did not acknowledge the cessation of brain activity as a sign of death, which meant that surgeons had to wait till a person's heart stopped before it could be used for transplantation. With no human heart available and left with little choice other than to let the patient die, the Mississippi surgeons decided on a surprising option. The lead knife bearer explained the situation:

> At this point there was sharp discussion among the members of the transplant team. We were all well aware that any transplantation of a heart in man would be followed by public consternation and major criticism. We also knew that the use of a chimpanzee ("monkey") heart would augment the criticism immeasurably. It was a profoundly sober moment for all, and an agonizing moment for some. There, I polled each of the five primary members of the transplant team individually, and their votes were recorded. Four voted to proceed with the transplantation, even though the chimpanzee heart had to be used. The fifth abstained. In view of the early success achieved with the chimpanzee kidney transplants ... I felt that this transplantation was morally justified: no human heart was available and the patient was being kept alive solely on the heart-lung machine.[25]

For the first hour, the chimpanzee's heart beat well, but it shortly proved too small to maintain the patient's blood pressure and he died. The decision to use an animal heart fell under immediate attack from both the public as well as those within the surgical community. "Evolution of a perfect subhuman species of organ donors appears remote," protested a colleague. "Perhaps the cardiac surgeon should pause while society becomes accustomed to resurrection of the mythological chimera."[26] As farfetched as the chimpanzee heart transplant operation appeared, it was an important step toward a successful human heart transplant. "This first clinical experience," wrote another cardiac surgeon, "clearly established the scientific feasibility of heart transplantation in man ... the field of clinical heart transplantation is certainly open to ethical exploration, and its future will be established in competent laboratories and clinics throughout the world."[27]

Three years later, the demesne of heart transplantation changed considerably. Knowledgeable observers believed that Norman Shumway, a surgeon at Stanford University, who had perfected an innovative technique for heart transplant in animals, and not the University of Mississippi team, would be the first to attempt a human-to-human heart transplant. Shumway, a graduate of Vanderbilt University School of Medicine, completed a surgical residency at the University of Minnesota before joining the surgical faculty at Stanford. Scholarly and reserved, he, along with his associates, was developing an impressive cocktail of immunosuppressive drugs to prevent a donor heart from being rejected by the recipient's body. Still, the profession of Medicine in general and surgeons in particular were unprepared for a startling announcement from South Africa.

On December 3, 1967, Christiaan Barnard, a cardiac surgeon at Groote Schuur Hospital in Cape Town, stunned the world. He successfully transplanted the heart of a young woman, who had died in a car crash into a middle-aged diabetic man suffering from a multiplicity of complications following a series of heart attacks. Barnard was a relative unknown in the world of cardiac surgery, but he was about to become a celebrity, lionized for his surgical daring, and the world's most eligible bachelor. This first human-to-human heart transplant was welcomed by some heart surgeons as establishing a needed precedent. Others were not so sanguine. Shumway and his team struggled in the laboratory to solve the problem of graft rejection and feared that surgeons would rush to replicate what they considered a premature surgical operation. In fact, Barnard had learned much about transplantation while visiting Shumway and was told that the Stanford team was not quite ready to proceed. Nevertheless, Barnard crafted a bold surgical statement and prompted a sprint by other cardiac surgeons to be the first to perform a heart transplant in their respective countries.

Even a hesitant Shumway could not resist the growing pressure. He completed his first human heart transplant in January 1968. With the Stanford team leading the way and lending a measure of legitimacy, the field of cardiac transplantation expanded rapidly with media coverage generating fame and fortune. In Barnard's case, journalists and photographers flew in from around the globe and encircled Groote Schuur Hospital. He was interviewed by all the major American TV networks, with guest appearances on *Face the Nation* and numerous talk shows along with a visit to President Johnson at his Texas ranch. "The line between life and death needs redefinition," asserted an editorial in the *New York Times*. "The [heart transplant] is one of the peaks of modern scientific achievement, fully comparable to the heights scaled earlier in such fields as space exploration or molecular biology."[28]

During the year that followed, over one hundred heart transplants were performed around the world; the vast majority of the patients were dead within one month. Cardiac surgeons were forced to confront the fact that they were too hasty in their chase for acclaim. The strain was even too much for Barnard, who was hospitalized with a bleeding stress ulcer. The editors of the *New York Times* revised their earlier optimistic views:

> Heart transplants are clearly not yet a miracle breakthrough promising new health and long life to millions suffering cardiac ailments. They are still extremely risky experimental procedures that offer limited hope of life prolongation. . . . Before these transplants can really become standard therapeutic procedures helping large numbers of people, much effort must be devoted to preventing the body's rejection of foreign organs, to finding better means of assuring tissue compatibility between donor and recipient, and to setting up the appropriate legal and medical procedures for securing more viable hearts for potential beneficiaries.[29]

Criticism grew over what was viewed as rash human experimentation. Many doctors felt that for the time being heart transplants should be performed only in centers where their surgeons and physicians had an extensive background of experimental work and broad experience in tissue typing and immunosuppressive therapy. The admonitions worked and the figure of one hundred heart transplants in 1968 dropped by 50 percent in 1969 and fell to just nine in 1971. By 1976, Shumway had the only ongoing program in cardiac transplantation in the United States.

Through the remainder of the 1970s and the early 1980s, the Stanford group continued its research. At the same time, federal and state legislative bodies began to pass laws defining "brain death" as a legal terminal event. The beating heart of a "brain-dead" individual could be obtained for transplant with a family's consent and without legal ramifications. The acquisition of donor hearts became better organized and the technique for removing hearts and transporting them underwent improvement. National and international registries were organized to match surgeons with patients in need of a heart transplant together with appropriate donors.

Above all, Shumway's efforts to better understand the immunology of rejection and his championing of cyclosporine, as a critical immunosuppressive drug, made heart transplants infinitely safer. Others followed his lead and, by the early 1990s, survival rates had significantly increased and fifty centers in the United States were carrying out heart transplants with long-term survival. Presently, America has the highest rate of heart transplantation of any country in the world, 3,552 procedures in 2019.*

Shumway continued his research into heart transplantation while serving as chairman of the Department of Cardiothoracic Surgery at Stanford. In 1993 he retired, and in 2006, at the age of eighty-three, he died from lung cancer. Barnard's surgical career was cut short by rheumatoid arthritis in 1983, although the media attention had increasingly distracted him from his work. Barnard's death in 2001 was caused by a severe asthma attack.

The success achieved from the combined efforts of scientists, physicians, and surgeons in the transplantation of human hearts represents one of the most remarkable triumphs in the history of surgery. The effort altered basic cultural and sociologic concepts about ourselves and led to a necessary redefinition of death. The pioneering heart surgeons were courageous and intrepid and stood apart from their surgical colleagues, because every heart operation was a matter of life or death. When a heart transplant is successful, everybody is overjoyed by the saving of a life. When the procedure fails, the cardiac surgeon has little choice but to return the next day and try again. This grim persistence in battling the body's own defenses is what made organ transplantation possible. Anything seemed doable. Surgeons could transplant not only hearts and kidneys successfully but also hands, intestines, livers, lungs, pancreases, penises, and even faces.

*   *   *

As I was completing work on this chapter, an obituary appeared in the news concerning the death of Connie Culp, the first face transplant recipient in the United States. Presently there have been approximately sixty face transplants performed

---

* The United States has led the world in the performance of organ transplants since statistics were first maintained in the 1980s. In 2019, over 40,000 organ transplants were completed, including 23,401 kidney, 8,896 liver, 3,552, heart, 2,714 lung, 872 kidney/pancreas, 143 pancreas, 81 intestine, and 45 heart/ lung.

worldwide, and Culp's near-total facial reconstruction in 2008 was, at the time, the most technically challenging ever performed. Her sad story was typical of face transplant patients, who are most often injured by burns or gunshot. In Culp's case, her face had been horribly disfigured when she was shot by her husband in his failed attempt at a murder/suicide. The wounds left her incapable of breathing or eating on her own. Culp's twenty-three-hour procedure allowed her to breathe and eat and smile and talk. However, like all transplant patients, she needed to take immunosuppressive drugs for the rest of her life. The drugs make any organ recipient more susceptible to infections and Culp's death, eleven and a half years following her procedure, was related to an overwhelming infection.

The selection criteria for facial transplantation are multifaceted and extend beyond surgical problem solving on to the psychosocial aftermath of major facial disfigurement. Thus, candidates for facial transplantation require an extensive evaluation by a team of experts, including plastic surgeons, transplant specialists, ophthalmologists, otolaryngologists, psychologists, psychiatrists, oral surgeons, and speech pathologists. In addition, a strong support network of family and friends is a critical requirement for success, especially when an often-blind individual, as are many facial transplant patients, is required to adhere to a strict daily regimen of immunosuppressive drugs. All of this occurs against the backdrop of profound emotional implications that result from an extensive reconstructive surgical operation and knowledge that one's new face is that of a dead person.

A facial transplantation consists of a series of operations (the patient's face is removed and replaced including the underlying blood vessels, bones, fat, muscles, and nerves) that requires rotating teams of surgical specialists and lasts anywhere from eight to thirty-six hours, followed by a two-week hospital stay. Issues including age, gender, hair color, skeletal shape/size, and skin tone present a level of difficulty in donor-recipient matching not found with other organ transplantations. For these and other reasons, despite numerous technical breakthroughs, facial transplantation remains an experimental procedure, a caution that must be acknowledged by the profession and the public.

Because organ transplantation raises issues at the intersection of ethics, law, psychology, surgery, and religion, its growth as a therapeutic procedure has brought a level of interdisciplinary cooperation not seen in other areas of Medicine. The transplantation of organs also stands out with its multiple interfaces as a candid reflection of political and sociocultural viewpoints not otherwise present in other fields of surgery. Organ transplants demonstrate that human beings are complex and dynamic organisms who must increasingly bring all manner of cultural, environmental, genetic, immunologic, and sociologic considerations into the surgical decision-making process.

Putting facial transplantation aside, other forms of replacement surgery are less controversial and, consequent to their widespread use, are arguably more important in treating society's surgical ills. Leading the list are orthopedic joint replacements—ankle, finger, hip, knee, and shoulder—the most commonly performed implant operations in the world. They not only are pain relieving but also dramatically improve daily function. As early as 1948, *Life* reported on a "radical new operation" that replaced diseased bone with "joints of steel and plastic."[30] In a study financed by the United States Office of Naval Research, a surgeon in Manhattan experimented with replacing the ball-and-socket of the hip joint as treatment for limbs damaged during the war. The work was preliminary and the operation did not become widely used until the 1970s, when a surgeon working in Manchester, England, realized that the body's fluids alone were not capable of lubricating steel sufficiently; the steel hip squeaked with every move. Steel was replaced with plastic and other artificial lubricants and the mechanical success of hip replacements spread worldwide. Currently, almost 1 million knee replacements are completed in America every year along with half a million hip replacements and one hundred thousand shoulder arthroplasties.

The technologic complexities of transplants established new benchmarks with regard to the performance of surgery. However, these yardsticks would themselves shortly undergo a revolution of change with the advent of novel forms of operations completed with minimally invasive techniques on an outpatient basis.

PART VI

THE PRESENT AND
THE FUTURE

19.

CHANGES

*Those surgeons of conscience (though perhaps relatively few in number) if
left unfettered in our free society, will in time leaven the entire profession.*

Everett Idris Evans, *Annals of Surgery*, 1949

*We should always let our judgments and recommendations be guided by
the fact that we operate on patients, not on diseases.*

Stanley O. Hoerr, *American Journal of Surgery*, 1962

In the late twentieth and early twenty-first centuries, the rise of minimally invasive surgery (aka Band-Aid, keyhole, or laparoscopic surgery) in conjunction with the advent of ambulatory surgery (aka outpatient or same-day surgery) represented a paradigmatic shift as noteworthy as any prior surgical development. Out were the foot-long, debilitating incisions of the classic/open approach to surgical operations. Gone were the unsightly raised scars and multiple-week recoveries, replaced by wounds measured in inches and healing at times within days. In was the endo- or laparoscope—a visualization tool consisting of a long, thin tube joined to a fiber-optic cable system with a camera and light—that allows surgeons to work in an almost bloodless field while the manipulation of tissue is displayed on a computer monitor. The high-definition screen is startling in its clarity. Shadows are eliminated and each member of the operating team has a crystal-clear view of the surgery.

Presently, the phrase "minimally invasive surgery" refers to any surgical procedure that is performed through a small incision rather than a large one. It is an inclusive concept and not limited to use of an endoscope. For example, repair of groin hernia through a three-inch incision is a form of minimally invasive surgery. The wide range of technologically refined procedures that constitute minimally invasive surgery and how the human body is manipulated during them is nothing short of astonishing.* Early on, two operations set the forward path for such outpatient surgery: the laparoscopic removal of gallbladders (aka laparoscopic cholecystectomy or "lap chole") and the ambulatory repair of groin hernias.

Laparoscopic cholecystectomy was developed in France and Germany in the late 1980s. By the mid-1990s, it was the prevailing operation in Europe and North America for the removal of uncomplicated gallstones. "In the history of surgery," declared a perceptive enthusiast, "few procedures have so rapidly changed the surgeon's custom of thinking and acting as has laparoscopic cholecystectomy. It has been the true detonator of the laparoscopic revolution."[1] Yet by characterizing the recent developments in laparoscopy as a "revolution," the surgeon overlooked almost one hundred years of endoscopic history.

During the late nineteenth century, the development of lenses, lights, and endoscopes allowed doctors to pioneer rudimentary laparoscopic approaches. Over the ensuing decades, these techniques were refined, but it took the invention of miniature computer chip–based cameras in the 1980s to widely open the field. This technologic innovation offered a way to project a magnified view of the operative field onto a large, high-resolution computer monitor, thus freeing the surgeon's hands and facilitating the performance of increasingly complex laparoscopic and thoracoscopic procedures.

Endoscopy rapidly became a central therapeutic measure of surgery. Prior to modern computer technology, it was a surgical approach with few applications; laparoscopy was used mostly by gynecologists for short, simple procedures such as tying

---

* Presently, endoscopy-based minimally invasive surgical procedures are available for a wide variety of conditions in each surgical specialty. For example: **General**—gallbladder, hernias, liver tumors, obesity surgery, pancreatic cancer, and varicose veins; **Cardiothoracic**—heart valves, lung, tumors, and esophageal diseases; **Colorectal**—rectal disease; **Gynecology**—cervical and uterine tumors, endometriosis, ovarian cysts, and hysterectomy; **Neurosurgery**—cervical disc hernias, spinal trauma, and skull base brain tumors; **Orthopedic**—carpal tunnel release, knee ligament repair, and lumbar disc hernias; **Otorhinolaryngology**—head and neck cancers and thyroid tumors; **Plastic**—brow lift, breast augmentation, and abdominoplasty or "tummy tucks"; and **Urology**—bladder tumors, kidney disorders, and prostate cancer. When an endoscopic operation is within the abdominal or pelvic cavities, it is termed "laparoscopy." If the procedure is performed within the chest cavity, then it is referred to as "thoracoscopy."

the fallopian tubes. In 1990, the development of a device to allow the easy passage of various surgical tools, especially clips and staples, through the laparoscope to help ligate bleeding blood vessels and aid in the dissection of tissue made surgeons more comfortable with the concept of laparoscopic cholecystectomies. The early prototype of this equipment was originally devised in Russia and introduced in America in the late 1950s, surrounded by a backstory of Cold War intrigue.

* * *

In 1958, Mark Ravitch, a surgeon at The Johns Hopkins Hospital, was asked to organize a goodwill trip to the Soviet Union sponsored by the United States National Research Council. In Kiev, he was to be apprised of Russian advances in blood banking, but the day's itinerary was altered when it became apparent that the Soviets, despite claims, had nothing to show. Instead, Ravitch's Intourist Russian guide, after an endless stream of "Nyets" regarding other surgical sites, agreed to accompany Ravitch and his group to an institute for chest surgery. There Ravitch encountered something unusual. "I was startled," he recalled, "to see a series of patients who had [portions of their lungs removed] with staples instead of sutures and saw the extraordinary simplicity and efficiency of the instruments."[2]

Ravitch, a seasoned surgeon—he graduated Phi Beta Kappa from the University of Oklahoma and completed medical school and general surgical and cardiothoracic surgical residencies at Johns Hopkins—was unfamiliar with a device that could safely staple together human flesh. The curious surgical instrument fascinated him and he tried to locate a Russian government office in Kiev where he could purchase a stapler, but his search proved fruitless. "I suppose," recalled Ravitch, "it was not unlike what might have happened if one had been at Fort Bragg in 1939 and seen a bazooka and said, 'That looked like a dandy little weapon, and how did one purchase one?'"[3]

Several cities later, Ravitch was dining at a crowded restaurant in Leningrad (presently St. Petersburg) when a young Russian couple asked if they could share the table. The conversation turned to why an American was visiting the country. Ravitch identified himself as a touring surgeon and mentioned that among the things most impressive to him was the stapling device. Serendipity took over as the young man said he was familiar with them and that they were manufactured at a Russian army factory located on the outskirts of the city. When told this, Ravitch recalled that earlier in the day, as he was being driven down Nevsky Prospect, one of Leningrad's main thoroughfares, he spotted a sign with gold Cyrillic letters hanging above a storefront that read: "Surgical Instruments and Apparatus." Ravitch's parents had immigrated from Russia and he was fairly conversant with the language.

An inquisitive Ravitch was puzzled by the presence of a retail business that sold the tools of a profession administered by the Communist government. The next morning, he visited the store and found it was true. They were selling surgical staplers but had only one in stock. "'Is it for sale?' he asked the clerk. 'Yes.' 'Is it for sale for cash?' 'Of course.' 'How much?' '440 rubles.' 'Could I buy it right now?' 'Naturally.' 'We are foreigners,' Ravitch said." The salesperson's reply was straightforward: "What of it?"[4] Ravitch left the store holding a thirteen-inch-long, one-and-a-half-pound metal stapler packaged in a black-velvet-lined birchwood box.

Back in Baltimore with his Cold War trophy, Ravitch demonstrated the stapler to an audience of Hopkins surgeons and started a process that would lead to America's multi-billion-dollar laparoscopic surgical business. Not unlike the initial negative reactions to the discovery of anesthesia and antisepsis, his conservative and cynical colleagues criticized the strange-looking device. They felt that the appliance was an affront to their operative skills. "Well, that's great," remarked one skeptic, "but it looks awfully big and heavy. Besides, I love to sew."[5] The act of suturing requires dexterity and patience and has long been the surgeon's trademark. As Ravitch explained, "Surgeons are proud of their art and reluctant to believe that an automatic instrument can do things as well as they can."[6] The surgical worrywarts warned that if the Russian-designed stapler was useful and supplanted suturing, surgeons would lose their deft finger-work abilities and be unable to manually sew in crucial situations where a stapler was not applicable.

Ravitch was an opinionated and strong-willed curmudgeon. He did not let his colleagues' opposition dissuade him and began to incorporate staplers into his clinical practice. As he thought, the tool helped save time in the operating room and produced results equal to hand-stitched sutures.* Less than a year later, Ravitch

---

* Starting in the 1990s, surgical clips, a sophisticated reconfiguration of staples, were developed (staples penetrate tissue while clips clasp). Most surgical clips and staples are currently made of titanium (absorbable kinds are also available) and, although dozens of these fasteners may be used during a surgical procedure to control bleeding, occlude ducts, or join tissues together, such as intestine, they remain inside the

presented his findings at a conference of leading American surgeons. "The principles involved in this apparatus have been applied to many types of operative procedures," he clarified. "There seems to be reason to believe that some of these instruments and their derivatives will find a permanent place in surgery."[7]

Ravitch found the stapling device so effective that he decided to pitch it to American manufacturing companies in the early 1960s. At first, the companies showed little interest. According to Ravitch, the belief among the manufacturers was that "[a] very special instrument of this kind could never recover the enormous costs involved in its development."[8] However, over the next two decades, the financial incentives for surgical device companies changed and they devoted larger amounts of capital to development, marketing, and research. This occurred as federally sponsored health care programs and the rise of the medical-industrial complex brought about spectacular growth in surgery.

During the 1970s, even after accounting for the large rise in population from the post–World War II baby boom, the number of cardiothoracic operations increased 99 percent, neurosurgery 65 percent, ophthalmology 40 percent, gynecology 32 percent, orthopedic 26 percent, urologic 20 percent, and general surgery 9 percent.[9] By 1980, almost 25 million surgical operations were being completed yearly in the United States. A decade and a half later, the annual growth continued, led by over 2 million cataract extractions and 858,000 cesarean sections.[10]

Surgical staplers appeared ever more appealing to the nation's medical manufacturers as they invested heavily in the new technology. The companies diversified and offered advanced product lines for a wide variety of operations on the abdomen and the chest. One surgical manufacturing company saw its patient base jump from twenty thousand in 1969 to seven hundred thousand a decade later. A reporter for *Time* noted how "American improvements on Russian designs are beginning to

---

patient's body after the operation is completed. Titanium clips and staples are entirely safe for the short and long term and do not interfere with medical examinations such as X-rays and CAT or MRI scans, nor will they trigger any safety devices at airports. The devices are tiny, usually less than a quarter of an inch in size, and do not show signs of decay or rust. The clips and staples are used in a wide variety of surgical operations, including those on delicate tissues such as the brain, heart, joints, and lungs. When titanium fasteners are used inside the body they do not need to be removed and simply become incorporated into the surrounding tissue. When skin is stapled versus hand-sutured (staples used on the skin are slightly larger in size than those used within the body), the staples must be removed. The skin staple remover is a small manual metal device that removes the staples effortlessly and painlessly.

bring automatic suturing into the operating room." According to the journalist, "the machines have already graduated from stitch work repairs to performing some of the most important stages of surgery."[11]

Among the critical new tools was a disposable tubelike device, called a trocar, which a surgeon inserted into a patient's abdomen through a puncture incision. This gadget served as a temporary portal into the body for miniaturized surgical instruments, including clip applicators, graspers, scalpels, scissors, and TV cameras. The internal access to the body's interior provided by this device heralded a new form of surgery and a basic transformation in surgical technique. In response, hospitals constructed operating rooms dedicated to laparoscopy and filled them with expensive state-of-the-art equipment. Corporate and hospital revenues shot up in conjunction with the number of laparoscopic operations. By the end of the 1990s, surgeons were routinely using laparoscopy for appendectomies, colon removals, hysterectomies, and other types of abdominal and pelvic surgery: greater than 90 percent of the 750,000 gallbladder removals performed in America in 2000 involved laparoscopic techniques.

* * *

Among the significant surgical prizes that laparoscopy would claim was the repair of groin or inguinal hernias.* The procedure is one of the most common abdominal operations—over eight hundred thousand a year in the United States alone—and the potential for worldwide profits was enormous. Knowing this, laparoscopic

---

* A hernia occurs when an organ or fatty tissue squeezes through a weak spot in a surrounding muscle or connective tissue of the abdominal wall. The most common types of hernia are inguinal (groin), umbilical (belly button), and incisional (resulting from a weak or poorly healed previous incision). In an inguinal hernia, a portion of either intestine, bladder, or fat protrudes through the abdominal wall into the groin's inguinal canal, where it can then extend into the scrotum. About 95 percent of all groin hernias are inguinal, and most occur in men because of a natural weakness in this area from the passage of the blood vessels and sperm duct that support the testicles. A femoral hernia is a type of groin hernia that occurs predominantly in women, especially those who are pregnant or obese, and occurs when a piece of intestine or fat drops into the upper thigh. In an umbilical hernia, part of the intestine passes through the abdominal wall near a defect in the navel. Umbilical hernias are most common in newborns. In an incisional hernia, the intestine pushes through the abdominal wall at the site of previous abdominal surgery where the incision has weakened or not fully healed. Of all hernias, 80 percent are inguinal or femoral, 5 to 10 percent are umbilical, 5 percent are incisional, and 5 percent are other types.

equipment manufacturers focused their public relations and advertising campaigns on the ubiquitous surgical procedure in an effort to change a century-old operative tradition.

The repair of a groin hernia is often referred to as the raison d'être of the surgeon. The procedure has many variations but, at its most basic, involves strengthening a weakness of the muscles and other soft tissues in the lower abdominal wall. Ravitch, in addition to his work with surgical staplers, was also considered a leading expert on hernia surgery. He remarked: "If no other field were offered to the surgeon for his activity than hernia repair, it would be worthwhile to become a surgeon and to devote an entire life to this service."[12] Ravitch based this observation on the fact that hernia surgery contains all the fundamental elements of a surgical operation: an understanding of functional anatomy; a knowledge of pathophysiology; familiarity with varying techniques of repair; and need for gentle handling and meticulousness in dissecting tissues. Due to the relatively straightforward nature of a hernia operation, surgical mentors favored the procedure as an ideal teaching tool for their novitiates.

The modern repair of groin hernias was first described in the late nineteenth century and variations of this basic technique endured through much of the twentieth century. The approach required general anesthesia, a six-to-eight-inch incision, and numerous tight sutures to close the rent in the groin. Ravitch, along with thousands of other surgeons, advocated for these methods: "It is the simplest operation," he explained, "which will consistently give satisfactory results without extensive dissection."[13]

While the repair was generally effective, it triggered severe discomfort in patients and required a lengthy period of recovery with weeks of disability. The caricature of the postoperative hernia patient in exquisite pain, unable to lift or walk, was part of American culture for decades. Yet surgeons who favored the sutured repair tended to dismiss postoperative discomfort as nothing more than a minor nuisance. According to Ravitch, the most annoying complications were only "hemorrhage . . . , displacement of the testis . . . , [and] infection."[14] Rarely mentioned were discomfort and disability. Ravitch, following a peripatetic career as professor of surgery at Columbia University, Johns Hopkins, the University of Chicago, and the University of Pittsburgh, died in 1989, an unremitted champion of the traditional sutured hernia repair. But for surgeons of his generation, disregard of postoperative difficulties was about to change.

Attitudes about hernia repair and postoperative discomfort and disability began to shift in the late 1980s. Surgeons conceived a new style of hernia repair based on a small incision (three inches in length), local anesthesia, and recovery as an outpatient. Leading the charge was Irving Lichtenstein, a California-based general surgeon who, according to a lengthy obituary in the *New York Times*, "transformed hernia surgery from an operation requiring hospitalization and long recuperation into an uncomplicated outpatient procedure."[15] Unlike many of the individuals who revolutionized aspects of surgical care, Lichtenstein was neither a well-known academician—he had a private surgical practice in Beverly Hills—nor extensively published. What set Lichtenstein apart was his ability to withstand pressure from the surgical establishment while championing bold and innovative surgical ideas.

Lichtenstein studied in Philadelphia at the University of Pennsylvania and Hahnemann Medical School (presently the Drexel University College of Medicine) and moved west to Los Angeles, where he completed a general surgical residency at Cedars of Lebanon Hospital (currently Cedars-Sinai Medical Center). Long active in the American Civil Liberties Union of Southern California, he often hosted receptions in his home for civil rights leaders—including one for the Reverend Martin Luther King Jr., where agents of the Federal Bureau of Investigation warned of a possible assassination attempt. Lichtenstein always enjoyed a good battle. In 1964, he weathered one when he stood in front of a thousand doctors attending the annual convention of the AMA in San Francisco and told them they were treating their hernia patients improperly.

Lichtenstein explained that it was not necessary to perform hernia surgery under general anesthesia, with extensive cutting and sewing, followed by two days of hospitalization and a week of bed rest. Instead, the repair could be completed using local anesthesia with minimal dissection and the patient driving home the next day.[16] Pandemonium broke out. "I was shocked," recalled Lichtenstein. "Physicians were shouting questions at me, criticizing me, challenging me. There was a great deal of confusion."[17] Subsequent developments in hernia surgery led Lichtenstein to routinely use a sterile swatch of inert plastic mesh to reinforce the tissue weakness. The mesh causes little reactivity with the body's immune system and simply becomes encased within a vigorous growth of scar tissue. Although his claims caused a furor, Lichtenstein's beliefs became widespread. By the late 1990s, the minimally invasive, mesh-based, same-day Lichtenstein Hernia Repair was widely praised, and it is now considered one of the gold standard operations due to its low complication rate, mild discomfort, and reduced risk of the hernia's recurring. Later in life, Lichtenstein suffered from severe Parkinson's disease and stopped operating in the mid-1980s; he died in 2000.

The use of mesh and outpatient hernia surgery quickly replaced the sutured repair with its two- or three-day hospital stay and onerous recovery. As mesh-based outpatient hernia repairs gained popularity, laparoscopic equipment makers worked to convince surgeons of the advantages of placing the mesh through a laparoscope. Beginning in the mid-1990s, they barraged doctors with advertising pamphlets and brochures. Salespeople stressed that a laparoscopic hernia repair left barely visible scars and returned an individual to normal activities in a short time. In an era of technologic wonders, it was not surprising that laparoscopic manufacturers steadily increased their market share of hernia repairs. By 2003, surgeons used laparoscopic technique for 15 percent of hernia operations; at present, the number approaches over 60 percent. Whether a laparoscopic or open hernia repair is superior to the other remains an open question.

*　*　*

In 1984, I joined the Lichtenstein bandwagon and abandoned my general surgical practice to concentrate solely on the same-day mesh-based repair of groin hernias. Although my use of mesh differed from Lichtenstein's approach and I employed epidural instead of local anesthesia, for the next two decades—until my retirement from clinical practice in 2004—I was a hernias-only general surgeon. I examined almost eleven thousand patients and performed close to five thousand minimally invasive repairs.[18] I am often asked to explain the rationale behind my decision. Why would I endure eleven years of medical school and surgical residency and limit myself to one operation shortly after the completion of my training? The answer is genuinely simple. My growing interest in studying and writing surgical history had overwhelmed my interest in practicing the whole gamut of general surgery.

More to the point, a rookie general surgeon does not have anything that resembles a fixed schedule, between consultations, emergencies, lengthy operations, and assisting other surgeons in the operating room. I wanted my days to be more flexible so I could immerse myself in reading and researching surgical history. By concentrating only on the elective repair of hernias (an operation that I enjoyed performing), I could easily set my operating schedule and allow ample time for my "outside" activity. Thus, the bottom-line reason I became a hernia surgeon was to provide myself the freedom to better understand the history of my profession—not simply its hagiography but the full breadth of the American surgical experience, from its economics to its operations to its sociologic underpinnings.

Within four years following my decision, I had authored a bibliography of surgery in nineteenth-century America,[19] edited a multi-authored work on the history of surgery in the United States,[20] written a series of history articles for surgical journals,[21] and began research for an illustrated coffee-table book on the evolution of surgery worldwide. I came to understand that the history of surgery remained poorly served by present-day historians.[22] Surgery is an arcane subject and difficult to understand and write about if an author has not lived and worked in surgery's house. Clearly, the boldness and ingenuity with which surgeons approached seemingly unsolvable clinical problems was a stirring, albeit unrecognized, chapter in American and world history.

*   *   *

The advent of robotic surgery is the next stage in the evolution of minimally invasive endoscopic surgery. In contrast to the utilization of robotics in industry, the surgical robot, first introduced in the mid-1990s, does not work autonomously but rather serves as a mechanical interface between surgeon and patient. Robotic technology allows surgeons to perform complex tasks that would exceed their abilities with traditional laparoscopic instrumentation. To use a surgical robot, the knife bearer sits at a console and employs his or her hands and feet to control movement of the robotic instruments within the patient's body. The robot's rods or arms are thinner than conventional laparoscopic equipment. They never tremble and can maneuver and cut and suture in deeper, tighter-fitting areas. Furthermore, laparoscopic surgery generally shows only a two-dimensional image on the computer screen while the robotic camera provides a three-dimensional picture of the surgical area—the surgeon views the site through a stereoscopic viewer attached to a computerized monitor.

Robotic surgery has also brought the idea of telesurgery to the profession. Theoretically, a surgeon can operate on a patient at great distance; trained personnel would still be required on-site to prepare the patient, insert the robot arms, change instruments, and assume charge if complications or unexpected findings occurred that could not be controlled robotically. The notion of long-distance robotic surgery is especially appealing as a method to treat wounded soldiers or to support patients in hostile environments, such as deep-sea exploration, outer space missions, and polar expeditions. Telesurgery remains mostly hypothetical, but robotic surgery systems have become widely used in gynecologic and urologic surgery and, to a lesser extent, in cardiac, general, and otolaryngologic surgery.

While surgical device makers extoll the use of laparoscopic and robot technology, they rarely dwell on the cost of the operation—in part, because it is expensive (having a laparoscopic or robot hernia repair adds several thousand dollars to a hospital bill). For robot surgery, there are specific drawbacks including the bulkiness and setup time for the equipment as well as a paucity of compelling data to demonstrate superiority of robotic operations over laparoscopic procedures. For example, various studies have failed to demonstrate the clinical benefits of robotic surgery over more traditional operative approaches in gallbladder removal, hernia repair, and excision of the large intestine. These concerns also include robotic operations for certain cancer procedures, including cervical malignancy, rectal tumors, and kidney growths.[23]

What equipment manufacturers fail to acknowledge, and surgeons must be aware of, is that by prematurely encouraging the utilization of economically unproven technologies, a company's profits are increased but at the possible expense of patient welfare. As a surgeon noted, "because the robot has been so heavily marketed, I know of instances where there's no real benefit, but surgeons insist on using it, in order to attract patients."[24] Certainly, laparoscopic, robotic, and other technologies will play a crucial role in the ongoing evolution of surgery. However, an emphasis on monetary gain can overshadow a technique's true surgical importance. These misleading values can foster a form of socioeconomic tyranny of surgical technology and create conflicts of interest that pit financial reward against clinical benefit.[25]

*   *   *

Surgery had always been a grand fraternity of men, but starting in the late twentieth century the profession underwent another type of revolution, the large-scale arrival of women as surgeons. The demographic makeover was transformative, although there had been females practicing the art of surgery in Europe and North America long before women started to receive formal medical degrees in the mid-nineteenth century. As far back as the early Middle Ages, so-called surgeonesses had a role in providing surgical services for their households or the poor. As long as these women were not seen as competitors for financial gain and did not appear to be making a substantive living from their surgical practice, they were allowed the autonomy to practice their craft.

With the expansion of the male-dominated Church in the sixteenth century, women were shunted aside and discouraged from practicing any form of surgical therapy. In 1540, when England's Henry VIII granted a charter to the Royal Commonality of Barber-Surgeons, he barred women from joining the organization and accused them of using "Sorceries and Witchcraft" and applying such treatments "unto the Diseased, as they were noyous" (i.e., annoying, vexatious, or harmful).[26] Fifty years later, a charter given to the Barber-Surgeons of Salisbury ordered "that no such woman, or any other, shall take or meddle with any cure of Chirurgery."[27] At the same time, the Barber-Surgeons of London willingly paid for the "arresting of wydowe Ebbes an abuser of the Arte of Surgery."[28] Despite the harassment, women continued to provide surgical care without formal education and training or evidence of personal recognition for the next several centuries.

Even with the advent of modern surgical training at the start of the twentieth century, the road for female surgeons remained difficult. The reasons for this were varied: attitudes from surgical professors who openly declared their aversion to teaching women; concern that women's presence in the profession would lead to declines in the autonomy, earnings, and status of male surgeons; men refusing to be treated by women; parents' reluctance to spend large sums of money to provide daughters a professional education; social expectations for women to be housewives; and societal norms that directed women toward other areas of health care, specifically nursing. Moreover, through the mid-twentieth century, only a handful of women had performed enough operative surgery to become skilled mentors. Without role models and with limited access to hospital positions, the ability of the few practicing female physicians to specialize in surgery seemed an impossibility. And there was the practical nature of surgical intervention. Women and their female "temperament" were not believed to be up to the physical task of opening human flesh. "In the case of a surgical operation," smugly explained a male surgeon:

> The man is satisfied with doing his level best, and if the patient died, he would think it could not have been helped. But a woman would

worry herself over it while operating, and even afterwards, and the consequence is that the next patient suffers also.[29]

Over the years, an occasional woman was admitted to the ACS, but few held any positions of authority or leadership in surgery until the 1970s, when social activists lobbied Congress and sued public institutions to deal with existing systemic discrimination against women. These efforts succeeded, resulting in equal-protection laws that women took advantage of. In 1972, the Title IX Education Amendments of the Higher Education Act banned discriminatory policies in admissions and salaries for any school receiving federal funding. Between 1972 and 1980, medical schools almost doubled the number of females that they accepted, from 15 to 28 percent. By 2005, the number of women entering medical school equaled the number of men.

Currently, females constitute almost 40 percent of the slightly more than 1 million active physicians in America. However, they make up less than 20 percent of surgeons. Although women are increasingly represented in surgery, the profession remains a male-dominated field. Moreover, there is a gender imbalance within the surgical specialties, ranging from a high in obstetrics/gynecology to a low in orthopedics. In 2020, the approximate numbers of active surgeons in the United States were:

Specialty	Total # of surgeons	Total # of Female surgeons
Obstetrics/Gynecology	43,000	25,000 (58%)
Ophthalmology	20,000	5,000 (25%)
General	26,000	5,400 (21%)
Otolaryngology	10,000	1,800 (18%)
Plastic	7,500	1,275 (17%)
Urology	10,000	900 (9%)
Neurological	6,000	500 (8%)
Cardiothoracic	4,750	375 (8%)
Orthopedic	20,000	1,200 (6%)

Despite inroads at the top of Medicine, in academic roles and policy-making circles, women still have a minority presence. Progress toward gender equality in surgery has been slow, although females have begun to assume leadership positions in most key surgical organizations. If one individual can be cited for encouraging women to enter the world of American surgery it was Olga Jonasson, a pioneer in the field of clinical transplantation. In 1987, when she was named chair of the department of surgery at Ohio State University College of Medicine, Jonasson became the first woman in the United States to head an academic surgery department—presently, there are approximately twenty-five women who hold such a position. "The decisions of the surgeon as team leader are final," she explained, "and men have simply been unwilling to accept women in that role of the all-powerful decision maker."[30]

Jonasson attended the University of Illinois College of Medicine where she also completed a general surgical residency. She followed this with surgical fellowships in transplantation immunobiology at the Walter Reed Army Institute of Research and Massachusetts General Hospital. More than anything, in educating and training surgical residents Jonasson showed that setting an example of aptitude and responsibility was more than important; it was the only thing that counted. Following her retirement from clinical practice, she served as Director of Education and Surgical Services at the ACS. Jonasson died from lymphoma in 2006.

Only four decades ago, the idea of a woman who chose to become a physician, let alone a surgeon, was viewed as a strange, if not aberrant, decision. For someone like Jonasson, to attain positions of leadership, she confronted prejudices that did not exist for her male counterparts. Today, biases that hinder women's progress—many still endure—are the only abnormal things about a female's place in the profession of surgery. The plain fact is that with over 50 percent of today's medical school students being women, it is imperative that female students be encouraged to become surgeons and allowed to rise to top academic and clinical leadership positions. Only in this way can the profession help the next generation of surgeons establish a culture of gender equity in the workplace.

*   *   *

During the 1970s, the dramatic rise in numbers of surgical procedures, coupled with the emergence of a strong consumers' movement, led to questions of over-usage of operations and concerns about the quality of surgical health care in America. Through these years, researchers documented significant numbers of fatal errors in surgical operations, large disparities in access to surgical care, and noticeable differences in surgical outcomes among institutions. As socioeconomic concerns assumed greater relevance, articles on the question of unnecessary surgery appeared throughout the lay press and in government publications and scientific journals.

Three reports were especially troubling and instigated fundamental changes in the manner in which surgeons evaluated and treated their patients. A 1973 article in the widely respected journal *Science* demonstrated extreme geographic variations in the per capita use of nine common surgical procedures dependent on the number of surgeons in an area.[31] The second report showed that the United States had twice as many surgeons per capita as England and twice the number of operations performed per population.[32] These two papers provided support to the concept that American surgeons performed surgery according to their own financial needs. It was construed that a portion of surgical procedures in the United States were completed solely for remunerative purposes, which would deem them unnecessary. The third report detailed an investigation that concerned presurgical screening consultations, commonly termed "second opinion programs."[33] By having a patient, previously recommended for elective surgery, undergo a second surgical opinion, it was found that almost one-quarter of surgical procedures cleared by one surgeon were not confirmed by the second surgeon.

The reaction to the third paper was overwhelming and centered on purported cost savings that could be realized by decreasing elective surgical rates through mandatory second opinion programs. In response, the federal government established an around-the-clock toll-free telephone hotline to answer questions and direct patients to a second opinion program. Medicare required that second opinions be obtained from a board-certified surgeon before any patient could be confirmed for elective surgery. At the state level, the nation's Blue Cross Blue Shield plans instituted compulsory second opinion consultations for their insured populations.

In early 1976, as socioeconomic pressures mounted, the matter of second opinion programs and unnecessary surgery was taken up in a congressional study, *Cost and Quality of Health Care: Unnecessary Surgery*. The conclusions staggered the nation's surgeons:

> [S]econd consultations before surgery can cut down on unnecessary surgical procedures . . . surgical payments by the fee-for-service mechanism encourage surgery in questionable situations . . . unnecessary surgery has deleterious effects upon the American public . . . there

were approximately 2.4 million unnecessary surgeries performed in 1974 at a cost to the American public of almost $4 billion, and . . . these unnecessary surgeries led to 11,900 deaths last year.[34]

At the same time, a five-part series of front-page articles in the *New York Times* featured sensational accusations of unnecessary and incompetent surgery:

> The American surgical profession, which is probably the best trained in the world, contains a number of unethical, incompetent and careless practitioners. . . . [There are] far more doctors doing surgery than are needed and too many new surgeons being trained each year, with the likely result that at least some surgeons "make work" for themselves by doing operations that are unnecessary.[35]

Despite a steady stream of unparalleled clinical triumphs, the closing decades of the twentieth century and the swirling questions of unnecessary surgery and inept surgeons were a confusing time for the nation's knife bearers. In an era of political and socioeconomic change, developments outside the surgeon's world appeared to endanger the profession's control of its own organization and standards of clinical judgment. Matters were even more confounded when the results of a five-year effort to investigate the delivery, financing, and organization of surgical services; ethical and legal issues; government relations; interprofessional relations; societal-surgeon relations; surgical manpower; and surgical research were released. The *Study on Surgical Services for the United States*, sponsored in part by the ACS, was intended to be the most introspective analysis in which any segment of American Medicine had engaged. It was massive in scope with over ten thousand surgeons questioned concerning their practice routines and work schedules. In addition, an in-depth analysis of surgery in four diverse geographic areas of the country was completed on another twenty-seven hundred surgeons. The three-volume, 2,782-page report was issued in the spring of 1976.

The findings were startling. Data on surgical manpower and workloads showed that one-half of the nation's surgeons carried out fewer than four operations per week. The conclusion was obvious; surgeons' operative work was more modest than originally thought. It was suggested that the number of surgical training programs be reduced and identified more closely with university centers. In addition, a recommendation called for the sum of individuals entering surgical practice to be decreased.

The unanticipated results were corroborated by other independent studies. In turn, these prompted stronger recommendations, closely paralleling those of the *Study on Surgical Services*, based on the assumption that costly and specialized surgical skills in the United States were underutilized. As proposals to place constraints on surgical manpower became louder, the research and recommendations of the *Study on Surgical Services* were soon questioned by—of all authorities—the ACS, its own parent. "Unreliable data such as those cited in the *Study on Surgical Services for the United States*," wrote an official of the College, "provide a poor basis for manpower estimates or for advanced planning."[36] Amid professional bitterness, Francis Moore, of kidney transplant fame and a lead editor of the *Study on Surgical Services*, viewed the supposed surgical surplus and question of unnecessary surgery as realistic problems that needed to be faced squarely "rather than adopting the juvenile view that surgeons are such wonderful people that one can never imagine a situation in which there are actually too many of them."[37]

Despite the fanfare associated with its publication, within twelve months of its release the *Study on Surgical Services* was an orphan in the world of surgical politics, disowned by its creator, and rendered incapable of having an impact on American surgery.* Why the surgical establishment refused to endorse the major findings of its

---

* The *Study on Surgical Services* is forgotten, but its section on "surgical research contributions" contains fascinating material for historians of surgery. Surgeons were asked to identify the most important advances made in their area of expertise during the twenty-five-year period from 1945 to 1970. The importance of each contribution was determined by reviewing scientific journals and seeking the opinions of board-certified surgical experts, using as a directive the applicability of a research contribution to the care of patients and the diagnosis and treatment of disease (M. J. Orloff, "Identification of Important Contributions of Surgical Research to Health Care from 1945 to 1970," in *Surgery in the United States: A Summary Report of the Study on Surgical Services for the United States*, 3 vols. [Chicago: American College of Surgeons & American Surgical Association, 1976], 2:1443–1497). Among the research contributions that general surgeons deemed important were: cardiopulmonary resuscitation using compression of the chest wall for cardiac arrest; effect of hormones on cancer; hemodialysis; intravenous feeding; kidney transplantation; replacement of arteries by synthetic grafts; surgery for peptic ulcer disease; and topical chemotherapy of burns. Among the other surgical specialties, neurosurgeons selected the use of shunts to relieve hydrocephalus along with the development of stereotactic surgery, a form of minimally invasive intervention that uses a three-dimensional coordinate system to locate small targets inside the brain. Orthopedic surgeons chose total hip replacement; urologists listed ileal conduits, a system of urinary

own study is cloaked in almost five decades of obscurity. However, in the 1970s, the issues that swirled around surgical manpower and the calls to decrease the number of the country's surgeons ran counter to established beliefs that there were not too many knife bearers but too many "other" individuals (i.e., non-board-certified surgeons and non–surgically trained general practitioners) who performed surgery. By the late 1990s, the concern had faded away. More than 95 percent of surgery completed in the United States was being done by board-certified surgeons. This occurred primarily due to: an expanding number of board-certified surgeons entering practice; increased strictness of hospital credentialing that required surgeons to have board certification; the inability of individuals to obtain surgical malpractice insurance unless they were board-certified in a surgical specialty; and the intensifying complexity of surgical operations that necessitated specialized residency education and training.

In addition, through death and retirement the older group of general practitioners—who viewed common surgical operations, especially gallbladder removal, repair of hernias, and tonsillectomy, as within their clinical purview—was decreasing in size. The natural attrition also came at a time when fewer than 10 percent of American medical school graduates were entering general practice. Generalists had a serious dilemma with few alternatives. Their competency was questioned, patients abandoned them, hospitals revoked their admitting privileges, and young doctors ignored them. General practitioners would have to redefine themselves or go extinct. They employed a timeless strategy: if you can't beat them, join them. Ironically, it was a path that would lead to their becoming specialists.

In 1947, a group of general practitioners organized the American Academy of General Practice. Through the years, leaders tried to persuade the rank and file that an association with the Academy equaled board certification. However, general practitioners found that the true litmus test for professionalism in Medicine after World War II was actual board certification; they would never be accepted as specialists without an "official" board certificate. In 1969, the American Board of Family Practice was organized as the nation's twentieth recognized medical and

---

drainage that uses a short segment of the small intestine to replace a bladder that has been removed; otorhinolaryngologists selected surgery for conductive deafness; ophthalmologists designated retinal laser photocoagulation, a procedure employed to treat leaking blood vessels in the retina as well as sealing retinal tears; and pediatric surgeons singled out combined therapy involving chemotherapy, radiation, and surgery for Wilms's tumor (aka nephroblastoma), the most common type of kidney cancer in children. An appendix in the study provides an extensive history of each research contribution (2:1687–2016).

surgical specialty: the longtime label of "general practitioner" was replaced with a new moniker, "family practitioner." By the standards of the Medical establishment and government and lay criteria, the field of family practice was officially a specialty.

The awarding of board certificates to family practitioners was a watershed event in the process of professionalization in America. From medical education through clinical practice, the concept of specialization triumphed as patients increasingly sought medical and surgical care from specialists. For surgeons, the organization of the American Board of Family Practice had special significance. In its formation, the Board eschewed surgery as part of the education and training of family practitioners. After centuries of professional disagreements over who had the right to practice surgery, family practitioners no longer competed for surgical patients.

Although family practitioners do not perform surgical operations, surgeons face a new form of competition brought on by a remarkable transformation in how American society views knife bearers and other physicians who work with their hands. For almost four millennia, stretching back to the time of Hammurabi of Babylon, lesser respect was accorded surgeons based on the principle that they were baser individuals who dirtied themselves by using their hands, in contrast to dutiful physicians.

Currently, the surgical profession is at a crossroads where innovation and socioeconomics have begun to influence the surgeon's conventional role of working with one's hands and the nature of who and what constitutes a scalpel wielder. In the past, technologic advances, whether Paré's development of ligatures and forceps to control bleeding during an amputation or Lister's discovery of antisepsis, led to increases in the complexity, extent, and number of surgical operations. Now progress in technology brings about fewer and tinier operations as high-tech surgical devices are further miniaturized and refined.

The shrinking number of open surgical operations reflects a sea change in the variety of possible procedures as many are replaced by nonsurgical treatments (aka minimally invasive interventional procedures). Moore termed the specialty fields that encroach on the areas previously occupied by surgeons as "almost surgical practice,"[38] exemplified by today's interventional cardiologists, gastroenterologists, and radiologists. For example, the treatment of arteriosclerotic heart disease by coronary artery bypass surgery has markedly decreased due to the development of stenting procedures to open up clogged arteries, while the removal of certain types of gallstones, previously accomplished through a large open incision, is achieved with an endoscope passed through the mouth into the duodenum.

In addition to interventional therapies, Moore's definition should also include other traditionally nonsurgical specialties that now employ the term "surgeon" in their training programs, such as "dermatologic surgeon." The reality is that for many patients, the best treatment often involves a combination of surgical procedures and nonsurgical interventions, but the rapid development of imaging technologies, mechanical devices, and types of therapies has led to ambiguity regarding a specialty's claim on techniques and treatments.

During these beginning years of the twenty-first century, the impact of technologic advances and socioeconomic factors has changed the deep-rooted definition of surgery and surgeons. The line-in-the-sand demarcation between surgical and nonsurgical treatments, and what surgeons do and what nonsurgeons do, has become an indistinct border. One thing is certain: the four-thousand-year-old prejudicial attitude against surgeons and working with one's hands no longer applies. In a reversal of long-held beliefs, doctors who work with their hands, surgeons and nonsurgeons alike, are now widely admired and encouraged in their activities. These individuals represent state-of-the-art American Medicine and will increasingly shape the future of health care. The surgeons and physicians who work with their hands are the beneficiaries of society's approbation and financial recompenses.

*　　*　　*

I conclude my history of surgery with a reemphasis of two points. First, the most remarkable story in the history of surgery is how modern surgery has decisively become an indispensable branch of Medicine for helping people live healthy and longer lives. For thousands of years, surgery was impotent in the face of serious disease. From the Greeks and Romans to World War I, surgery's tasks were straightforward: contend with lethal diseases, physical infirmities, and wound management. However, surgeons performed these with minimal success, which often left patients wary of the surgeon's scalpel. Today the opposite is true. Few in the industrialized world escape having an illness that does not call for a surgeon's know-how. The ease and safety of modern surgery has changed the lives of billions of human beings.

Second, throughout its evolution, the art of surgery has been largely characterized by its tools and the manual aspects of the craft. It is clear that the impact of recent technologic change on the surgical profession, notably the miniaturization of its tools and the minimization of the invasiveness of procedures, is an advance that is as significant as any in surgery's evolution. It is also apparent that progress in technology has altered the definition of surgery and who performs it. As developments unfold, surgeons will reinvent themselves in a manner that affects their professional identity and redefines their profession's limits and its capabilities. The possibilities are endless, especially with the advent of artificial intelligence, innovative automation, and surgical robots. One hundred years from now, a "surgeon," perhaps one already born as life expectancies lengthen, will relate the history of surgery. Of course, the closing decades of their story will depend on how much the world of Medicine maintains room for those who work with their hands. After all, according to *The Oxford English Dictionary*, that is ultimately the definition of a surgeon: "One who practices the art of healing by manual operation."[39]

20.
PROSPECTS

I am just laboring in the vineyard. I am at the operating table, and I make my rounds. I believe there is a cross-fertilization between writing and surgery. If I withdraw from surgery, I would not have another word to write. Having become a writer makes me a better doctor.

Richard Selzer, quoted in the *New York Times*,
September 28, 1979, page C24

Narrative history is easiest to compose when the primary story has a recognizable ending. However, the history of surgery in America and worldwide has no such finish and attempting to predict tidy conclusions about its future is a Sisyphean task. Nevertheless, five thousand years of recorded history provide some insights about where surgery has been and where it may go. If the study of surgical history offers any lesson, it is that progress can always be expected, at least relative to the technology of a given era, and will lead to increasingly sophisticated surgical operations with better results. For example, in the present era, artificial intelligence and automation will undoubtedly robotize the surgeon's hand for a vast number of surgical procedures. Even with this type of radical transformation, the surgical sciences still retain a recognition of their historical roots as fundamentally a manually based art and craft.

Such a reflection and understanding of the past is important because the relationship that surgeons have to the history of their field is vastly different from other professions. The architect finds inspiration in Greek and Roman aesthetics. The engineer looks to structural designs from the nineteenth century to better understand the construction of bridges and buildings. The lawyer follows a chain of case law that dates back hundreds of years.

For the surgeon, there is little of practical value before the 1930s, a time that is a rough turning point between premodern and modern surgery. The advances after that era have not come without political and socioeconomic costs. These social dilemmas often dwarf clinical triumphs, and this suggests that going forward, the surgeon's most difficult challenges may not be in the clinical realm but, instead, in better understanding the cultural forces that affect the practice of surgery. Indeed, recent decades mark the beginnings of a schizophrenic existence for surgeons: newly devised complex and lifesaving operations are met with innumerable accolades, while criticisms of the economic and social aspects of surgery portray the surgeon as an egocentric financially driven individual.

Although this perspective appears counterintuitive, the dramatic and theatrical features of surgery—which make surgeons conquerors and heroes from one perspective and symbols of greed and mendacity from the opposite point of view—are the very reasons why society demands so much of them. There is the definitive and precise nature of surgical intervention, the expectation of success that surrounds every operation, the short time frame in which outcomes are realized, the high income levels of surgeons, and the inquisitiveness of lay individuals about every aspect of consensually cutting into another human's flesh. These truths, ever more sensationalized in this age of instantaneous communication with mass media and social media, make surgeons seem more accountable than their medical colleagues and emblematic of the best and worst in American Medicine.

For knife bearers, surgery has become an arena of trade-offs, a balance between costs, expectations, organization, and technology. There is no denying that surgeons bring huge responsibilities to the care of patients: scalpel wielders can cause irreparable harm or astonishing miracles with one slice of their blade. However, the rise of new technologies brings a slew of additional concerns, not the least of which is ensuring that the public understands the devices are intended to extend the capabilities of surgeons, not to replace them. Likewise, surgeons must not alienate or distance themselves from patients. The human element of a surgeon's touch remains an essential ingredient in the surgical care of another human being. Treating patients with empathy and understanding will ensure that a surgeon's services are irreplaceable in the coming age of artificial intelligence and robotics.

Much as surgeons will have to change their attitudes and perceptions, patients have to confront the reality that no matter how advanced surgery becomes, it cannot solve all the health-related problems in life. The public grows frustrated not only with these administrative and financial difficulties but also because modern surgery has fostered a gap between expectations and realities. Surgeons, in their embrace of science, learned to cure numerous common ailments and created an impression that surgery had many answers. However, society will need to come to terms with where ethical lines should be drawn on everything from face transplants to robotized surgery to gene therapy for surgical diseases. The ultimate question remains: How can the interface of ethics, science, and surgery be brought together in the gray area between individual rights and the greater good?

The optimistic outlook is that surgery will overcome many of the challenges it currently faces. Imagine walking into a superspecialized surgeon's office—there will be hybrid surgical specialties, novel surgical specialties, and surgical subspecialties, all with cross-fertilization—and deposit samples of blood, feces, hair, saliva, and urine. One hour later, you receive a printout of your surgical needs matched to your genetic profile. You are also handed a vial with digestible computer chips—genomic testing is expected to be central to the future of surgery—which will wirelessly relay your genetic reports to surgeons who could be thousands of miles away.

This team of knife bearers will have diagnostic tools that dwarf current technologies. Body scanners in the future will not only have greater resolution and higher magnification, but they will also measure biochemical activity in tissues and correlate it with changes in an organ's anatomy, all the way down to the cellular level. Imagine an "intelligent" surgical cautery/scalpel where an electrical current heats tissue to make an incision with minimal blood loss while the instrument contains a futuristic miniature mass spectrometer that analyzes the vaporized tissue/smoke to detect cellular elements coming from the incision. This new "smart" scalpel will be able to identify whether tissue is malignant and inform a surgeon where to dissect in real time, contrasted with waiting for the results of a tissue biopsy.

Once your surgical team processes this diagnostic information, they will have a myriad of startling clinical options available. Gene therapy will allow them to replace the faulty genes that cause surgical illnesses at the most basic of cellular building blocks. Genetic-based therapies will take the place of many operative treatments, including the repair of bodily malformations and the treatment of chronic surgical problems. In cases where operations are necessary, such as organ transplantations and trauma, robotic surgery will handle much of the burden. Robots will perform procedures that require greater-than-human precision, including face transplants and the replacement of body parts once thought impossible.

Surgical robots can dramatically increase an operation's precision, but the real breakthrough will come with entirely autonomous robots in the operating rooms. Because human surgical performance is dictated by numerous mental, physical, social, and technical variables, surgical consistency is difficult to both qualify and quantify. Current surgical robots possess clear advantages over humans (i.e., not affected by fatigue, more precise movement, and resistant to tremor), which have been shown to produce higher success rates and lower mortality figures for certain procedures. In the future, Artificial Intelligence (AI) combined with the advantages of surgical robots may further maximize surgical practice by completely removing or greatly reducing the potential for human error.

Political, scientific, and socioeconomic issues will act as a catalyst for further development and refinement of autonomous AI surgical robots. Such devices will allow the rapid dissemination of surgical skills via the Internet or other mobile platforms, making surgical care available to all and standardizing surgical outcomes apart from geographic and socioeconomic constraints. A clinically capable AI surgical robot will be able to deliver care in environments where surgeons are not found, for example, aboard a spacecraft rocketing to Mars or in war zones where danger lurks. All of this will probably take decades, if not centuries, to achieve, but it seems a surety that completely autonomous AI-based machine surgeries will be part of mankind's future.

The three-dimensional bio-printing of organs is also expected to play a key role in surgery. This involves layering living cells on top of each other to eventually create an artificial living tissue. Since this process creates tissues and organs derived from the cells of the patient requiring a transplant, it eliminates the likelihood of rejection and the need for lifelong immunosuppressive drugs. The availability of three-dimensional bio-printed organs might bring about a shift from requiring human participants in research trials and end experimentation on animals. The accessibility of three-dimensional printing and other simulation techniques will aid in the planning of complicated and risky surgeries. Surgeons have already printed a full-sized three-dimensional replica of the heart of an infant born with a congenital defect. They were then able to strategize on how to best perform an extremely complicated surgical operation on the tiny heart. The newborn survived with little to no lasting ill effects.

There will be novel training tools, including augmented reality, which adds digital elements to a live view or virtual reality with its complete immersion experience that shuts out the physical world. These distinctive features (i.e., augmented reality users do not lose touch with reality, while virtual reality puts information into an individual's eyesight and brain as fast as possible) have a huge potential in assisting surgeons to become more adept at surgeries. Augmented reality-backed surgical operations can help surgeons visualize the three-dimensional anatomy of a patient during surgery; it is as if the knife bearer had X-ray vision with great accuracy, safety, and operating efficiency. In the same way, virtual reality can elevate the teaching and learning experience in surgery to a whole new level, replacing the need of surgeons-to-be to peek over a surgeon's shoulder during an operation. In fact, surgeons have begun to stream operations using virtual reality that allowed observers to "be in" the operating room using their virtual reality goggles. These tools will offer greater standardization in surgical residencies and let inexperienced surgeons train remotely and rehearse procedures in a controlled and safe environment.

If what I've written sounds like a Jules Verne adventure novel, a report that I read recently (July 15, 2021) from the *New England Journal of Medicine* should remove any doubts that the previously impossible will not become possible.[1] Researchers described an approach that combined a brain-computer interface and machine learning models that allowed them to generate text from the electrical activity of a patient's brain paralyzed due to a stroke and unable to speak. It was literally the reading of one's mind. The incredible is fast becoming imaginable in the surgeon's world; it is just a matter of time before surgery will be performed on the brain with real-time feedback coming from the brain itself about how the procedure is going.

Much of this inventiveness will require new learning curves and bring additional challenges and complexities to becoming a surgeon. There are the concerns related to the implementation of this technology. The regulation of data and protection of a patient's privacy will demand new guidelines and governance. The ethics of artificial intelligence and the autonomy of machines will bring unforeseen issues around their use. Who will be responsible for the action of fully or partially autonomous artificially intelligent surgical systems? Surgeons? Regulators? The public?

Of course, this is a picture of future life divorced from the realities of contemporary problems. New ideas might encourage better care that is coordinated and efficient or worse care that is bloated and superfluous. All of these futuristic biotechnologies—cellular scanning, gene therapies, nanotechnology, robotic surgeries, three-dimensional printing of organs, wireless surgical monitoring—will cost much more than the most sophisticated treatments we have currently. Policymakers will have to implement measures to curb runaway health inflation for these surgical breakthroughs if they are to become commonplace. Certainly, some advanced surgical procedures with prohibitive costs will be available only to the rich in wealthier countries. This will force poorer populations to do things the old-fashioned way, without robots and virtual reality and three-dimensional printing. Such inequities will need to be addressed and surgeons must be in the forefront of the decision-making.

If history teaches us anything, it is that surgery will advance and grow inexorably. Americans will be best served to face the economic, political, and social challenges of present-day surgery head-on while acknowledging that it is impossible to predict where the future of surgical science will lead us. The surgical crystal ball is a cloudy one at best. To study the fascinating history of my profession, with its magnificent personalities and outstanding scientific achievements, may not necessarily help us accurately predict the future of surgery. However, to understand surgery's past does shed some light on current and future clinical practices.

If scalpel wielders in the future wish to be regarded as more than mere technicians, then members of the profession need to better appreciate the value of its past glories. It is hardly necessary to dwell on the heuristic value that an appreciation of history provides in encouraging adjunctive humanistic, literary, and philosophic tastes. I would argue that, for a surgeon, the study of surgical history makes the everyday learning process more pleasurable and provides constant invigoration. To trace the evolution of what one does on a daily basis and understand it from a historical perspective is an enviable goal. To study the humanities and social sciences as they relate to surgery provides more than just valuable preparation for an empathetic bedside manner. An appreciation of anthropology, art, history, literature, philosophy, et cetera, sheds light on healing and suffering. Recall that ancient and early modern thinkers believed that Medicine was not entirely divergent from theology or the philosophic study of nature and the physical universe: imbalances in the physical body or its external environment disturbed the soul and brought about illness.

For younger surgeons, it is a magnificent adventure to appreciate what they are learning within the context of past cultural and socioeconomic institutions. The older practitioner will find that to study the history of their profession affords a ready escape from the mental stagnation that can accompany the ennui of decade upon decade of a busy and smothering clinical practice. In reality, there is no way to separate present-day surgery and one's own practice from the experiences of all the surgeons and all the years that have passed. I firmly believe that if surgery was taught with a greater emphasis on an appreciation of the profession's history, knife bearers would be better situated to cope with the clinical problems they face daily.

The public and the profession must study surgery's history and appreciate its past and not allow its rich heritage to be forgotten. More than ever, to understand surgery's story is an invitation to learn and marvel. It is an invitation no individual, be they patient, surgeon, or otherwise, should turn down.

ACKNOWLEDGMENTS

Few works on history stand alone and *Empire of the Scalpel* draws guidance and inspiration from a four-millennia body of writing on surgery's story. Beginning with Hammurabi's *Code* through works by Nuland, hundreds of authorities (as listed in the Bibliography, Notes, and References) are acknowledged for their research and thoughts on this fascinating topic.

In 1997, I first spoke with Eric Simonoff. He is a literary agent extraordinaire. A decade later, I began to work with Colin Harrison, an editor who stands above all others. Without their counsel and persuasion this project (as well as others) would not have seen the light of day. I thank Barbara Wild, the copyeditor, and Jason Chappell, the production editor, for their efforts as well as members of the marketing and publicity departments at Scribner. I especially want to acknowledge Emily Polson, Colin's assistant, who is a cheery voice at the other end of the Internet and telephone.

I give countless thanks to some dear friends: Laurie and Larry Sussman, who provide balance and cheer to my sometimes-erratic writing schedule; Jill and Al Sommer are always there and special gratitude to Al for his review of the manuscript; Jane and David Oshinsky, for their interest and encouragement; Diane and Harvey Ruben, whose steadfastness and steadiness are welcomed; Sue and Ray Helfand, who keep me laughing; and Dennis Meyers, a lifelong friend. Finally, to Barbara and Jimmy Kusisto, Eric Carlson, and Apple Hotaling, for ensuring that everything works.

To my immediate family, you are the glue of my life. To my wonderful wife, Beth, you are special and without your love and support I would accomplish little. To my daughter, Lainie, her husband, Adam, their amazing child, Alex; and my son, Eric, his wife, Elizabeth, and incredible little Benjamin, your inspiration illuminates my every thought.

NOTES

Author's Note

1. T. G. Weiser, A. B. Haynes, G. Molina, et al., "Size and Distribution of the Global Volume of Surgery in 2012," *Bulletin of the World Health Organization* 94 (2016): 201–209.

Chapter 1. Genesis

1. C. H. W. Johns, *The Oldest Code of Laws in the World: The Code of Laws Promulgated by Hammurabi, King of Babylon B.C. 2285–2242* (Edinburgh: T. & T. Clark, 1903), v.

2. Ibid., 45–46.

3. J. H. Breasted, *The Edwin Smith Surgical Papyrus*, 2 vols. (Chicago: University of Chicago Press, 1930), 1:xiii.

4. Ibid.

5. J. P. Allen, *The Art of Medicine in Ancient Egypt* (New York: Metropolitan Museum of Art, 2005), 75.

Chapter 2. Exodus

1. F. H. Garrison, *An Introduction to the History of Medicine* (Philadelphia: W.B. Saunders, 1914), 66.

2. F. Adams, *The Genuine Works of Hippocrates*, (London: Sydenham Society, 1849), 2:475–476.

3. N. Arikha, *Passions and Tempers: A History of the Humours* (New York: Ecco, 2007), 308.

Chapter 3. Prolific Pens

1. Celsus, *Celsus on Medicine*, books 7–8, with an English translation by W. G. Spencer, 3 vols. (Cambridge, MA: Harvard University Press, 1938), 3:295.

2. V. Robinson, "Galen and Greek Medicine," *Medical Review of Reviews* 18 (1912): 778–779.

3. A. J. Brock, *Greek Medicine: Being Extracts Illustrative of Medical Writers from Hippocrates to Galen* (London: J.M. Dent & Sons, 1929), 158.

4. Galen, *Galen on the Usefulness of the Parts of the Body*, 2 vols., trans. Margaret T. May (Ithaca, NY: Cornell University Press, 1968), 1:119.

5. Quoted in C. Gill, T. Whitmarsh, and J. Wilkins, *Galen and the World of Knowledge* (Cambridge: Cambridge University Press, 2009), 295.

Chapter 4. Darkness, Then Daylight

1. F. Adams, *The Seven Books of Paulus Aegineta*, 3 vols. (London: Sydenham Society, 1844), 1: xviii, xix.

2. M. S. Spink and G. L. Lewis, *Albuscasis on Surgery and Instruments* (Berkeley: University of California Press, 1973), 2.

3. P. Prioreschi, *A History of Medicine*, 6 vols., *Medieval* (Omaha, NE: Horatius Press, 2003), 5:287.

4. J. F. Malgaigne, *Surgery and Ambroise Paré*, translated from the French by Wallace B. Hamby, M.D. (Norman: University of Oklahoma Press, 1965), 36–37.

5. T. C. Allbutt, "The Historical Relations between Surgery and Medicine," *British Medical Journal* 2 (1904), 790.

6. Ibid.

7. Quoted in L. M. Zimmerman and I. Veith, *Great Ideas in the History of Surgery* (Baltimore: Williams & Wilkins, 1961), 138–139.

Chapter 5. The Human Road Map

1. Quoted in R. Porter, *The Greatest Benefit to Mankind: A Medical History of Humanity* (New York: W. W. Norton, 1997), 202.

2. Quoted in T. Dormandy, *The Worst of Evil: The Fight against Pain* (New Haven: Yale University Press, 2006), 92–93.

3. Ibid., 175–176.

4. J. B. de C. M. Saunders and C. D. O'Malley, *The Illustrations from the Works of Andreas Vesalius of Brussels* (Cleveland: World Publishing Company, 1950), 14.

5. A. Vesalius, *On the Fabric of the Human Body: A Translation of De Humani Corporis Fabrica Libri Septem*, book 1, *The Bones and Cartilages*, trans. William F. Richardson and John B. Carman (San Francisco: Norman, 1998), liii–liv.

6. Ibid., xlvii–l.

Chapter 6. To Stop the Flow

1. J. Malgaigne, *Surgery and Ambroise Paré*, trans. W. B. Hamby (Norman: University of Oklahoma Press, 1965), 397, 402.

2. Quoted in A. H. Buck, *The Growth of Medicine from the Earliest Times to about 1800* (New Haven: Yale University Press, 1917), 509.

3. A. Paré, *The Workes of That Famous Chirurgion, Ambrose Parey, translated out of Latine and compared with the French*, trans. Tho Johnson (London: Th. Cotes and R. Young, 1634), 767.

4. Quoted in Buck, *The Growth of Medicine*, 502–503.

5. R. Walsh, E. Littell, and J. J. Smith, "From the Retrospective Review, the Workes of That Famous Chirurgion, Ambrose Parey," *Museum of Foreign Literature and Science* 10 (1827): 160–161.

6. Quoted in S. Paget, *Ambroise Paré and His Times, 1510–1590* (New York: G.P. Putnam's Sons, 1897), 36.

7. Quoted in F. R. Packard, *Life and Times of Ambroise Paré* (New York: Paul B. Hoeber, 1921), 175.

8. A. Paré, *La Méthode de Traicter les Playes Faictes par Hacquebutes* (Paris: Chés viuant Gaulterot, 1545), 2.

9. Paré, *The Workes of That Famous Chirurgion*, "To the Reader."

10. Quoted in Packard, *Life and Times of Ambroise Paré*, 186, 189.

11. Quoted in Paget, *Ambroise Paré and His Times*, 173–174.

12. Quoted in ibid., 191.

13. Quoted in ibid., 202.

14. Quoted in Malgagnie, *Surgery and Ambroise Paré*, 305.

Chapter 7. The Circle

1. D. Power, *William Harvey* (London: T. Unwin Fisher, 1897), 26–27.

2. J. Aubrey, *'Brief Lives,' Chiefly of Contemporaries, Set Down by John Aubrey between the Years 1669 & 1696*, vol. 1, *A–H*, ed. Andrew Clark (Oxford: Clarendon Press, 1898), 301–302.

3. W. Harvey, *An Anatomical Dissertation upon the Movement of the Heart and Blood in Animals, Being a Statement of the Discovery of the Circulation of Blood*, trans. G. Moreton (Canterbury, UK: privately printed, 1894), 49.

4. W. Munk, *The Roll of the Royal College of Physicians of London, Comprising Biographical Sketches*, vol. 1 (London: By the College, Pall Mall East, 1878), 136.

Chapter 8. Emergence

1. J. H. Reveille-Parise, *Lettres de Guy Patin* (Paris: Chez JB Baillière, 1846), 2:327–328.

2. J. A. Le Roi, *Journal de la Santé du Roi Louis XIV, de l'Année 1647 a l'Année 1711* (Paris: August Durand, 1862), 171.

3. Ibid., 395.

4. Ibid., 401.

5. Ibid., 402.

6. Louis XIV, *Déclaration du Roy portant que les démonstrateurs établis au Jardin tinueront leurs leçons et exercises . . . 20 Janvier, 1673*, 5.

7. J. F. Blondel, *Architecture Françoise, ou Recueil des Plans, Elevations, Coupes et Profils*, 4 vols. (Paris: Charles-Antoine Jombert, 1752), 2:87.

8. J. W. D. Maury, "The Department of Surgery," *Columbia University Quarterly* 11 (1908–1909): 163.

9. G. Brice, *Description nouvelle de la Ville de Paris*, 2 vols. (Paris: Nicholas le Gras, 1698), 2:179–180.

10. F. Quesnay, *Memoires de l'Academie Royale de Chirurgie* (Paris: Charles Osmont, 1743), xxxii–xxxiii.

11. Louis XV, "Declaration du Roy," quoted in *Recherches Critiques et Historiques sur l'Origine, sur les Divers Etats et sur les Progrés de la Chirurgie en France* (Paris: Charles Osmont, 1744), 521.

12. *Memoirs of the Royal Academy of Surgery, at Paris: Containing a Great Variety of Cases*, translated from the original (London: E. Cave, 1750), xx.

13. J. F. South, *Memorials of the Craft of Surgery in England* (London: Cassell, 1886), 253.

14. "Our Great Ones of the Past: Men of the British School; William Cheselden, F.R.S.," *Medical Times and Gazette* 314 (1856): 424.

15. W. Cheselden, *The Anatomy of the Human Body*, 5th ed. (London: William Bowyer, 1740), 333–334.

16. T. Gataker, trans., *The Operations in Surgery of Mons. Le Dran* (London: C. Hitch & R. Dodsley, 1749), 472–473.

Chapter 9. Transition

1. Quoted in S. Paget, *John Hunter, Man of Science and Surgeon* (London: T. Fisher Unwin, 1897), 27.

2. F. T. Ranson, *Men and Events in Surgery* (n.p.: private printing, n.d.), 65.

3. Paget, *John Hunter*, 27.

4. D. Ottley, *The Life of John Hunter, F.R.S.* (London: Longman, Rees, Orme, Brown, Green & Longman, 1835), 29.

5. Ibid., 31–32.

6. Quoted in S. D. Gross, *Lives of Eminent American Physicians and Surgeons of the Nineteenth Century* (Philadelphia: Lindsay & Blakiston, 1861), 359.

7. Paget, *John Hunter*, 87–89.

8. J. Hunter, *A Treatise on Venereal Disease* (London: private printing, 1786), 327.

9. Paget, *John Hunter*, 150.

10. E. J. Wood, *Giants and Dwarfs* (London: Richard Bentley, 1868), 158.

11. Ibid., 159.

12. M. S. Guttmacher, "John Hunter and His Friends," *Bulletin of the Johns Hopkins Hospital* 45 (1929): 32.

13. Quoted in J. A. Bondeson, *A Cabinet of Medical Curiosities* (New York: W. W. Norton, 1997), 195–196.

14. Wood, *Giants and Dwarfs*, 163.

15. Paget, *John Hunter*, 120.

16. Quoted in J. Dobson, *John Hunter* (Edinburgh: E. & S. Livingstone, 1969), 344.

Chapter 10. Pain-Free

1. F. Burney, letter dated March 22, 1812, from Frances Burney to her sister, Esther, in the Henry W. and Albert A. Berg Collection, New York Public Library, New York.

2. P. Huguet, *The Consoling Thoughts of St. Francis de Sales* (Dublin: M. H. Gill & Son, 1877), 217–218.

3. A. Velpeau, quoted in N. P. Rice, *Trials of a Public Benefactor, As Illustrated in the Discovery of Etherization* (New York: Pudney & Russell, 1859), 81.

4. H. Davy, *Researches, Chemical and Philosophical; Chiefly Concerning Nitrous Oxide, or Dephlogisticated Nitrous Air, and Its Respiration* (London: J. Johnson, 1800), 556.

5. H. Bigelow, "A History of the Discovery of Modern Anaesthesia," in Edward Clarke, Henry Bigelow, Samuel Gross, et al., *A Century of American Medicine, 1776–1876* (Philadelphia: Henry C. Lea, 1876), 80.

6. *Hartford Daily Courant*, December 10, 1844, 3.

7. J. M. Riggs, quoted in M. E. Soifer, "Historical Notes on Horace Wells," *Bulletin of the History of Medicine* 9 (1941): 109.

8. R. Hodges, *A Narrative of Events Connected with the Introduction of Sulphuric Ether into Surgical Use* (Boston: Little, Brown, 1891), 12.

9. H. Wells, *A History of the Discovery of the Application of Nitrous Oxide Gas, Ether, and Other Vapors, to Surgical Operations* (Hartford: J. Gaylord Wells, 1847), 6.

10. W. M. Cornell, "Letter to the Editor," *Medical and Surgical Reporter* 11 (1864): 326.

11. H. Wells, quoted in Rice, *Trials of a Public Benefactor*, 145.

12. Quoted in Hodges, *A Narrative of Events*, 30–31.

13. Quoted in J. Wales, *Discovery by the Late Dr. Horace Wells, of the Applicability of Nitrous Oxyd Gas, Sulphuric Ether and Other Vapors, in Surgical Operations, Nearly Two Years before the Patented Discovery of Drs. Charles T. Jackson and W.T.G. Morton* (Hartford: Elihu Geer, 1852), 49.

14. Quoted in E. Warren, *The Life of John Collins Warren, M.D. Compiled Chiefly from His Autobiography and Journals*, 2 vols. (Boston: Ticknor & Fields, 1860), 1:381.

15. Quoted in "William Thomas Green Morton, Inventor and Revealer of Anaesthetic Inhalation," *Industrial News* 2 (1881): 114.

16. J. C. Warren, "Inhalation of Ethereal Vapor for the Prevention of Pain in Surgical Operations," *Boston Medical and Surgical Journal* 35 (1846): 376.

17. *Boston Daily Journal*, October 17, 1846, 2.

18. H. O. McCrillis, "The Conquest of Pain," *New England Magazine* 38 (1908): 252.

19. H. J. Bigelow, "Insensibility during Surgical Operations Produced by Inhalation," *Boston Medical and Surgical Journal* 35 (1846): 309, 317.

20. Quoted in R. Reynolds, "A Lay Sermon," *British Medical Journal* 2 (1895): 915.

21. M. J. Morton, "Memoranda Relating to the Discovery of Surgical Anesthesia, and Dr. William T.G. Morton's Relation to This Event," *Post-Graduate* 20 (1905): 337.

22. Quoted in J. R. V. Barker, *The Brontës* (London: Weidenfeld & Nicolson, 1994), 519.

23. "Insensibility during Surgical Operations, by Inhalation," *New York Journal of Medicine* 8 (1847): 122.

24. "Insensibility during Surgical Operations Produced by Inhalation," *Medical Examiner* 2 (1846): 720.

25. W. H. Atkinson, "Discussion of Anaesthesia," *Transactions of the Dental Society of the State of New York*, minutes of the tenth annual meeting, (1878): 44.

26. W. T. Smith, "On the Utility and Safety of the Inhalation of Ether," *Lancet* 1 (1847): 378.

27. "The War—from a Correspondent," *Lancet* 2 (1854): 223.

28. G. A. Otis and D. L. Huntington, "Anaesthetics," in *The Medical and Surgical History of the War of the Rebellion*, part 3 (Washington, DC: Government Printing Office, 1883), 2:887.

29. H. H. Smith, *A System of Operative Surgery: Based Upon the Practice of Surgeons in the United States* (Philadelphia: Lippincott, Grambo, 1852), 22.

30. "Prizes Awarded by the French Academy for 1847 and 1848," *Boston Medical and Surgical Journal* 42 (1850): 278–279.

31. Quoted in Hodges, *A Narrative of Events*, 128.

32. *New York Times*, November 15, 1858, 2.

Chapter 11. They're Alive

1. J. Bell, *The Principles of Surgery, As They Relate to Wounds, Ulcers, and Fistulas*, 3 vols. (London: Longman, Hurst, Rees, Orme, and Brown, Paternoster-Row; and Cadell and Davies, Strand, 1815), 1:655–658.

2. Z. Hertzveld, "Remarks on Some Appearances of Cases in So Called Purulent Poisoning of the Blood," *Monthly Journal of Medical Science* 7 (1847): 702.

3. T. S. Wells, "Some Causes of Excess Mortality after Surgical Operations," *British Medical Journal* 2 (1864): 386.

4. R. J. Godlee, *Lord Lister* (London: Macmillan, 1917), 14.

5. R. Liston, quoted in R. Reynolds, "A Lay Sermon," *British Medical Journal* 2 (1895): 915.

6. Quoted in Godlee, *Lord Lister*, 16.

7. J. R. Leeson, *Lister As I Knew Him* (London: Baillière, Tindall & Cox, 1927), 58.

8. C. E. Douglas, "Reminiscences of 'the Chief,'" In *Joseph, Baron Lister, Centenary Volume, 1827–1927*, ed. A. L. Turner (London: Oliver and Boyd, 1927), 148–149.

9. R. H. Russell, "Reminiscences of 'the Chief,'" in Turner, *Joseph, Baron Lister*, 157.

10. J. Stewart, "Reminiscences of 'the Chief,'" in Turner, *Joseph, Baron Lister*, 143.

11. F. M. Caird, "Reminiscences of 'the Chief,'" in Turner, *Joseph, Baron Lister*, 138.

12. G. T. Wrench, *Lord Lister, His Life and Work* (London: T. Fisher Unwin, 1913), 8.

13. Stewart, "Reminiscences," 143.

14. Quoted in Wrench, *Lord Lister*, 35.

15. T. Gibson, "Lister–the Man," *Queen's Quarterly* 34 (1926): 432.

16. Quoted in Wrench, *Lord Lister*, 82.

17. J. Lister, "On a New Method of Treating Compound Fracture, Abscess, Etc., with Observations on the Conditions of Suppuration," *Lancet* 1 (1867): 327.

18. J. Lister, "Illustrations of the Antiseptic System of Treatment in Surgery," *Lancet* 2 (1867): 669.

19. A. Jacobi, "Proceedings of Societies, Medical Society of the County of New York, Stated Meeting, March 1, 1869," *New York Medical Journal* 9 (1869): 159.

20. "Professor Lister in Germany," *Lancet* 2 (1875): 868.

21. S. Gross, "A Century of American Surgery," *American Journal of the Medical Sciences* 142 (1876): 483.

22. Quoted in Jacobi, "Proceedings of Societies," 156.

23. "Letter from Philadelphia," *Boston Medical and Surgical Journal* 95 (1876): 369.

24. Ibid., 366.

25. T. E. Satterthwaite, "The Present Condition of the Evidence concerning 'Disease-Germs,'" in *Transactions of the International Medical Congress of Philadelphia, 1876*, ed. John Ashhurst (Philadelphia: printed for the Congress, 1877), 1028.

26. W. Canniff, "Discussion on Dr. Hodgen's paper," in Ashhurst, *Transactions of the International Medical Congress of Philadelphia*, 532.

27. F. H. Hamilton, "Discussion on Dr. Hodgen's paper," in Ashhurst, *Transactions of the International Medical Congress of Philadelphia*, 532.

28. J. Lister, "Section on Surgery," in Ashhurst, *Transactions of the International Medical Congress of Philadelphia*, 537.

29. Ibid.

30. "Meeting of the International Medical Congress," *Boston Medical and Surgical Journal* 95 (1876): 327.

31. "Letter from Philadelphia," 367.

32. R. Kinloch, "Discussion on Dr. Hodgen's Paper," in Ashhurst, *Transactions of the International Medical Congress of Philadelphia*, 533.

33. R. Weir, "Discussion on Dr. Hodgen's Paper," in Ashhurst, *Transactions of the International Medical Congress of Philadelphia*, 534.

34. A. Howe, "International Medical Congress," *Eclectic Medical Journal* 36 (1876): 481.

35. "Letter from Philadelphia," 366.

36. T. E. Satterthwaite, "Discussion on Mr. Lister's Address," in Ashhurst, *Transactions of the International Medical Congress of Philadelphia*, 542.

37. G. Shrady, "The New York Hospital," *Medical Record* 13 (1878): 113.

38. J. Lister, "The Antiseptic Method of Dressing Open Wounds, a Clinical Lecture," *Medical Record* 11 (1876): 695.

39. Ibid., 696.

40. H. Cameron, *Joseph Lister, the Friend of Man* (London: William Heinemann, 1949), 117.

41. Quoted in Wrench, *Lord Lister*, 393.

42. G. Shrady, "Antiseptic Surgery," *Medical Record* 15 (1879): 206.

43. Quoted in L. M. Zimmerman and I. Veith, *Great Ideas in the History of Surgery* (Baltimore: Williams & Wilkins, 1961), 466–467.

44. "Antiseptic Surgery," *Lancet* 2 (1875): 597.

45. A. Flaneur, "Antiseptic Surgery," *Lancet* 1 (1878): 36.

46. Quoted in Wrench, *Lord Lister*, 519.

47. Quoted in R. B. Fisher, *Joseph Lister, 1827–1912* (New York: Stein and Day, 1977), 294.

Chapter 12. Scientific Progress

1. W. Welch, "In Memoriam—William Stewart Halsted," *Bulletin of the Johns Hopkins Hospital* 36 (1925): 38.

2. J. S. Billings, "American Inventions and Discoveries in Medicine, Surgery, and Practical Sanitation," in *Annual Report of the Board of Regents of the Smithsonian Institution, Showing the Operations, Expenditures, and Condition of the Institution to July, 1892* (Washington, DC: Government Printing Office, 1893), 618.

3. W. G. MacCallum, *William Stewart Halsted, Surgeon* (Baltimore: Johns Hopkins Press, 1930), 23.

4. W. S. Halsted, "The Training of the Surgeon," *Bulletin of the Johns Hopkins Hospital* 15 (1904): 271.

5. Welch, "In Memoriam," 37.

6. Quoted in MacCallum, *William Stewart Halsted*, 42.

7. Quoted in ibid., viii.

8. W. Halsted, "Practical Comments on the Use and Abuse of Cocaine; Suggested by Its Invariably Successful Employment in More Than a Thousand Minor Surgical Operations," *New York Medical Journal* 42 (1885): 294.

9. W. Burket, *Surgical Papers by William Stewart Halsted*, 2 vols. (Baltimore: Johns Hopkins Press, 1924), 1:167.

10. P. Olch, "William S. Halsted and Local Anesthesia: Contributions and Complications," *Anesthesiology* 42 (1975): 483.

11. S. Flexner and J. Flexner, *William Henry Welch and the Heroic Age of American Medicine* (New York: Viking, 1941), 159.

12. B. M. Bernheim, *The Story of the Johns Hopkins: Four Great Doctors and the Medical School They Created* (New York: Whittlesey House, 1948), 20.

13. H. Cushing, *The Life of Sir William Osler*, 2 vols. (Oxford: Clarendon Press, 1925), 1:325.

14. Quoted in J. S. Rankin, "William Stewart Halsted: A Lecture by Dr. Peter D. Olch," *Annals of Surgery* 243 (2006): 424.

15. Halsted, "Training," 273.

16. Ibid., 272.

17. G. F. Shrady, "American Achievements in Surgery," *The Forum* 17 (1894): 170–171.

Chapter 13. The Shock of Technology

1. H. H. Grant, "Amputation of the Breast for Malignant Disease," *American Practitioner and News* 13 (1892): 399.

2. W. C. Röntgen, "On a New Kind of Rays," *Science* 3 (1896): 230.

3. H. Cattell, "Application of the X-rays to Surgery," *Science* 3 (1896): 345.

4. M. H. Richardson, "The Practical Value of the Roentgen Ray in the Routine Work of Surgical Office Practice," *Medical News* 69 (1896): 686.

5. E. F. Stevens, *The American Hospital of the Twentieth Century* (New York: Architectural Record, 1921), 106.

6. C. Seiler, *Handbook of the Diagnosis and Treatment of Diseases of the Throat, Nose, and Naso-Pharynx* (Philadelphia: Henry C. Lea's Son, 1883), 23.

7. T. Maijgren, quoted in "New York, Meeting—April 1921," *Transactions of the Illuminating Engineering Society* 16 (1921): 70.

8. G. F. Shrady, "American Achievements in Surgery," *The Forum* 17 (1894): 167–178.

9. E. H. Pratt, "A Surgical Talk upon the Orifices of the Body." *The Medical Era* 3 (1886): 268–269.

10. S. D. Gross, *A System of Surgery; Pathological, Diagnostic, Therapeutic, and Operative*, 2 vols. (Philadelphia: Blanchard & Lea, 1859), 1:434.

11. *New York Times Magazine*, January 2, 1916, 9.

12. G. Crile, *George Crile: An Autobiography*, 2 vols. (Philadelphia: J. B. Lippincott, 1947), 1:37.

13. F. H. Martin, *The Joy of Living: An Autobiography*, 2 vols. (Garden City, NY: Doubleday, Doran, 1933), 1:462.

14. G. W. Crile, *Hemorrhage and Transfusion: An Experimental and Clinical Research* (New York: D. Appleton, 1909), 535.

15. L. Pilcher, "The Influence of War Surgery upon Civilian Practice," *Transactions of the American Surgical Association* 37 (1919): 12.

16. Crile, *George Crile*, 1:302.

17. I. M. Rutkow, "The Letters of William Halsted and Erwin Payr," *Surgery, Gynecology & Obstetrics* 161 (1985): 81–82.

18. V. Vaughan, "The Promotion of Periodic Health Examinations by the Medical Profession," *American Medical Association Bulletin* 16 (1923): 297.

19. Editorial, "An Artist in Surgery," *New York Times*, January 8, 1943, 19.

Chapter 14. Mass Appeal

1. S. S. Bishop, *Diseases of the Ear, Nose, and Throat and Their Accessory Cavities* (Philadelphia: F. A. Davis, 1901), 407.

2. *Physical Defects: The Pathway to Correction* (New York: American Child Health Association, 1934), 80–96.

3. J. G. Mumford, *The Practice of Surgery* (Philadelphia: W.B. Saunders, 1910), 17.

4. M. Tinker, "America's Contribution to Surgery," *Johns Hopkins Hospital Bulletin* 13 (1902): 212.

5. R. H. Fitz, "Perforating Inflammation of the Vermiform Appendix; with Special Reference to Its Early Diagnosis and Treatment," *Transactions of the American Association of Physicians* (1886): 135.

6. S. H. Adams, "Modern Surgery," *McClure's Magazine* 24 (1905): 484.

7. R. T. Morris, *Fifty Years a Surgeon* (New York: E. P. Dutton, 1936), 183.

8. J. Deaver, "Appendicitis," *Philadelphia Medical Journal* 10 (1902): 21.

9. S. Lewis, *Arrowsmith* (New York: Harcourt, Brace, 1925), 210.

10. F. L. Stanton, *Songs from Dixie Land* (Indianapolis: Bobbs-Merrill, 1900), 91.

11. Workers Health Posters, *Public Health Reports* 59 (1944): 1414.

12. W. Osler, *The Principles and Practice of Medicine* (New York: D. Appleton, 1895), 440.

13. "Valentino Stricken; Goes under Knife," *New York Times*, August 16, 1926, 1.

14. "Valentino Rallies; Crisis in Three Days," *New York Times*, August 17, 1926, 1.

15. "Surgeon Explains Valentino's Death," *New York Times*, September 4, 1926, 3.

16. "Valentino Better; Passes the Crisis," *New York Times*, August 20, 1926, 2.

17. "Valentino Sinking; Second Crisis Near; Pleurisy Spreads," *New York Times*, August 23, 1926, 1.

18. Ibid.

19. Editorial, "Death of Valentino and Yellow Journalism," *The Nation*, September 8, 1926, 207.

20. "Thousands in Riot at Valentino Bier," *New York Times*, August 25, 1926, 1.

21. H. Lilienthal, "Resection of the Lung for Suppurative Infections with a Report Based on 31 Operative Cases in Which Resection Was Done or Intended," *Annals of Surgery* 65 (1922): 257.

22. W. Meyer, "Anesthesia in Differential Pressure Chambers, Cabinets, and Other Apparatus for Thoracic Surgery," in *Surgery, Its Principles and Practice*, 8 vols., ed. W. W. Keen (Philadelphia: W.B. Saunders, 1913), 6:955.

23. Quoted in E. D. Churchill, "Evarts Graham, Early Years and the Hegira," *Annals of Surgery* 136 (1952): 5.

24. "Death of a Surgeon," *Time*, March 18, 1957, 42.

25. T. B. Ferguson, "Evarts A. Graham, M.D.: The Father of Chest Surgery," *Outlook Magazine*, Autumn 1981, 5.

26. L. Brock, "Evarts A. Graham," *Annals of Thoracic Surgery* 9 (1970): 278.

27. Ferguson, "Evarts A. Graham," 8.

28. "Death of a Surgeon," 42.

29. "Brainman," *Time*, April 17, 1939, 38.

30. "A Family of Doctors," *New York Times*, June 24, 1934, "Editorials," 4.

31. "Dr. Cushing's Diary of Lights and Shadows in the War." *New York Times*, May 24, 1936, Book Review, 5.

32. H. Cushing, "The Special Field of Neurological Surgery after Another Interval," *Archives of Neurology and Psychiatry* 4 (1920): 611–612.

33. Quoted in I. M. Rutkow, "The Unpublished Letters of William Halsted and Harvey Cushing," *Surgery, Gynecology & Obstetrics* 166 (1988): 371.

34. Ibid., 373.

35. Ibid., 374.

36. H. Cushing, "The Special Field of Neurological Surgery: Five Years Later," *Bulletin of the Johns Hopkins Hospital* 21 (1910): 339.

37. H. Cushing, *From a Surgeon's Journal* (Boston: Little, Brown, 1934), 197.

38. Ibid.

39. E. G. Reid, *The Great Physician: A Short Life of Sir William Osler* (London: Oxford University Press, 1931), 290.

40. J. F. Fulton, *Harvey Cushing: A Biography* (Springfield, IL: Charles C. Thomas, 1946), 590.

Chapter 15. Professionalization

1. W. Rogers, *Ether and Me, or "Just Relax"* (New York: G. P. Putnam's Sons, 1929), 22.

2. H. Bowditch, "Report of Committee on Medical Ethics," *Transactions of the American Medical Association* 19 (1868): 91.

3. *Code of Ethics of the American Medical Association, Adopted May 1847* (Philadelphia: T.K. and P.G. Collins, 1848), 15–16.

4. J. Homberger, *Batpaxomyomaxia: A Fight on "Ethics"* (New Orleans: private printing, 1869), 17.

5. H. H. Smith, *A System of Operative Surgery: Based upon the Practice of Surgeons in the United States: And Comprising a Bibliographical Index and Historical Record of Many of Their Operations, during a Period of Two Hundred Years* (Philadelphia: Lippincott, Grambo, 1852), xxiii.

6. A. E. Hertzler, *The Horse and Buggy Doctor* (New York: Harper & Brothers, 1938), 27.

7. N. S. Davis, "Address on the Present Status and Future Tendencies of the Medical Profession in the United States," *Journal of the American Medical Association* 1 (1883): 38.

8. D. H. Storer, "Presidential Address," *Transactions of the American Medical Association* 17 (1866): 64.

9. Quoted in T. Bonner, *The Kansas Doctor: A century of pioneering* (Lawrence: University of Kansas Press, 1959), 68.

10. C. Herrick, *Railway Surgery: A Handbook on the Management of Injuries* (New York: William Wood, 1899), 3.

11. R. H. Reed, "Railway Surgery—Its Present Status and Importance," *Railway Age and Northwestern Railroader* 18 (1893): 522.

12. F S D, "The Missouri Pacific Hospital at St. Louis," *Railway Surgeon* 3 (1897): 514.

13. Herrick, *Railway Surgery*, 17.

14. F. H. Davenport, "Specialism in Medical Practice; Its Present Status and Tendencies," *Boston Medical and Surgical Journal* 145 (1901): 82.

15. B. Holmes, "The Hospital Problem," *Journal of the American Medical Association* 47 (1906): 320.

16. L. Davis, *Fellowship of Surgeons: A History of the American College of Surgeons* (Springfield, IL: Charles C. Thomas, 1960), 444.

17. F. Martin, *The Joy of Living: An Autobiography*, 2 vols. (Garden City, NY: Doubleday, Doran, 1933), 1:330.

18. Davis, *Fellowship of Surgeons*, 3.

19. Martin, *Joy*, 1:397.

20. Ibid., 398.

21. Ibid., 404.

22. *Philadelphia Inquirer*, November 11, 1911, 1.

23. Martin, *Joy*, 1:409.

24. Anon., "Editorial, The American College of Surgeons," *Journal of the Michigan State Medical Society* 12 (1913): 338.

25. Martin, *Joy*, 1:414.

26. P. Jones, "The American Royal College of Surgeons-J.B.M.," *California State Journal of Medicine* 11 (1913): 176.

27. Martin, *Joy*, 1:445.

28. "Hospital Standardization," *Bulletin of the American College of Surgeons* 6 (1922): 3.

29. Ibid.

30. W. Shepherd, "The New Control of Surgeons," *Harper's Magazine*, February 1924, 303, 311.

31. H. Daniel, "Better Hospitals for Everybody," *The World's Work*, June 1920, 208.

32. J. Dodson, "The Fifth, or Intern, Year," *Journal of the American Medical Association* 73 (1919): 471–472.

33. Council on Medical Education and Hospitals, "Hospitals Furnishing Acceptable Internships," *Journal of the American Medical Association* 75 (1920): 409.

34. Council on Medical Education and Hospitals, "Hospitals Approved for Advanced Internships and Residencies," *Journal of the American Medical Association* 88 (1927): 828.

35. Quoted in J. Barr, "The Education of American Surgeons and the Rise of Surgical Residencies, 1930–1960," *Journal of the History of Medicine and Allied Sciences* 73 (2018): 12.

36. Quoted in P. Olch, "Evarts A. Graham, the American College of Surgeons, and the American Board of Surgery," *Journal of the History of Medicine and Allied Sciences* 27 (1972): 252.

37. E. Graham, "What Is Surgery?," *Southern Medical Journal* 18 (1925): 865.

38. E. Archibald, "Address of the President—Higher Degrees in the Profession of Surgery," *Annals of Surgery* 102 (1935): 481.

39. Quoted in Olch, "Evarts A. Graham," 257.

40. I. M. Rutkow, "William Stewart Halsted and the Germanic Influence on Education and Training Programs in Surgery," *Surgery, Gynecology & Obstetrics* 147 (1978): 602–606; I. M. Rutkow, "William Halsted and Theodor Kocher: 'An Exquisite Friendship,'" *Annals of Surgery* 188 (1978): 630–637; I. M. Rutkow "Valentine Mott (1785–1865), the Father of American Vascular Surgery: A Historical Perspective," *Surgery* 85 (1979): 441–450; I. M. Rutkow, "William Halsted and Rudolph Matas: Their Unique Alliance," *Surgery* 87 (1980): 524–538; I. M. Rutkow, "The Letters of William Halsted and Anton von Eiselsberg," *Archives of Surgery* 115 (1980): 993–1001; I. M. Rutkow, "The Letters of

William Halsted and Alexis Carrel," *Surgery, Gynecology & Obstetrics* 151 (1980): 676–688; I. M. Rutkow, B. G. Rutkow, and C. B. Ernst, "Letters of William Halsted and Rene Leriche: 'Our Friendship Seems So Deep,'" *Surgery* 88 (1980): 806–825.

Chapter 16. The Blood of War

1. F. G. Slaughter, *The New Science of Surgery* (New York: Julian Messner, 1946), 3.

2. B. A. Schneider, "The New Science of Surgery," *Quarterly Review of Biology* 22 (1947): 95.

3. R. Shryock, *American Medical Research, Past and Present* (New York: Commonwealth Fund, 1947), 293.

4. "Penicillin Saves Flier on First Use in Rumania," *New York Times*, September 11, 1944, 6.

5. P. H. Long, "Medical Progress and Medical Education During the War," *Journal of the American Medical Association* 130 (1946): 984.

6. W. Mauldin, *Up Front* (New York: Henry Holt, 1945), 37.

7. "Medical Officers Get Point System," *New York Times*, August 10, 1945, 16.

8. B. Fantus, "The Therapy of the Cook County Hospital," *Journal of the American Medical Association* 109 (1937): 128.

9. "Blood Transfusion Betterment Association," *Bulletin of the New York Academy of Medicine* 6 (1930): 682.

10. "Plans Are Laid to Get Blood for British," *New York Times*, August 12, 1940, 18.

11. "19 Members of Family Donate Blood to Britain," *New York Times*, December 17, 1940, 6.

12. D. Stetten, "The Blood Plasma for Great Britain Project," *Bulletin of the New York Academy of Medicine* 17 (1941): 29.

13. Ibid., 33.

14. Ibid., 36.

15. Quoted in S. Love, *One Blood: The Death and Resurrection of Charles R. Drew* (Chapel Hill: University of North Carolina Press, 1996), 104.

16. Ibid., 124.

17. Ibid., 105.

18. Ibid., 120.

19. J. Scudder, "Practical Genetic Concepts in Modern Medicine," *Journal of the National Medical Association* 51 (1959): 267.

20. D. Bull and C. Drew, "Symposium on Fluid and Electrolyte Needs of Surgical Patients: The Preservation of Blood," *Annals of Surgery* 112 (1940): 501.

21. Quoted in Love, *One Blood*, 149.

22. Stetten, "The Blood Plasma," 37.

23. Quoted in D. B. Kendrick, *Medical Department, United States Army, Surgery in World War II, Blood Program in World War II* (Washington, DC: Office of the Surgeon General, 1964), 102.

24. Quoted in Love, *One Blood*, 152.

25. Quoted in Charles R(ichard) Drew, *Current Biography Yearbook* (New York: H.W. Wilson, 1944), 180.

26. "Red Cross Bans Negro Blood!," *Cleveland Call & Post*, December 27, 1941, 1.

27. "Red Cross Rejects Negro Blood Donors," *PM*, December 22, 1941, 10.

28. G. Brooks, "Negro Hero (to Suggest Dorie Miller)," *Common Ground* 5 (1945): 45.

29. J. E. Rankin, "Labeling of Blood Banks," *Appendix to the Congressional Record* (Washington, DC: Government Printing Office, 77th Congress, 2nd session, [May 28,] 1942), 88[9]: A1985.

30. Quoted in Love, *One Blood*, 165.

31. Ibid., 169.

32. Quoted in D. L. Nahrwold and P. J. Kernahan, *A Century of Surgeons and Surgery: The American College of Surgeons, 1913–2012* (Chicago: American College of Surgeons, 2012), 127.

33. Quoted in M. Fishbein, *A History of the American Medical Association, 1847 to 1947* (Philadelphia: W.B. Saunders, 1947), 742.

34. A. D. Bevan, "The Over-crowding of the Medical Profession," *Journal of the American Association of Medical Colleges* 11 (1936): 377–384.

35. *New York Times*, March 31, 1944, 23.

36. C. R. Drew, "Negro Scholars in Scientific Research," *Journal of African American History* 35 (1950): 135–136.

Chapter 17. The Center of Things

1. "Major Operation to Save a Life Put on Network TV for First Time," *New York Times*, June 11, 1952, 1.

2. Ibid., 20.

3. Ibid.

4. "March of Medicine," *Variety*, June 18, 1952, 33.

5. "Doctors Say President Can Run; Condition 'Most Satisfactory'; Hospital Stay Is Put at 15 Days," *New York Times*, June 10, 1956, 1.

6. "Surgeon Relates Operation Story," *New York Times*, June 10, 1956, 1.

7. "Johnson Is 'Doing Well' after 2-Hour Operation to Remove Gall Bladder," *New York Times*, October 9, 1965, 1.

8. "Two Operations for the Price of One," *Life*, October 29, 1965, 104.

9. S. Paget, *The Surgery of the Chest* (Bristol, UK: John Wright, 1896), 121.

10. E. E. Derby, *The Iliad of Homer Rendered into English Blank Verse* (London: John Murray, 1865), 2:23.

11. H. C. Dalton, "Stab Wound of Pericardium—Resection of Rib—Suture of Pericardium—Recovery," *St. Louis Medical and Surgical Journal* 68 (1895): 164.

12. D. H. Williams, "Stab Wound of the Heart and Pericardium—Suture of the Pericardium—Recovery—Patient Alive Three Years Afterward," *Medical Record* 51 (1897): 439.

13. Ibid., 437.

14. Quoted in "Dwight Harken, 83, the Pioneer of Surgery on the Heart, Is Dead," *New York Times*, August 29, 1993, 36.

15. "13 GI's Still Alive with 'Fatal' Hurts," *New York Times*, April 29, 1945, 19.

16. D. E. Harken and A. C. Williams, "Foreign Bodies in and in Relation to the Thoracic Vessels and Heart," *American Journal of Surgery* 72 (1946): 80–90.

17. J. H. Gibbon Jr., "The Development of the Heart-Lung Apparatus," *American Journal of Surgery* 135 (1978): 608.

18. Ibid., 609.

19. Ibid., 615.

20. J. H. Gibbon Jr., "The Development of the Heart-Lung Apparatus," *Review of Surgery* 27 (1970): 236.

21. "The Last Field," *Time*, September 26, 1949, 42.

22. Quoted in S. Johnson, *The History of Cardiac Surgery, 1896–1955* (Baltimore: Johns Hopkins Press, 1970), 149.

23. Quoted in A. Romaine-Davis, *John Gibbon and His Heart-Lung Machine* (Philadelphia: University of Pennsylvania Press, 1991), 121.

24. "Heart's Job Done by New Apparatus," *New York Times*, May 8, 1953, 31.

25. "Historic Operation," *Time*, May 18, 1953, 48.

26. Editorial, "Machine Hearts," *New York Times*, May 10, 1953, section 4, 10.

27. J. H. Gibbon Jr., "The Development of the Heart-Lung Apparatus," 239.

28. "Surgery's New Frontier," *Time*, March 25, 1957, 66–77.

29. "Heart Surgery," *Variety*, May 14, 1958, 40.

30. J. A. Younger, "Open Heart Surgery," *Appendix to the Congressional Record* (Washington, DC: Government Printing Office, 104th Congress, 2nd session, [July 28,] 1958), 104[12]: A6746.

31. I. M. Rutkow, "Thoracic and Cardiovascular Operations in the United States, 1979 to 1984," *Journal of Thoracic and Cardiovascular Surgery* 92 (1986): 184.

Chapter 18. Out with the Old

1. The Nobel Assembly at Karolinska Institute, The Nobel Prize in Physiology or Medicine 1990 Press Release, www.nobelprize.org/prizes/medicine/1990/press-release.

2. T. Starzl, *The Puzzle People: Memoirs of a Transplant Surgeon* (Pittsburgh: University of Pittsburgh Press, 1992), 71.

3. "The Best Hope of All," *Time*, May 3, 1963, 60.

4. Ibid., the cover.

5. F. D. Moore, *A Miracle and a Privilege: Recounting a Half Century of Surgical Advance* (Washington, DC: Joseph Henry Press, 1995), 19.

6. "The Best Hope," 58.

7. Moore, *A Miracle*, 155.

8. "A Pair of Life Savers," *Time*, October 22, 1990, 62.

9. T. Starzl, "Joseph E. Murray, MD, FACS, Opened Doors for Transplant Surgeons," *Bulletin of the American College of Surgery* 98 (2013): 63.

10. Moore, *A Miracle*, 166.

11. F. D. Moore, *Transplant: The Give and Take of Tissue Transplantation* (New York: Simon & Schuster, 1972), 84.

12. J. Merrill, J. Murray, J. H. Harrison, and W. R. Guild, "Successful Homotransplantation of the Human Kidney between Identical Twins," *Journal of the American Medical Association* 160 (1956): 278.

13. Moore, *Transplant*, 100.

14. Ibid.

15. Quoted in J. Fenster, *Mavericks, Miracles, and Medicine: The Pioneers Who Risked Their Lives to Bring Medicine into the Modern Age* (New York: Barnes & Noble Books, 2003), 277.

16. Quoted in J. Thorwald, *The Patients* (New York: Harcourt Brace Jovanovich, 1971), 137.

17. Moore, *A Miracle*, 172.

18. J. E. Murray, "The Fight for Life: The Pioneering Surgeon of the World's First Successful Human Organ Transplant Reflects on the Gift of Life," *Harvard Medicine*, Summer 2011.

19. Moore, *A Miracle*, 173.

20. "Twin Gains in Operation," *New York Times*, December 28, 1954, 25.

21. J. P. Merrill, J. E. Murray, J. H. Harrison, et al., "Successful Homotransplantation of the Kidney between Non-identical Twins," *New England Journal of Medicine* 262 (1960): 1251–1260; J. E. Murray, J. P. Merrill, G. I. Dammon, et al., "Kidney Transplantation in Modified Recipients," *Annals of Surgery* 156 (1962): 337–355.

22. Moore, *Transplant*, 109.

23. J. P. Merrill, J. E. Murray, F. Takacs, et al., "Successful Transplantation of Kidney from a Human Cadaver," *Journal of the American Medical Association* 185 (1963): 347–353; J. E. Murray, J. P. Merrill, J. H. Harrison, et al., "Prolonged Survival of Human Kidney Homografts by Immunosuppressive Drug Therapy," *New England Journal of Medicine* 268 (1963): 1315–1323.

24. Moore, *A Miracle*, 184.

25. J. D. Hardy, *The World of Surgery, 1945–1985: Memoirs of One Participant* (Philadelphia: University of Pennsylvania Press, 1986), 275.

26. N. E. Shumway and R. R. Lower, "Special Problems in Transplantation of the Heart," *Annals of the New York Academy of the Sciences* 120 (1964): 776.

27. J. D. Hardy and C. M. Chavez, "The First Heart Transplant in Man," *American Journal of Cardiology* 22 (1968): 780.

28. "Historic Heart Experiment," *New York Times*, December 5, 1967, 46.

29. "A Year of Heart Transplants," *New York Times*, December 2, 1968, 46.

30. "Joints of Steel and Plastic," *Life*, April 12, 1948, 127.

Chapter 19. Changes

1. J. Perissat, "Laparoscopic Cholecystectomy: The French Experience," in *Laparoscopic Surgery: An Atlas for General Surgeons*, ed. G. C. Vitale, J. S. Sanfilippo, and J. Perissat (Philadelphia: J. B. Lippincott, 1995), 147.

2. M. M. Ravitch, "Historical Perspective and Personal Viewpoint," in *Current Practice of Surgical Stapling*, ed. M. M. Ravitch, F. Steichen, and R. Welter (Philadelphia: Lea & Febiger, 1991), 3.

3. Quoted in E. Vitone, "The Surgical Curmudgeon," *Pittmed*, Spring 2013, 22.

4. Ibid.

5. Ibid.

6. Ibid., 6.

7. M. M. Ravitch, I. W. Brown, and G. F. Daviglus, "Experimental and Clinical Use of the Soviet Bronchus Stapling Instrument," *Surgery* 46 (1959): 108.

8. Quoted in Vitone, "The Surgical Curmudgeon," 6.

9. I. M. Rutkow, "Rates of Surgery in the United States: The Decade of the 1970s," *Surgical Clinics of North America* 62 (1982): 559–578.

10. I. M. Rutkow, "Surgical Operations in the United States, Then (1983) and Now (1994)," *Archives of Surgery* 132 (1997): 983–990.

11. "A Stitch to Save Nine," *Time*, September 2, 1966, 61.

12. Mark Ravitch, *Repair of Hernias* (Chicago: Year Book Medical Publishers, 1969), 7.

13. Ibid., 28.

14. Ibid., 82–84.

15. "Irving Lichtenstein, Pioneer in Hernia Surgery, Dies at 80," *New York Times*, June 25, 2000, 35.

16. I. L. Lichtenstein, "Local Anesthesia for Hernioplasty, Immediate Ambulation and Return to Work: A Preliminary Report," *California Medicine* 100 (1964): 106–109.

17. "Irving Lichtenstein," 35.

18. I. M. Rutkow, "The PerFix Plug Repair for Groin Hernias," *Surgical Clinics of North America*. 83 (2003): 1079–1098.

19. I. M. Rutkow, *The History of Surgery in the United States, 1775–1900*, vol. 1, *Textbooks, Monographs and Treatises* (San Francisco: Norman, 1988).

20. I. M. Rutkow, ed., "History of Surgery in the United States," *Surgical Clinics of North America* (Philadelphia: W.B. Saunders, December1987).

21. I. M. Rutkow, "The Letters of William Halsted and Erwin Payr," *Surgery, Gynecology & Obstetrics* 161 (1985): 75–87; I. M. Rutkow, "The Letters of William Stewart Halsted and William Williams Keen," *Surgery* 100 (1986): 550–561; I. M. Rutkow, "The Letters of William Stewart Halsted and Johns Chalmers DaCosta," *American Journal of Surgery* 154 (1987): 320–332; I. M. Rutkow, "Reference Works Related to United States Surgical History: A Chronologic Bibliography of American Textbooks, Monographs, and Treatises

Relating to the Surgical Sciences, 1775–1899," *Surgical Clinics of North America* 67 (1987): 1127–1152; I. M. Rutkow, "American Surgical Biographies," *Surgical Clinics of North America* 67 (1987): 1153–1180; I. M. Rutkow, "A History of *The Surgical Clinics of North America*," *Surgical Clinics of North America* 67 (1987): 1217–1239; I. M. Rutkow, "The *Surgical Clinics* during the 1920s; Including Biographies of William Mayo, George Crile, Frank Lahey, Allan Kanavel, Sumner Koch, and William Babcock," *Surgical Clinics of North America* 67 (1987): 1241–1328; I. M. Rutkow and K. Hempel, "An Experiment in Surgical Education, the First International Exchange of Residents: The Letters of Halsted, Küttner, Heuer, and Landois, *Archives of Surgery* 123 (1988): 115–121; I. M. Rutkow, "John Syng Dorsey (1783–1818)," *Surgery* 103 (1988): 45–55; I. M. Rutkow, "The Unpublished Letters of William Halsted and Harvey Cushing," *Surgery, Gynecology & Obstetrics* 166 (1988): 370–382.

22. I. M. Rutkow, "The Value of Surgical History," *Archives of Surgery* 126 (1991): 953–956.

23. K. H. Sheetz, J. Claflin, and J. B. Dimick, "Trends in the Adoption of Robotic Surgery for Common Surgical Procedures," *Journal of the American Medical Association, Network Open*, 2020; 3(1): e1918911, doi:10.1001/jamanetworkopen.2019.18911.

24. Quoted in D. T. Max, "Dr. Robot," *The New Yorker*, September 30, 2019, 27.

25. I. M. Rutkow, "Laparoscopic Hernia Repair: The Socioeconomic Tyranny of Surgical Technology," *Archives of Surgery* 127 (1992): 1271.

26. Quoted in A. Clark, *Working Life of Women in the Seventeenth Century* (New York: Harcourt, Brace & Howe, 1920), 259.

27. Ibid.

28. S. Young, *The Annals of the Barber-Surgeons of London* (London: Blades, East & Blades, 1890), 392.

29. Quoted in C. Brock, "Women in Surgery: Patients and Practitioners," in *The Palgrave Handbook of the History of Surgery*, ed. T. Schlich (London: Palgrave Macmillan, 2018), 138.

30. Quoted in "Olga Jonasson, 72, Surgeon and a Role Model for Women," *New York Times*, September 13, 2006, C13.

31. J. Wennberg and A. Gittelsohn, "Small Area Variations in Health Care Delivery," *Science* 182 (1973): 1102–1108.

32. J. Bunker, "Surgical Manpower: A Comparison of Operations and Surgeons in the United States and in England and Wales," *New England Journal of Medicine* 282 (1970): 135–141.

33. E. G. McCarthy and G. W. Widmer, "Effects of Screening by Consultants on Recommended Elective Surgical Procedures," *New England Journal of Medicine* 291 (1974): 1331–1336.

34. "Cost and Quality of Health Care: Unnecessary Surgery," *Subcommittee on Oversight and Investigations of the Committee on Interstate and Foreign Commerce* (Washington, DC: United States Government Printing Office, 1976), 49.

35. J. E. Brody, "Incompetent Surgery Is Found Not Isolated," *New York Times*, January 27, 1976, 1, 24.

36. J. N. Haug, "Misconceptions on Surgical Residency Positions," *Bulletin of the American College of Surgeons* 61 (1976): 11.

37. F. D. Moore, "Medical and Surgical Manpower and Economic Phenomena," *Surgery* 95 (1984): 374.

38. F. D. Moore, "Surgical Manpower: Past and Present Reality, Estimates for 2000," *Surgical Clinics of North America* 62 (1982): 585.

39. J. A. H. Murray, H. Bradley, W. A. Craigie, and C. T. Onions, *A New English Dictionary on Historical Principles*, vol. 9 (Oxford: At the Clarendon Press, 1919), part 2, SU-TH, 235.

Chapter 20. Prospects

1. D. A. Moses, S. L. Metzger, J. R. Liu, et al., "Neuroprosthesis for Decoding Speech in a Paralyzed Person with Anarthria," *New England Journal of Medicine* 385 (2021): 217–227.

BIBLIOGRAPHY

Allbutt, T. C. *The Historical Relations of Medicine and Surgery to the End of the Sixteenth Century*. London: Macmillan, 1905.

Bankoff, G. *The Story of Surgery*. London: Arthur Barker, 1947.

Billings, J. S. "The History and Literature of Surgery." In *System of Surgery*, 4 vols., edited by F. S. Dennis, 1:17–144. Philadelphia: Lea Brothers, 1895.

Bishop, W. J. *The Early History of Surgery*. London: Robert Hale, 1960.

Buck, A. H. *The Dawn of Modern Medicine*. New Haven: Yale University Press, 1920.

———. *The Growth of Medicine from the Earliest Times to about 1800*. New Haven: Yale University Press, 1917.

Cartwright, F. F. *The Development of Modern Surgery from 1830*. London: Arthur Barker, 1967.

Clarke, E. H., H. J. Bigelow, S. D. Gross, et al. *A Century of American Medicine, 1776–1876*. Philadelphia: Henry C. Lea, 1876.

Cope, Z. *A History of the Acute Abdomen*. London: Oxford University Press, 1965.

———. *Pioneers in Acute Abdominal Surgery*. London: Oxford University Press, 1939.

Earle, A. S. *Surgery in America: From the Colonial Era to the Twentieth Century*. New York: Praeger, 1983.

Edmondson, J. M. *American Surgical Instruments: An Illustrated History of Their Manufacture and a Directory of Instrument Makers to 1900*. San Francisco: Norman, 1997.

Ellis, H. *Famous Operations*. Media, PA: Harwal, 1984.

———. *A History of Surgery*. London: Greenwich Medical, 2001.

———. *Surgical Case-Histories from the Past*. London: Royal Society of Medicine Press, 1994.

Fenster, J. M. *Mavericks, Miracles, and Medicine: The Pioneers Who Risked Their Lives to Bring Medicine into the Modern Age*. New York: Barnes & Noble, 2003.

Fisher, G. J. "A History of Surgery." In *The International Encyclopedia of Surgery*, 6 vols., edited by J. Ashhurst, 6:1146–1202. New York: William Wood, 1886.

Gawande, A. "Two Hundred Years of Surgery." *New England Journal of Medicine* 366 (2012): 1716–1723.

Glaser, H. *The Road to Modern Surgery*. London: Lutterworth, 1960.

Graham, H. *The Story of Surgery*. New York: Doubleday & Doran, 1939.

Haeger, K. *The Illustrated History of Surgery*. New York: Bell Publishing, 1988.

Henderson, V. J., and C. H. Organ. *Noteworthy Publications by African-American Surgeons*. Oakland, CA: Claude H. Organ, Jr., 1995.

Hollingham, R. *Blood and Guts: A History of Surgery*. New York: Thomas Dunne, 2008.

Hurwitz, A., and G. A. Degenshein. *Milestones in Modern Surgery*. New York: Hoeber-Harper, 1958.

Kirkup, J. *The Evolution of Surgical Instruments: An Illustrated History from Ancient Times to the Twentieth Century*. Novato, CA: historyofscience.com, 2006.

Lawrence, C., ed. *Medical Theory, Surgical Practice: Studies in the History of Surgery*. London: Routledge, 1992.

Lawrence, C. "Surgery (Traditional)." In *Companion Encyclopedia of the History of Medicine*, 2 vols., edited by W. F. Bynum and R. Porter, 2:961–983. London: Routledge, 1993.

Leonardo, R. A. *History of Surgery*. New York: Froben, 1943.

———. *Lives of Master Surgeons*. New York: Froben, 1948.

———. *Lives of Master Surgeons* (Supplement 1). New York: Froben, 1949.

Malgaigne, J. F. *Surgery and Ambroise Paré*. Translated from the French and edited by W. B. Hamby. Norman: University of Oklahoma Press, 1965.

Meade, R. H. *A History of Thoracic Surgery*. Springfield, IL: Charles C. Thomas, 1961.

———. *An Introduction to the History of General Surgery*. Philadelphia: W.B. Saunders, 1968.

Moore, F. D. "Surgery." In *Advances in American Medicine: Essays at the Bicentennial*, 2 vols., edited by J. Z. Bowers and E. F. Purcell, 2:614–684. New York: Josiah Macy Jr. Foundation, 1976.

Mukherjee, S. *The Emperor of All Maladies: A Biography of Cancer*. New York: Scribner, 2010.

Mumford, J. G. *A Narrative of Medicine in America*. Philadelphia: J. B. Lippincott, 1903.

———. "Narrative of Surgery; a Historical Sketch." In *Surgery, Its Principles and Practice*, 8 vols., edited by W. W. Keen, 1:17–78. Philadelphia: W.B. Saunders, 1909.

———. *Surgical Memoirs and Other Essays*. New York: Moffat, Yard, 1908.

Nuland, S. B. *Doctors: The Biography of Medicine*. New York: Knopf, 1988.

Organ, C., and M. M. Kosiba. *A Century of Black Surgeons: The USA Experience*. 2 vols. Norman, OK: Transcript Press, 1987.

Porter, R. *The Greatest Benefit to Mankind: A Medical History of Humanity*. New York: W. W. Norton, 1997.

Power, D. *A Mirror for Surgeons: Selected Readings in Surgery*. Boston: Little, Brown, 1939.

———. *A Short History of Surgery*. London: John Hale, 1933.

Ranson, F. T. *Men and Events in Surgery*. N.p., circa 1940.

Richardson, R. *The Story of Surgery: An Historical Commentary*. Shrewsbury, UK: Quiller Press, 2004.

Richardson, R. G. *Surgery: Old and New Frontiers*. New York: Charles Scribner's Sons, 1968.

Riedman, S. R. *Masters of the Scalpel: The Story of Surgery*. Chicago: Rand McNally, 1962.

Rutkow, E. *American Canopy: Trees, Forests, and the Making of a Nation*. New York: Scribner, 2012.

———. *The Longest Line on the Map: The United States, the Pan-American Highway, and the Quest to Link the Americas*. New York: Scribner, 2019.

Rutkow, I. *James A. Garfield*. New York: Times Books/Henry Holt, 2006.

———. *Seeking the Cure: A History of Medicine in America*. New York: Scribner, 2010.

Rutkow, I. M. *American Surgery: An Illustrated History*. Philadelphia: Lippincott-Raven, 1998.

———. *Bleeding Blue and Gray: Civil War Surgery and the Evolution of American Medicine*. New York: Random House, 2005.

———. *The History of Surgery in the United States, 1775–1900*. 2 vols. San Francisco: Norman, 1988 and 1992.

———. "The Origins of Modern Surgery." In *Surgery: Basic Science and Clinical Evidence*, edited by J. A. Norton, R. R. Bollinger, and A. E. Chang, 3–19. New York: Springer-Verlag, 2001.

———. "The Rise of Modern Surgery: An Overview." In *Sabiston Textbook of Surgery: The Biological Basis of Modern Surgical Practice*, edited by C. M. Townsend, R. D. Beauchamp, B. M. Evers, et al., 1–12. Philadelphia: W.B. Saunders, 2001.

———, ed. *Socioeconomics of Surgery*. St. Louis: Mosby, 1989.

———. *Surgery: An Illustrated History*. St. Louis: Mosby–Year Book, 1993.

Schlich, T., ed. *The Palgrave Handbook of the History of Surgery*. London: Palgrave, 2018.

——— and C. Crenner, eds. *Technological Change in Modern Surgery: Historical Perspectives on Innovation*. Rochester, NY: University of Rochester Press, 2017.

Schneider, D. *The Invention of Surgery: A History of Modern Medicine: From the Renaissance to the Implant Revolution*. New York: Pegasus Books, 2020.

Schwartz, S. *Gifted Hands: America's Most Significant Contributions to Surgery*. Amherst, NY: Prometheus Books, 2009.

Seelig, M. G. *Medicine: An Historical Outline*. Baltimore: Williams & Wilkins, 1925.

Smith, S. "The Evolution of American Surgery." *In American Practice of Surgery: A Complete System of the Science and Art of Surgery by Representative Surgeons of the United States and Canada*, 8 vols., edited by J. D. Bryant and A. H. Buck, 1:3–67. New York: William Wood, 1906.

Temkin, O. "The Role of Surgery in the Rise of Modern Medical Thought." *Bulletin of the History of Medicine* 25 (1951): 248–259.

Thompson, C. J. S. *The History and Evolution of Surgical Instruments*. New York: Schuman's, 1942.

Thorwald, J. *The Century of the Surgeon*. New York: Pantheon, 1956.

———. *The Triumph of Surgery*. New York: Pantheon, 1960.

Tilney, N. L. *Invasion of the Body*. Cambridge, MA: Harvard University Press, 2011.

Tröhler, U. "Surgery (Modern)." *In Companion Encyclopedia of the History of Medicine*, 2 vols., edited by W. F. Bynum and R. Porter, 2:984–1028. London: Routledge, 1993.

Van de Laar, A. *Under the Knife: A History of Surgery in 28 Remarkable Operations*. New York: St. Martin's Press, 2018.

Wangensteen O. H., and S. D. Wangensteen. *The Rise of Surgery, from Empiric Craft to Scientific Discipline*. Minneapolis: University of Minnesota Press, 1978.

Whipple, A. O. *The Evolution of Surgery in the United States*. Springfield, IL: Charles C. Thomas, 1963.

Young A. *Scalpel: Men Who Made Surgery*. New York: Random House, 1956.

Zimmerman, L. M., and I. Veith. *Great Ideas in the History of Surgery*. Baltimore: Williams & Wilkins, 1961.

REFERENCES

The major works that shaped my thinking are listed for each chapter.

Prelude

Bosk, C. L. *Forgive and Remember: Managing Medical Failure*. Chicago: University of Chicago Press, 1979.

Byrne, J. J. *A History of the Boston City Hospital, 1905–1964*. Boston: Sheldon Press, 1965.

Cheever, D. W., A. L. Mason, G. W. Gay, and J. B. Blake. *A History of the Boston City Hospital, from its Foundation until 1904*. Boston: Municipal Printing Office, 1906.

Evans, R. J. *In Defence of History*. New York: W. W. Norton, 1999.

Friedman E. "Annual Discourse—the Boston City Hospital: A Tale of Three 'Cities.'" *New England Journal of Medicine* 289 (1973): 503–506.

Glickman R. "House-Staff Training—the Need for Careful Reform." *New England Journal of Medicine* 318 (1988): 780–781.

Goldman L., and A. I. Schafer. *Goldman-Cecil Medicine*. 2 vols. Philadelphia: Elsevier/Saunders, 2016.

Lee, C. "Federal Regulation of Hospital Resident Work Hours: Enforcement with Real Teeth." *Journal of Health Care Law and Policy* 9 (2006): 162–216.

Rutkow, I. M. "An Evaluation of the Application Procedure for Surgical House Officership." *Annals of Surgery* 182 (1975): 130–134.

Tosh, J. *The Pursuit of History*. London: Routledge, 2015.

Townsend, C. M. *Sabiston Textbook of Surgery*. Philadelphia: Elsevier/Saunders, 2022.

PART I—BEGINNINGS

Chapter 1. Genesis

Bakay, L. *An Early History of Craniotomy: From Antiquity to the Napoleonic Era*. Springfield, IL: Charles C. Thomas, 1985.

Buck, A. H. *The Growth of Medicine from the Earliest Times to about 1800*. New Haven: Yale University Press, 1917.

Buckland, A. W. "Surgery and Superstition in Neolithic Times." *Journal of the Anthropological Institute of Great Britain and Ireland* 11 (1882): 7–21.

Daland, J. "Depressed Fracture and Trephining of the Skull by the Incas of Peru." *Annals of Medical History* 7 (1935): 550–558.

Davies, W. W. *The Code of Hammurabi and Moses*. Cincinnati: Jennings and Graham, 1905.

Elsberg, C. A. "The Edwin Smith Surgical Papyrus." *Annals of Medical History* 3 (1931): 271–279.

Jastrow, M. "Babylonian-Assyrian Medicine." *Annals of Medical History* 1 (1917): 231–257.

Horrax, G. *Neurosurgery: An Historical Sketch*. Springfield, IL: Charles C. Thomas, 1952.

Major, R. H. "The Papyrus Ebers." *Annals of Medical History* 2 (1930): 547–555.

Moorad, P. J. "A Comparative Study of Medicine among the Ancient Races of the East: Egypt, Babylonia, and Assyria." *Annals of Medical History* 9 (1937): 155–167.

O'Connor, D. C., and A. E. Walker. "Prologue." In *A History of Neurological Surgery*, edited by A. E. Walker, 1–22. Baltimore: Williams & Wilkins, 1951.

Rogers, L. "The History of Craniotomy." *Annals of Medical History* 2 (1930): 495–514.

Rogers, S. L. *Primitive Surgery: Skills before Science*. Springfield, IL: Charles C. Thomas, 1985.

Sachs, E. *The History and Development of Neurological Surgery*. New York: Paul B. Hoeber, 1952.

Saul, F. P., and J. M. Saul. "Trepanation: Old World and New World." In *A*

History of Neurosurgery, edited by S. H. Greenblatt, 29–35. Park Ridge, IL: American Association of Neurological Surgeons, 1997.

Chapter 2. Exodus

Cawadias, A. P. "From Epidauros to Galenos, the Principal Currents of Greek Medical Thoughts." *Annals of Medical History* 3 (1931): 501–514.

Chance, B. "On Hippocrates and the Aphorisms." *Annals of Medical History* 2 (1930): 31–46.

Edelstein, L. *The Hippocratic Oath: Text, Translation and Interpretation.* Baltimore: Johns Hopkins Press, 1943.

El-Abbadi, M. *Life and Fate of the Ancient Library of Alexandria.* Paris: UNESCO, 1992.

Galdston, I. "The Decline and Resurgence of Hippocratic Medicine." *Bulletin of the New York Academy of Medicine* 44 (1968): 1237–1256.

"Hippocrates." *Medical Classics* 3 (1938): iii–381.

Jones, W. H. S. *Philosophy and Medicine in Ancient Greece.* Baltimore: Johns Hopkins Press, 1946.

Longrigg, James. *Greek Rational Medicine: Philosophy and Medicine from Alcmaeon to the Alexandrians.* New York: Routledge, 1993.

Lund, F. B. "The Life and Writings of Hippocrates." *Boston Medical and Surgical Journal* 191 (1924): 1009–1014.

Lloyd, G. E. R., ed. *Hippocratic Writings.* Translated by J. Chadwick and W. N. Mann. London: Penguin Books, 1983.

Manjo, G. *The Healing Hand: Man and Wound in the Ancient World.* Boston: Harvard University Press, 1975.

Mirko, D. G. *Diseases in the Ancient Greek World.* Baltimore: Johns Hopkins University Press, 1991.

Schiff, S. *Cleopatra: A Life.* New York: Little, Brown, 2010.

Sigerist, H. E. "On Hippocrates." *Bulletin of the Johns Hopkins Institute of the History of Medicine* 2 (1934): 190–214.

Chapter 3. Prolific Pens

Allbutt, C. *Greek Medicine in Rome.* London: Macmillan, 1921.

Brain, P. *Galen on Bloodletting.* Cambridge: Cambridge University Press, 1986.

Burr, C. W. "Galen." *Annals of Medical History* 3 (1931): 209–217.

Finlayson, J. "Celsus." *Glasgow Medical Journal* 37 (1892): 321–348.

Fisher, G. J. "Aurelius Cornelius Celsus, B.C. 25—A.D. 40(?)." *Annals of Anatomy and Surgery* 5 (1882): 177–185, 224–227, 280–291.

Garrison, F. H. "New Views of Max Wellman on the Authorship of Celsus." *Annals of Medical History* 8 (1926): 203–207.

Jackson, R. *Doctors and Diseases in the Roman Empire*. Norman: University of Oklahoma Press, 1988.

Johnston, I. *Galen on Diseases and Symptoms*. Cambridge: Cambridge University Press, 2006.

Malloch, A. "Galen." *Annals of Medical History* 8 (1926): 61–68.

Milne, J. S. *Surgical Instruments in Greek and Roman Times*. Oxford: Clarendon, 1907.

Moon, R. O. "The Relation of Galen to the Philosophy of His Time." *British Medical Journal* 4 (1908): 1449–1451.

Nutton, V. "Galen in the Eyes of His Contemporaries." *Bulletin of the History of Medicine* 58 (1984): 315–324.

Prendergast, J. S. "The Background of Galen's Life and Activities and Its Influence on His Achievements." *Proceedings of the Royal Society of Medicine* 21 (1930): 1131–1148.

Sarton, G. *Galen of Pergamon*. Lawrence: University of Kansas Press, 1954.

Scarborough, J. *Roman Medicine*. Ithaca, NY: Cornell University Press, 1969.

Temkin, O. *Galenism: Rise and Decline of a Medical Philosophy*. Ithaca, NY: Cornell University Press, 1973.

Toledo-Pereyra, L. H. "Galen's Contribution to Surgery." *Bulletin of the History of Medicine* 28 (1973): 357–375.

Walsh, J. "Galen's Discovery and Promulgation of the Function of the Recurrent Laryngeal Nerves." *Annals of Medical History* 8 (1926): 176–184.

———. "Galen's Writings and Influences Inspiring Them." *Annals of Medical History* 6 (1934): 1–30, 143–149; 7 (1935): 428–437, 570–589; 8 (1936): 65–90; 9 (1937): 34–61; and 10 (1939): 525–537.

———. "Refutation of the Charges of Cowardice Made against Galen." *Annals of Medical History* 3 (1931): 195–208.

Chapter 4. Darkness, Then Daylight

Allbutt, T. C. *The Historical Relations of Medicine and Surgery to the End of the Sixteenth Surgery*. London: Macmillan, 1905.

Bishop, W. J. *The Early History of Surgery*. London: Robert Hale, 1960.

Buck, A. H. *The Growth of Medicine from the Earliest Times to about 1800*. New Haven: Yale University Press, 1917.

Campbell, D. *Arabian Medicine and Its Influence on the Middle Ages*. 2 vols. London: Kegan, Paul, Trench, Trübner, 1926.

Castiglioni, A. "The School of Salerno." *Bulletin of the History of Medicine* 6 (1938): 883–898.

Corner, G. W. "On Early Salernitan Surgery and Especially the 'Bamberg Surgery.'" *Bulletin of the History of Medicine* 5 (1937): 1–32.

———. "The Rise of Medicine at Salerno in the Twelfth Century." *Annals of Medical History* 3 (1931): 1–16.

Gottfried, R. S. *Doctors and Medicine in Medieval England, 1340–1530*. Princeton: Princeton University Press, 1986.

Harington, J. *The School of Salernum*. New York: Hoeber, 1920.

Leonardo, R. A. *History of Surgery*. New York: Froben Press, 1943.

Pouchelle, M. C. *The Body & Surgery in the Middle Ages*. Translated by Rosemary Morris. New Brunswick, NJ: Rutgers University Press, 1990.

Reichborn-Kjennerud, I. "The School of Salerno and Surgery in the North during the Saga Age." *Annals of Medical History* 9 (1937): 321–337.

Riesman, D. *The Story of Medicine in the Middle Ages*. New York: PB Hoeber, 1935.

Rosenman, L. D. *The Chirurgia of Roger Frugard*. Philadelphia: Xlibris, 2002.

Sa'di, L. "Reflection of Arabian Medicine at Salerno and Montpellier." *Annals of Medical History* 5 (1933): 215–225.

Walsh, J. J. *Medieval Medicine*. London: A & C Black, 1920.

PART II—FOUNDATIONS

Chapter 5. The Human Road Map

Buck, A. H. *The Growth of Medicine, from the Earliest Times to about 1800*. New Haven: Yale University Press, 1917.

Castiglione, A. "Three Pathfinders of Science in the Renaissance." *Bulletin of the Medical Library Association* 31 (1903): 203–207.

Cazort, M., M. Kornell, and K. B. Roberts. *The Ingenious Machine of Nature.* Ottawa: National Gallery of Canada, 1996.

Chen, P. W. *Final Exam: A Surgeon's Reflections on Mortality.* New York: Knopf, 2007.

Dawson, P. M. "The Heritage of Paracelsus." *Annals of Medical History* 10 (1928): 258–269.

Edelstein, L. "Andreas Vesalius, the Humanist." *Bulletin of the History of Medicine* 14 (1943): 547–561.

Fisch, M. H. "Vesalius and His Book." *Bulletin of the Medical Library Association* 31 (1943): 208–221.

Garrison, F. H. "In Defense of Vesalius." *Bulletin of the Society of Medical History of Chicago* 1 (1916): 47–65.

Haggard, H. W. *Devils, Drugs, and Doctors: The Story of the Science of Healing.* New York: Blue Ribbon Books, 1929.

Keele, K. D. "Leonardo da Vinci's Influence on Renaissance Anatomy." *Medical History* 8 (1964): 360–370.

Klebs, A. C. "Leonardo da Vinci and His Anatomical Studies." *Bulletin of the Society of Medical History of Chicago* 1 (1916): 66–83.

Mayor, A. H. *Artists and Anatomists.* New York: Artist's Limited Edition/ Metropolitan Museum of Art, 1984.

Nuland, S. B. *Doctors: The Biography of Medicine.* New York: Knopf, 1988.

O'Malley, C. D. *Andreas Vesalius of Brussels, 1514–1564.* Berkeley: University of California Press, 1964.

O'Malley, C. D., and J. B. de C. M. Saunders, eds. *Leonardo da Vinci on the Human Body.* New York: Schuman, 1952.

Pagel, W. *Paracelsus: An Introduction to Philosophical Medicine in the Era of the Renaissance.* Basel: Karger, 1958.

Roberts, K. B., and J. D. W. Tomlinson. *The Fabric of the Body: European Traditions of Anatomical Illustration.* Oxford: Clarendon, 1992.

Rolleston, H. "Harvey's Predecessors and Contemporaries." *Annals of Medical History* 10 (1928): 323–337.

Sawday, J. *The Body Emblazoned: Dissection and the Human Body in Renaissance Culture.* London: Routledge, 1995.

REFERENCES

Sigerist, H. E. "Commemorating Andreas Vesalius." *Bulletin of the History of Medicine* 14 (1943): 541–546.

Siraisi, N. G. *Medieval and Early Renaissance Medicine.* Chicago: University of Chicago, 1990.

———. "Medieval and Renaissance Medicine: Continuity and Diversity." *Journal of the History of Medicine and Allied Sciences* 41 (1986): 391–394.

Wear, A., R. K. French, and I. M. Lonie. *The Medical Renaissance of the Sixteenth Century.* Cambridge: Cambridge University Press, 1985.

Webster, C. *Health, Medicine and Mortality in the Sixteenth Century.* Cambridge: Cambridge University Press, 1979.

———. *Paracelsus: Medicine, Magic, and Mission at the End of Time.* New Haven: Yale University Press, 2008.

Zilboorg, G. "Psychological Sidelights on Andreas Vesalius." *Bulletin of the History of Medicine* 14 (1943): 562–575.

Zimmerman, L., and I. Veith. *Great Ideas in the History of Surgery.* Baltimore: Williams & Wilkins, 1961.

Chapter 6. To Stop the Flow

Bagwell, C. E. "Ambroise Paré and the Renaissance of Surgery." *Surgery, Obstetrics and Gynecology* 152 (1981): 350–354.

Baskett, T. F. "Ambroise Paré and the Arrest of Haemorrhage." *Resuscitation* 62 (2004): 133–135.

Carbonnier, J. *A Barber-Surgeon: A Life of Ambroise Paré, Founder of Modern Surgery.* New York: Pantheon, 1965.

Cumston, C. G. "A Brief Résumé of the Life and Work of Ambroise Paré." *Boston Medical and Surgical Journal* 145 (1901): 395–400, 431–435, 464–468.

Doe, J. *A Bibliography of the Works of Ambroise Paré: Premier Chirurgien & Conseiller du Roy.* Chicago: University of Chicago Press, 1937.

Donaldson, I. M. L. "Ambroise Paré's Accounts of New Methods for Treating Gunshot Wounds and Burns." *Journal of the Royal Society of Medicine* 108 (2015): 457–461.

Dowling, K., and J. T. Goodrich. "Two Cases of 16th Century Head Injuries Managed in Royal European Families." *Neurological Focus* 41 (2016): E2.

"Editorials: Addenda to Miss Janet Doe's Bibliography of Ambroise Paré." *Annals of Medical History* 2 (1940): 443–444.

Gross, S. D. "A Sketch of the Life, Character, and Services of Ambroise Paré." *North American Medico-Chirurgical Review* 5 (1861): 1059–1083.

Hamby, W. B. *Ambroise Paré: Surgeon of the Renaissance*. St. Louis: Warren H. Green, 1967.

———, ed. *The Case Reports and Autopsy Records of Ambroise Paré*. Springfield, IL: Charles C. Thomas, 1960.

Keynes, G., ed. *The Apologie and Treatise of Ambroise Paré Containing the Voyages Made into Divers Places with Many of His Writings upon Surgery*. London: Falcon Educational Books, 1951.

Meyer-Steineg, T. "Treatment of Gunshot Wounds and the Improvement Thereof by Ambroise Paré in the Campaign of Francis I against Charles V (1536–1544)." *Lancet* 211 (1928): 840–842.

Norwich, I. "A Consultation between Andreas Vesalius and Ambroise Paré at the Deathbed of Henri II, King of France, 15 July 1559." *South African Medical Journal* 80 (1991): 245–247.

Nuland, S. B. *Doctors: The Biography of Medicine*. New York: Alfred A. Knopf, 1988.

Paré, A. *On Monsters and Marvels*. Translated by J. L. Pallister. Chicago: University of Chicago Press, 1982.

Singer, D. W. *Selections from the Works of Ambroise Paré with Short Biography and Explanatory and Bibliographical Notes*. London: John Bale, Sons & Danielson, 1924.

Siraisi, N. G. "Medieval and Renaissance Medicine: Continuity and Diversity." *Journal of the History of Medicine and Allied Sciences* 41 (1986): 391–394.

Wear, A., R. K. French, and I. M. Lonie. *The Medical Renaissance of the Sixteenth Century*. Cambridge: Cambridge University Press, 1985.

Young, A. *Scalpel: Men Who Made Surgery*. New York: Random House, 1956.

Zanellog, M., P. Charlier, R. Corns, et al. "The Death of Henry II, King of France (1519–1559): From Myth to Medical and Historical Fact." *Acta Neurochirurgica* 157 (2015): 145–149.

Zimmerman, L. M., and I. Veith. *Great Ideas in the History of Surgery*. Baltimore: Williams & Wilkins, 1961.

Chapter 7. The Circle

Bradbury, S. *The Evolution of the Microscope*. Oxford: Pergamon Press, 1967.

Bylebyl, J. *William Harvey and His Age: The Professional and Social Context of the Discovery of Circulation*. Baltimore: Johns Hopkins Press, 1979.

Cohn, A. E. "The Development of the Harveian Circulation." *Annals of Medical History* 1 (1929): 16–36.

Edgar, I. I. "Elizabethan Conceptions of the Physiology of the Circulation." *Annals of Medical History* 8 (1936): 359–370, 456–465.

Fulton, J. F. *Michael Servetus, Humanist and Martyr*. New York: Herbert Reichner, 1953.

Herringham, W. "The Life and Times of Dr. William Harvey." *Annals of Medical History* 4 (1932): 109–125, 249–272, 347–363, 491–502, 575–589.

Keele, K. D. *William Harvey: The Man, the Physician, and the Scientist*. London: Thomas Nelson & Sons, 1965.

Keynes, G. L. *The Life of William Harvey*. Oxford: Oxford University Press, 1966.

Krumbhaar, E. B. "Bibliographical Matters Pertaining to the Discovery of the Circulation of Blood." *Annals of Medical History* 4 (1932): 57–86.

Macleod, J. J. R. "Harvey's Experiments on Circulation." *Annals of Medical History* 10 (1928): 338–348.

Pagel, W. *New Light on William Harvey*. Basel: Karger, 1976.

———. *William Harvey's Biological Ideas*. London: Karger, 1967.

Ratner, H. A. "William Harvey, M.D., Modern or Ancient Scientist?" *The Thomist: A Speculative Quarterly Review* 24 (1961): 26–27.

Rolleston, H. "Harvey's Predecessors and Contemporaries." *Annals of Medical History* 10 (1928): 323–337.

Roy, P. S. "Historical Development of Our Knowledge of the Circulation and Its Disorders." *Annals of Medical History* 1 (1917): 141–154.

Whitteridge, G. *William Harvey and the Circulation of the Blood*. London: MacDonald, 1971.

Wright, T. *William Harvey: A Life in Circulation*. Oxford: Oxford University Press, 2012.

Chapter 8. Emergence

Allbutt, T. C. *The Historical Relations of Medicine and Surgery to the End of the Sixteenth Century*. London: Macmillan, 1905.

Baker, F. "The Faculty of Paris in the Seventeenth Century." *New York Medical Journal* 98 (1913): 115–121.

Beier, L. M. "Seventeenth-Century English Surgery: The Casebook of Joseph Binns." In *Medical Theory, Surgical Practice: Studies in the History of Surgery*, edited by C. Lawrence, 48–84. London: Routledge, 1992.

Bodemer, C. W. "France, the Fundament, and the Rise of Surgery." *Diseases of the Colon and Rectum* 26 (1983): 743–750.

Cope, Z. *The Royal College of Surgeons of England: A History*. London: Anthony Blond, 1959.

———. *William Cheselden*. London: E. & S. Livingstone, 1953.

———. "William Cheselden and the Separation of the Barbers from the Surgeons." *Annals of the Royal College of Surgeons* 12 (1953): 1–13.

Dobson, J. *Barbers and Barber-Surgeons of London*. London: Blackwell Scientific, 1979.

Ellis, H. *A History of Bladder Stone*. Oxford: Blackwell Scientific, 1969.

Gelfand T. "The 'Paris Manner' of Dissection: Student Anatomical Dissection in Early Eighteenth-Century Paris." *Bulletin of the History of Medicine* 46 (1972): 99–130.

———. *Professionalizing Modern Medicine: Paris Surgeons and Medical Science and Institutions in the 18th Century*. Westport, CT: Greenwood Press, 1980.

Larson, M. *The Rise of Professionalism*. Berkeley: University of California Press, 1977.

Lindemann, M. *Medicine and Society in Early Modern Europe*. Cambridge: Cambridge University Press, 2010.

Nichols, J. *Literary Anecdotes of the Eighteenth Century, Comprising Biographical Memoirs of William Bowyer*. 6 vols. 4:613–624. London: private printing, 1812.

Packard, F. R. "Guy Patin and the Medical Profession in Paris in the Seventeenth Century." *Annals of Medical History* 4 (1922): 136–165, 215–240, 357–385.

Parker, G. *The Early History of Surgery in Great Britain*. London: A & C Black, 1920.

Power, D. A. "Evolution of the Surgeon in London." *St. Bartholomew's Hospital Journal* 19 (1912): 83–99.

Rolleston, H. "History of Medicine in the City of London." *Annals of Medical History* 3 (1941): 1–17.

Weiner, D. B., and M. J. Sauter. "The City of Paris and the Rise of Clinical Medicine." *Osiris* 18 (2003): 23–42.

Young, S. *The Annals of the Barber-Surgeons of London, Compiled from Their Records and Other Sources*. London: Blades, East & Blades, 1890.

Chapter 9. Transition

Adams, J. *Memoirs of the Life and Doctrines of the Late John Hunter*. London: W Thorn, 1817.

Bergland, R. M. "New Information concerning the Irish Giant." *Journal of Neurosurgery* 23 (1965): 265–269.

Burnett, F. L. "John Hunter." *Boston Medical and Surgical Journal* 156 (1912): 359–364.

Dobson, J. "John Hunter's Practice." *Annals of the Royal College of Surgeons (England)* 38 (1966): 181–190.

Foot, J. *The Life of John Hunter*. London: T. Becket, 1794.

Gross, S. D. *John Hunter and His Pupils*. Philadelphia: Presley Blakiston, 1881.

Jacyna, S. "Physiological Principles in the Surgical Writings of John Hunter." In *Medical Theory, Surgical Practice: Studies in the History of Surgery*, edited by C. Lawrence, 135–152. London: Routledge, 1992.

Kobler, J. *The Reluctant Surgeon: The Life of John Hunter*. London: Heinemann, 1960.

Moore, W. *The Knife Man: Blood, Body-Snatching, and the Birth of Modern Surgery*. London: Bantam, 2005.

Mumford, J. G. "John Hunter, 1728 to 1793." In *Surgery: Its Principles and Practice*, 8 vols., edited by W. W. Keen, 1:40–54. Philadelphia: W.B. Saunders, 1906.

Nuland, S. *Doctors: The Biography of Medicine*, 171–199. New York: Alfred A. Knopf, 1988.

Palmer, J. *The Works of John Hunter, F.R.S.* 4 vols. London: Longman, Rees, Orme, Brown, Green, and Longman, 1835.

Parker, G. *The Early History of Surgery in Great Britain.* London: A & C Black, 1920.

Peachey, G. C. *A Memoir of William & John Hunter.* Plymouth, UK: Brendon, 1924.

Porritt, A. "John Hunter, Distant Echoes." *Annals of the Royal College of Surgeons (England)* 41 (1967): 1–24.

Qvist, G. *John Hunter, 1728–1793.* London: W. Heinemann, 1981.

Stevenson, L. G. "John Hunter, Surgeon-General, 1790–1793. *Journal of the History of Medicine* 19 (1964): 239–266.

Wall, C. *The History of the Surgeon's Company, 1745–1800.* London: Hutchinson's, 1937.

PART III—REVOLUTIONS

Chapter 10. Pain-Free

Brown, M. "Surgery and Emotion: The Era before Anaesthesia." In *The Palgrave Handbook of the History of Surgery*, edited by T. Schlich, 327–347. London: Palgrave Macmillan, 2018.

Cohen, E. *The Modulated Scream: Pain in Late Medieval Culture.* Chicago: University of Chicago Press, 2009.

Cole, F. *Milestones in Anesthesia: Readings in the Development of Surgical Anesthesia, 1665–1940.* Lincoln: University of Nebraska Press, 1965.

Corretti, C., and S. P. Desai. "The Legacy of Eve's Curse: Religion, Childbirth Pain, and the Rise of Anesthesia in Europe: C. 1200-1800s." *Journal of Anesthesia History* 4 (2018): 182–190.

Duncum, B. M. *The Development of Inhalation Anaesthesia.* London: Wellcome Historical Medical Museum/Oxford University Press, 1947.

Faulconer, A., and T. E. Keys. *Foundations of Anesthesiology.* 2 vols. Springfield, IL: Charles C. Thomas, 1965.

Fenster, J. M. *Ether Day: The Strange Tale of America's Greatest Medical Discovery and the Haunted Men Who Made It.* New York: HarperCollins, 2001.

Fülöp-Miller, R. *Triumph over Pain.* New York: Literary Guild of America, 1938.

REFERENCES

Fulton, J. F., and M. E. Stanton. *The Centennial of Surgical Anesthesia: An Annotated Catalogue of Books and Pamphlets Bearing on the Early History of Surgical Anesthesia*. New York: Henry Schuman, 1946.

Greene, N. M. "Anesthesia and the Development of Surgery." *Anesthesia and Analgesia* 58 (1979): 5–12.

Keys, T. E. *The History of Surgical Anesthesia*. New York: Schuman's, 1945.

Ludovici, L J. *The Discovery of Anaesthesia*. New York: Thomas Y. Crowell, 1961.

MacQuitty, B. *Victory over Pain: Morton's Discovery of Anaesthesia*. New York: Taplinger, 1969.

Meek, H. "Frances Burney's Mastectomy Narrative and Discourses of Breast Cancer in the Late Eighteenth Century." *Literature and Medicine* 35 (2017): 27–45.

Metcalfe, N. H. "The Influence of the Military on Civilian Uncertainty about Modern Anaesthesia between Its Origins in 1846 and the End of the Crimean War in 1856." *Anaesthesia* 60 (2005): 594–601.

Nuland, S. *Doctors: The Biography of Medicine*, 263–303. New York: Alfred A. Knopf, 1988.

Pernick, M. S. *A Calculus of Suffering: Pain, Professionalism, and Anesthesia in Nineteenth-Century America*. New York: Columbia University Press, 1985.

Snow, S. J. *Blessed Days of Anaesthesia: How Anaesthetics Changed the World*. Oxford: Oxford University Press, 2008.

———. "Surgery and Anaesthesia: Revolutions in Practice." In *The Palgrave Handbook of the History of Surgery*, edited by T. Schlich, 195–214. London: Palgrave Macmillan, 2018.

Thernstrom, M. *The Pain Chronicle: Cures, Myths, Mysteries, Prayers, Diaries, Brain Scans, Healing, and the Science of Suffering*. New York: Farrar, Straus and Giroux, 2010.

Walmsley, D. M. *Anton Mesmer*. London: Robert Hale, 1967.

Wolfe, R. J. *Tarnished Idol: William Thomas Green Morton and the Introduction of Surgical Anesthesia. A Chronicle of the Ether Controversy*. San Anselmo, CA: Norman, 2001.

Young, A. *Scalpel: Men Who Made Surgery*, 134–155. New York: Random House, 1961.

Chapter 11. They're Alive

Brown, J. N. E. "Syme and his Son-in-law." *Annals of Medical History* 3 (1941): 18–35.

Carter, K. C. "The Development of Pasteur's Concept of Disease Causation and the Emergence of Specific Causes in Nineteenth-Century Medicine." *Bulletin of the History of Medicine* 65 (1991): 528–548.

Debré, P. *Louis Pasteur.* Translated by Elborg Forster. Baltimore: Johns Hopkins University Press, 1998.

Dubos, R. *Pasteur and Modern Science.* London: Heinemann, 1960.

Edgar, I. I. "Modern Surgery and Lord Lister." *Journal of the History of Medicine* 16 (1961): 193–214.

Farley, J., and G. L. Geison. "Science, Politics and Spontaneous Generation in Nineteenth-Century France: The Pasteur-Pouchet Debate." *Bulletin of the History of Medicine* 48 (1974): 161–198.

Farmer, L. *Master Surgeon: A Biography of Joseph Lister.* New York: Harper & Row, 1962.

Fitzharris, L. *The Butchering Art: Joseph Lister's Quest to Transform the Grisly World of Victorian Medicine.* New York: Scientific American/Farrar, Straus and Giroux, 2017.

Gaw, J. L. *A Time to Heal: The Diffusion of Listerism in Victorian Britain.* Philadelphia: American Philosophical Society, 1999.

Geison, G. L. "Pasteur, Louis." In *Dictionary of Scientific Biography*, 18 vols., edited by C. C. Gillispie, 10:350–416. New York: Charles Scribner's Sons, 1974.

Guthrie, D. *Lord Lister, His Life and Doctrine.* Edinburgh: E. & S. Livingstone, 1949.

Judd, C. C. W. "The Life and Work of Lister." *Bulletin of the Johns Hopkins Hospital* 21 (1910): 293–304.

Keim, A., and L. Lumet. *Louis Pasteur.* Translated by Frederic Cooper. New York: Frederick A. Stokes, 1914.

Kelley, E. C., ed. "Joseph Lister." *Medical Classics* 2 (1937): 4–101.

Latour, B. *The Pasteurization of France.* Boston: Harvard University Press, 1988.

Lawrence, C., and R. Dixey. "Practising on Principle: Joseph Lister and the Germ Theories of Disease." In *Medical Theory, Surgical Practice: Studies in the History of Surgery*, edited by C. Lawrence, 153–215. London: Routledge, 1992.

Nuland, S. B. *Doctors: The Biography of Medicine*, 343–385. New York: Alfred A. Knopf, 1988.

Porter, J. R. "Louis Pasteur: Achievements and Disappointments." *Bacteriological Reviews* 25 (1961): 389–403.

Porter, R. *The Greatest Benefit to Mankind: A Medical History of Humanity.* New York: HarperCollins, 1997.

Richmond, P. A. "American Attitudes toward the Germ Theory of Disease (1860–1880)." *Journal of the History of Medicine* 9 (1954): 428–454.

Robbins, L. *Louis Pasteur and the Hidden World of Microbes.* New York: Oxford University Press, 2001.

Rutkow, I. "Joseph Lister and His 1876 Tour of America." *Annals of Surgery* 257 (2013): 1181–1187.

Schechter, D. C., and H. Swan. "Jules Lemaire: A Forgotten Hero of Surgery." *Surgery* 49 (1961): 817–826.

Thomson, S. C. "A House-Surgeon's Memory of Joseph Lister." *Annals of Medical History* 2 (1919): 93–108.

Truax, R. *Joseph Lister, Father of Modern Surgery.* Indianapolis: Bobbs Merrill, 1944.

Wangensteen, O. H., and S. D. Wangensteen. "Lister, His Books, and Evolvement of His Antiseptic Wound Practices." *Bulletin of the History of Medicine* 48 (1974): 100–128.

Worboys, M. "The History of Surgical Wound Infections: Revolution or Evolution?" In *The Palgrave Handbook of the History of Surgery*, edited by T. Schlich, 215–233. London: Palgrave Macmillan, 2018.

———. "Joseph Lister and the Performance of Antiseptic Surgery." *Notes and Records of the Royal Society* 67 (2013): 199–209.

Young, A. *Scalpel: Men Who Made Surgery*, 165–193. New York: Random House, 1965.

Chapter 12. Scientific Progress

Absolon, K. B. *The Surgeon's Surgeon, Theodor Billroth, 1829–1894.* 3 vols. Lawrence, KS: Coronado Press, 1979, 1981, and 1987.

Carter, B. N. "The Fruition of Halsted's Concept of Surgical Training." *Surgery* 32 (1952): 518–527.

Chesney, A. M. *The Johns Hopkins Hospital and the Johns Hopkins University School of Medicine: A Chronicle.* Vol. 1, *Early Years, 1867–1893,* 1943, vol. 2, *1893–1905,* 1958; vol. 3, *1905–1914,* 1963. Baltimore: Johns Hopkins Press.

Colp, R. "Notes on Dr. William S. Halsted." *Bulletin of the New York Academy of Medicine* 60 (1974): 876–887.

Crowe, S. J. *Halsted of Johns Hopkins, the Man and His Men.* Springfield, IL: Charles C. Thomas, 1957.

Dumont, A. E. "Halsted at Bellevue—1883–1887." *Annals of Surgery* 172 (1970): 929–935.

Garrison, F. H. *John Shaw Billings: A Memoir.* New York: G.P. Putnam's Sons, 1915.

Harvey, A. M. *Research and Discovery in Medicine: Contributions from Johns Hopkins.* Baltimore: Johns Hopkins University Press, 1976–1981.

Harvey, A. M., G. H. Brieger, S. L. Abrams, and V. A. McKusick. *A Model of Its Kind.* Vol. 1, *A Centennial History of Medicine at Johns Hopkins;* vol. 2, *A Pictorial History of Medicine at Johns Hopkins.* Baltimore: Johns Hopkins University Press, 1989.

Hughes, E. F. X. "Halsted and American Surgery." *Surgery* 75 (1974): 169–177.

Imber, G. *Genius on the Edge: The Bizarre Double Life of Dr. William Stewart Halsted.* New York: Kaplan, 2010.

Mukherjee, S. *The Emperor of All Maladies: A Biography of Cancer.* New York: Scribner, 2010.

Nuland, S. B. *Doctors: The Biography of Medicine.* New York: Alfred A. Knopf, 1988.

Olch, P. D. "William S. Halsted's New York Period, 1874–1886." *Bulletin of the History of Medicine* 40 (1966): 495–510.

Patey, D. H. "Halsted's Influence upon British Surgery." *Surgery* 32 (1952): 528–529.

Penfield, W. "Halsted of Johns Hopkins." *Journal of the American Medical Association* 210 (1969): 214–218.

Rutkow, I. M. *American Surgery: An Illustrated History.* Philadelphia: Lippincott-Raven, 1998.

———. "An Experiment in Surgical Education—the First International Exchange of Residents." *Archives of Surgery* 123 (1988): 115–121.

———. "William Halsted and Theodor Kocher: 'An Exquisite Friendship.'" *Annals of Surgery* 188 (1978): 630–637.

———. "William Halsted, His Family, and 'Queer Business Methods.'" *Archives of Surgery* 131 (1996): 123–127.

———. "William Stewart Halsted." *Archives of Surgery* 135 (2000): 1478.

———. "William Stewart Halsted (1852–1922)." *Hernia* 1 (1997): 61–63.

———. "William Stewart Halsted and the Germanic Influence on Education and Training Programs in Surgery." *Surgery, Gynecology & Obstetrics* 147 (1978): 602–606.

Tucker, A. *It Happened at Hopkins: A Teaching Hospital.* Baltimore: Johns Hopkins Hospital, 1973.

Turner, T. B. *Heritage of Excellence: The Johns Hopkins Medical Institutions, 1914–1917.* Baltimore: Johns Hopkins University Press, 1974.

Young, A. *Scalpel: Men Who Made Surgery.* New York: Random House, 1956.

Chapter 13. The Shock of Technology

Adams, A. "Surgery and Architecture: Spaces for Operating." In *The Palgrave Handbook of the History of* Surgery, edited by T. Schlich, 261–279. London: Palgrave Macmillan, 2018.

Barr, J., L. C. Cancio, D. J. Smith, et al. "From Trench to Bedside: Military Surgery during World War I upon Its Centennial." *Military Medicine* 184 (2019): 214–220.

Brecher, R., and E. Brecher. *The Rays: A History of Radiology in the United States and Canada.* Baltimore: Williams & Wilkins, 1969.

English, P. C. *Shock, Physiological Surgery, and George Washington Crile: Medical Innovation in the Progressive Era.* Westport, CT: Greenwood, 1980.

Freebert, E. *The Age of Edison: Electric Light and the Invention of Modern America.* New York: Penguin, 2014.

Glasser, O. *William Conrad Röntgen and the Early History of the Roentgen Rays.* Springfield, IL: Charles C. Thomas, 1934.

Howell, J. *Technology in the Hospital: Transforming Patient Care in the Early Twentieth Century.* Baltimore: Johns Hopkins Press, 1995.

Lane, W. A. "Remarks on the Operative Treatment of Chronic Constipation." *British Medical Journal* 1 (1908): 126–130.

Malinin, T. I. *Surgery and Life: The Extraordinary Career of Alexis Carrel.* New York: Harcourt Brace Jovanovich, 1979.

Millham, F. H. "A Brief History of Shock." *Surgery* 148 (2010): 1026–1037.

Morton, W. J., and E. W. Hammer. *The X Ray or Photography of the Invisible and its Value in Surgery.* New York: American Technical Book Company, 1896.

Nathoo, N., F. L. Lautzenheiser, and G. H. Barnett. "The First Direct Human Blood Transfusion: The Forgotten Legacy of George W. Crile." *Neurosurgery* 64 (2009): [Suppl. 3] 20–27.

Pasveer, B. "Knowledge of Shadows: The Introduction of X-ray Images in Medicine." *Sociology of Health and Illness* 11 (1989): 360–381.

Perkowitz, S. *Empire of Light: A History of Discovery in Science and Art.* Washington, DC: Joseph Henry Press, 1998.

Rosenberg, C. E. *The Care of Strangers: The Rise of America's Hospital System.* New York: Basic Books, 1987.

Rutkow, E. I., and I. M. Rutkow. "George Crile, Harvey Cushing, and the Ambulance Américaine: Military Medical Preparedness in World War One." *Archives of Surgery* 139 (2004): 678–685.

Rutkow, I. M. "Edwin Hartley Pratt and Orificial Surgery: Unorthodox Surgical Practice in Nineteenth Century United States." *Surgery* 114 (1993): 558–563.

———. "How American Surgeons Introduced Radiology into U.S. Medicine." *American Journal of Surgery* 165 (1993): 252–257.

———. "Orificial Surgery." *Archives of Surgery* 136 (2001): 1088.

Sarton, G. "The Discovery of X-rays." *Isis* 26 (1937): 349–364.

Schivelbusch, W. *Disenchanted Night: The Industrialization of Light in the Nineteenth Century.* Berkeley: University of California Press, 1988.

Warwick, A. "X-rays as Evidence in German Orthopedic Surgery, 1895–1900." *Isis* 96 (2005): 1–24.

Wexler, A. "The Medical Battery in the United States (1870–1920): Electrotherapy at Home and in the Clinic." *Journal of the History of Medicine and Allied Sciences* 72 (2017): 166–192.

Young, A. *Scalpel: Men Who Made Surgery,* 287–301. New York: Random House, 1956.

PART IV—BAPTISMS

Chapter 14. Mass Appeal

Aboud, F. C., and A. C. Verghese. "Evarts Ambrose Graham, and the Dawn of Clinical Understanding of Negative Intrapleural Pressure." *Clinical Infectious Diseases* 34 (2002): 198–203.

Aldrich, M. "Train Wrecks to Typhoid Fever: The Development of Railroad Medicine Organizations, 1850 to World War I." *Bulletin of the History of Medicine* 75 (2001): 254–289.

Ballance, C. A. *A Glimpse into the History of the Surgery of the Brain.* London: Macmillan, 1922.

Barber, Mueller C. *Evarts A. Graham: The Life, Lives and Times of the Surgical Spirit of St. Louis.* Hamilton, ON: B.C. Decker, 2002.

Baue, A. E. "Evarts A. Graham and the First Pneumonectomy." *Journal of the American Medical Association* 251 (1984): 261–264.

Bliss, M. *Harvey Cushing: A Life in Surgery.* New York: Oxford University Press, 2005.

Brock, C. "Risk, Responsibility and Surgery in the 1890s and Early 1900s." *Medical History* 57 (2013): 317–337.

Brooks, S. M. *McBurney's Point: The Story of Appendicitis.* South Brunswick, NJ: A. S. Barnes, 1969.

Cartwright, F. F. *The Development of Modern Surgery.* London: Arthur Barker, 1967.

Cope, Z. *A History of the Acute Abdomen.* London: Oxford University Press, 1965.

Ellenberger, A. R. *The Valentino Mystique: The Death and Afterlife of the Silent Film Idol.* Jefferson, NC: McFarland, 2005.

Ferguson, T. B. "Evarts A. Graham—the Man." *Journal of Thoracic Surgery* 88 (1984): 803–826.

Frampton, S. "Opening the Abdomen: The Expansion of Surgery." In *The Palgrave Handbook of the History of Surgery*, edited by T. Schlich, 175–194. London: Palgrave Macmillan, 2018.

Gavrus, D. "Opening the Skull: Neurosurgery as a Case Study of Surgical Specialization." In *The Palgrave Handbook of the History of Surgery*, edited by T. Schlich, 435–455. London: Palgrave Macmillan, 2018.

Graham, E. A., and J. J. Singer. "Successful Removal of an Entire Lung for Carcinoma of the Bronchus." *Journal of the American Medical Association* 101 (1933): 1371–1374.

Greenblatt, S. H. "The Image of the 'Brain Surgeon' in American Culture: The Influence of Harvey Cushing." *Journal of Neurosurgery* 75 (1991): 808–811.

Grob, G. N. "The Rise and Decline of Tonsillectomy in Twentieth-Century America." *Journal of the History of Medicine and Allied Sciences* 62 (2007): 383–421.

Harvey, S. C. "The Story of Harvey Cushing's Appendix." *Surgery* 32 (1952): 501–514.

Hochberg, L. A. *Thoracic Surgery before the 20th Century*. New York: Vantage Press, 1960.

Horrax, G. *Neurosurgery: An Historical Sketch*. Springfield, IL: Charles C. Thomas, 1952.

Howell, J. *Technology in the Hospital: Transforming Patient Care in the Early Twentieth Century*, 60–61, 207–221. Baltimore: Johns Hopkins Press, 1995.

Keys, T. E. *The History of Surgical Anesthesia*. New York: Schuman's, 1945.

Meade, R. H. "The Evolution of Surgery for Appendicitis." *Surgery* 55 (1964): 741–752.

———. *A History of Thoracic Surgery*. Springfield, IL: Charles C. Thomas, 1961.

———. *An Introduction to the History of General Surgery*. Philadelphia: W.B. Saunders, 1968.

Olch, P. D. "Evarts A. Graham: Pivotal Figure in American Surgery." *Perspectives in Biology and Medicine* 26 (1983): 472–485.

———. "Evarts A. Graham in World War I: The Empyema Commission and Service in the American Expeditionary Forces." *Journal of the History of Medicine and Allied Sciences* 44 (1989): 430–436.

Oschner, A. "History of Thoracic Surgery." *Surgical Clinics of North America* 46 (1966): 1355–1376.

Ravitch, M. M. *A Century of Surgery*. 2 vols. Philadelphia: J. B. Lippincott, 1981.

Richardson, R. *The Story of Surgery: An Historical Commentary.* Shrewsbury, UK: Quiller Press, 2004.

Rutkow, E., and I. Rutkow. "Harvey Cushing and the Battle of Boston Common: Military Medical Preparedness for World War One." *Annals of Surgery* 251 (2010): 191–198.

Rutkow, E. I., and I. M. Rutkow. "George Crile, Harvey Cushing, and the Ambulance Américaine: Military Medical Preparedness in World War One." *Archives of Surgery* 139 (2004): 678–685.

Sachs, E. *The History and Development of Neurological Surgery.* London: Cassell, 1952.

Smith, D. C. "Appendicitis, Appendectomy, and the Surgeon." *Bulletin of the History of Medicine* 70 (1996): 414–441.

Thomson, E. H. *Harvey Cushing: Surgeon, Author, Artist.* New York: Henry Schuman, 1950.

Ullman, S. G. *Valentino As I Knew Him.* New York: Macy-Masius, 1926.

Williams, G. R. "A History of Appendicitis with Anecdotes Illustrating Its Importance." *Annals of Surgery* 197 (1983): 495–506.

Chapter 15. Professionalization

Aldrich, M. "Train Wrecks to Typhoid Fever: The Development of Railroad Medicine Organizations, 1850 to World War I." *Bulletin of the History of Medicine* 75 (2001): 254–289.

Barr, J., and T. N. Pappas. "The Role of the American Board of Surgery in the Development of Surgical Residencies in Post–World War II America." *American Surgeon* 85 (2019): 245–251.

Burrow, J. G. *Organized Medicine in the Progressive Era: The Move Toward Monopoly.* Baltimore: Johns Hopkins University Press, 1977.

Derbyshire, R. C. *Medical Licensure and Discipline in the United States.* Baltimore: Johns Hopkins Press, 1969.

Donabedian, A. "The End Results of Health Care: Ernest Codman's Contribution to Quality Assessment and Beyond." *Milbank Quarterly* 67 (1989): 233–256.

Firor, W. M. "Residency Training in Surgery. Birth, Decay, and Recovery." *Review of Surgery* 22 (1965): 153–157.

Kernahan, P. "Surgery Becomes a Specialty: Professional Boundaries and Surgery." *The Palgrave Handbook of the History of Surgery*, edited by T. Schlich, 95–113. London: Palgrave Macmillan, 2018.

Kernahan, P. J. "A Condition of Development: Muckrakers, Surgeons, and Hospitals, 1890–1920." *Journal of the American College of Surgeons* 206 (2008): 376–384.

Lederer, S. "Surgery and Popular Culture: Situating the Surgeon and the Surgical Experience in Popular Media." In *The Palgrave Handbook of the History of Surgery*, edited by T. Schlich, 349–367. London: Palgrave Macmillan, 2018.

Nahrwold, D. L., and P. J. Kernahan. *A Century of Surgeons and Surgery: The American College of Surgeons 1913–2012*. Chicago: American College of Surgeons, 2012.

Olch, P. D. "Evarts A. Graham: Pivotal Figure in American Surgery." *Perspectives in Biology and Medicine* 26 (1983): 472–485.

Rodman, J. S. *History of the American Board of Surgery, 1937–1952*. Philadelphia: J. B. Lippincott, 1956.

Rosen, G. "Changing Attitudes of the Medical Profession to Specialization." *Bulletin of the History of Medicine* 12 (1942): 343–354.

Rutkow, I. "The American Medical Association's Section on Surgery: The Beginnings of the Organization, Professionalization, and Specialization of Surgery in the United States." *Annals of Surgery* 265 (2017): 227–233.

———. "The Education, Training, and Specialization of Surgeons: Turn-of-the-Century America and Its Postgraduate Medical Schools." *Annals of Surgery* 258 (2013): 1130–1136.

———. "Edward Bermingham and the *Archives of Clinical Surgery*: America's First Surgical Journal." *Annals of Surgery* 261 (2015): 812–819.

Rutkow, I., and K. D. Lillemoe. "American Exceptionalism and the American Surgical Association: The Rise of Surgery in the United States." *Annals of Surgery* 267 (2018): 789–795.

Rutkow, I. M. "Railway Surgery, Traumatology and Managed Health Care in 19th-Century United States." *Archives of Surgery* 128 (1993): 458–463.

Starr, P. *The Social Transformation of American Medicine*. New York: Basic Books, 1982.

Stephenson, G. W. *American College of Surgeons at 75*. Chicago: American College of Surgeons, 1990.

Stevens, R. *American Medicine and the Public Interest*. New Haven: Yale University Press, 1971.

Snyder, C. "Julius Homberger, M.D." *Archives of Ophthalmology* 68 (1962): 875–878.

Weisz, G. *Divide and Conquer: A Comparative History of Medical Specialization*. Oxford: Oxford University Press, 2006.

Yagoda, B. *Will Rogers: A Biography*. New York: Alfred A. Knopf, 1993.

PART V—TRIUMPHS

Chapter 16. The Blood of War

Barr, J. *Of Life and Limb: Surgical Repair of the Arteries in War and Peace, 1880–1960*. Rochester, NY: University of Rochester Press, 2019.

Barr, J., K. J. Cherry, and N. M. Rich. "Vascular Surgery in the Pacific Theaters of World War II: The Persistence of Ligation amid Unique Military Medical Conditions." *Annals of Surgery* 269 (2019): 1054–1058.

———. "Vascular Surgery in World War II: The Shift to Repairing Arteries." *Annals of Surgery* 263 (2016): 615–620.

Barr, J., and S. H. Podolsky. "A National Medical Response to Crisis—the Legacy of World War II." *New England Journal of Medicine*, April 29, 2020, https://doi.org/10.1056/NEJMp2008512.

Chester, R. K. "'Negroes' Number One Hero': Doris Miller, Pearl Harbor, and Retroactive Multiculturalism in World War II Remembrance." *American Quarterly* 65 (2013): 31–61.

Churchill, E. D. *Surgeon to Soldiers: Diary and Records of the Surgical Consultant Allied Force Headquarters, World War II*. Philadelphia: J. B. Lippincott, 1972.

———. "The Surgical Management of the Wounded in the Mediterranean Theater at the Time of the Fall of Rome." *Annals of Surgery* 120 (1944): 268–283.

Cutler, E. C. "Military Surgery—United States Army—European Theater of Operations, 1944–1945." *Surgery, Gynecology & Obstetrics* 82 (1946): 261–274.

DeBakey, M. E. *Medical Department, United States Army, Surgery in World War II.* Vol. 2, *General Surgery.* Washington, DC: Office of the Surgeon General, 1955.

———. "Military Surgery in World War II—a Backward Glance and a Forward Look." *New England Journal of Medicine* 236 (1947): 341–350.

Dougherty, P. J., P. R. Carter, D. Seligson, et al. "Orthopaedic Surgery Advances Resulting from World War II." *Journal of Bone and Joint Surgery* 86 (2004): 176–181.

Duke, M. "Frank Gill Slaughter: Physician and Writer." *Hektoen International: A Journal of Medical Humanities* 9 (Spring 2017).

Eben, A. "World War II Neurosurgery." *Journal of Neurosurgery* 93 (2000): 901–904.

Guglielmo, T. A. "'Red Cross, Double Cross': Race and America's World War II–Era Blood Donor Service." *Journal of American History* 97 (2010): 63–90.

Hardaway, R. M. "Wound Shock: A History of Its Study and Treatment by Military Surgeons." *Military Medicine* 169 (2004): 265–269.

Hardwick, R. *Charles Richard Drew: Pioneer in Blood Research.* New York: Scribner's, 1967.

Lederer, S. E. *Flesh and Blood: Organ Transplantation and Blood Transfusion in Twentieth-Century America.* New York: Oxford University Press, 2008.

Lewis, P. "Frank Slaughter, Novelist of Medicine, Is Dead at 93." *New York Times*, May 23, 2001, C19.

Organ, C., and M. M. Kosiba. *A Century of Black Surgeons: The USA Experience.* 2 vols. Norman, OK: Transcript Press, 1987.

O'Shea, J. S. "Louis T. Wright and Henry W. Cave: How They Paved the Way for Fellowships for Black Surgeons." *Bulletin of the American College of Surgeons* 90 (2005): 26.

Robinson, G. C. *American Red Cross Blood Donor Service during World War II, Its Organization and Operation.* Washington, DC: American Red Cross, 1946.

Rutkow, I. "The American Medical Association's Section on Surgery: The Beginnings of the Organization, Professionalization, and Specialization of Surgery in the United States. *Annals of Surgery* 265 (2017): 227–223.

Rutkow, I. M. "Arthur Dean Bevan." *Archives of Surgery* 131 (1996): 845.

Schneider, W. H. "Blood Transfusions between the Wars." *Journal of the History of Medicine and Allied Sciences* 58 (203): 216–224.

Slaughter, F. G. "How to Be an Expert on Anything." *The Writer* 90 (1977): 11–13.

———. "When the Scalpel Sharpens the Pen." *Journal of the American Medical Association* 200 (1967): 19–22.

Starr, D. *Blood: An Epic History of Medicine and Commerce*. New York: Little, Brown, 1999.

Wynes, C. *Charles Richard Drew: The Man and the Myth*. Urbana: University of Illinois, 1988.

Chapter 17. The Center of Things

Alivizatos, P. "Dwight Emery Harken, MD, an All-American Surgical Giant: Pioneer Cardiac Surgeon, Teacher, Mentor." *Baylor University Medical Center Proceedings* 31 (2018): 554–557.

Barr, J., and T. N. Pappas. "President Eisenhower and His Bowel Obstruction." *Bulletin of the American College of Surgeons* 102 (2017): 57–58.

Buckler, H. *Doctor Dan, Pioneer in American Surgery*. New York: Little, Brown, 1954.

Fenster, J. M. *Mavericks, Miracles, and Medicine: The Pioneers Who Risked Their Lives to Bring Medicine into the Modern Age*. New York: Barnes & Noble Books, 2003.

Forrester, J. S. *The Heart Healers: The Misfits, Mavericks and Rebels Who Created the Greatest Medical Breakthrough of Our Lives*. New York: St. Martin's Press, 2015.

Gonzalez-Crussi, F. *Carrying the Heart: Exploring the World within Us*. New York: Kaplan, 2009.

Harken, D. E. "The Emergence of Cardiac Surgery: I. Personal Recollections of the 1940s and 1950s." *Journal of Thoracic and Cardiovascular Surgery* 98 (1989): 805–813.

Johnson, S. *The History of Cardiac Surgery, 1896–1955*. Baltimore: Johns Hopkins Press, 1970.

Lederer, S. "Surgery and Popular Culture: Situating the Surgeon and the Surgical Experience in Popular Media." In *The Palgrave Handbook of the*

History of Surgery, edited by T. Schlich, 349–367. London: Palgrave Macmillan, 2018.

Miller, B. J. "The Development of Heart Lung Machines." *Surgery, Gynecology & Obstetrics* 154 (1982): 403–414.

Monagan, D. *Journey into the Heart: A Tale of Pioneering Doctors and Their Race to Transform Cardiovascular Medicine.* New York: Gotham Books, 2007.

Pappas, T. N. "President Eisenhower's Bowel Obstruction: The Story of His Surgeons and Their Decision to Operate." *Annals of Surgery* 258 (2013): 192–197.

Richardson, R. *The Story of Surgery: An Historical Commentary.* Shrewsbury, UK: Quiller Press, 2004.

Rutkow, I. M. "Surgical Operations in the United States: Then (1983) and Now (1994)." *Archives of Surgery* 132 (1997): 983–990.

Serlin, D. "Performing Live Surgery on Television and the Internet since 1945." In *Imagining Illness: Public Health and Visual Culture,* edited by D. Serlin, 233–244. Minneapolis: University of Minnesota Press, 2010.

Shumacker, H. B. *A Dream of the Heart: The Life of John H. Gibbon, Jr., Father of the Heart–Lung Machine.* Santa Barbara, CA: Fithian Press,1999.

———. *The Evolution of Cardiac Surgery.* Bloomington: Indiana University Press, 1992.

Chapter 18. Out with the Old

Baumgartner, W. A., B. A. Reitz, V. L. Gott, et al. "Norman E. Shumway, MD, PhD: Visionary, Innovator, Humorist." *Journal of Thoracic and Cardiovascular Surgery* 137 (2009): 269–277.

Bordley, J., and A. M. Harvey. *Two Centuries of American Medicine, 1776–1976.* Philadelphia: W.B. Saunders, 1976.

Cooper, D. K. C. "Christiaan Barnard—the Surgeon Who Dared: The Story of the First Human-to-Human Heart Transplant." *Global Cardiology Science and Practice,* 2018, 11, https://doi.org/10.21542/gcsp.2018.11.

Fenster, Julie. *Mavericks, Miracles, and Medicine: The Pioneers Who Risked Their Lives to Bring Medicine into the Modern Age.* New York: Barnes & Noble Books, 2003.

REFERENCES

Hamilton, D. *A History of Organ Transplantation: Ancient Legends to Modern Practice*. Pittsburgh: University of Pittsburgh Press, 2012.

Hollingham, R. *Blood and Guts: A History of Surgery*. New York: Thomas Dunne Books/St. Martin's Press, 2008.

Lederer, S. E. *Flesh and Blood: Organ Transplantation and Blood Transfusion in Twentieth-Century America*. Oxford: Oxford University Press, 2008.

McRae, D. *Every Second Counts: The Race to Transplant the First Human Heart*. New York: G.P. Putnam's Sons, 2006.

Moore, F. D. "A Nobel Award to Joseph E. Murray, MD: Some Historical Perspectives." *Archives of Surgery* 127 (1992): 627–632.

Murray, J. E. *Surgery of the Soul: Reflections on a Curious Career*. Canton, MA: Science History Publications, 2001.

Nuland, Sherwin. *Doctors: The Biography of Medicine*. New York: Alfred A. Knopf, 1988.

Obrecht, S. "Transplantation Surgery: Organ Replacement between Reductionism and Systemic Approaches." In *The Palgrave Handbook of the History of Surgery*, edited by T. Schlich, 411–433. London: Palgrave Macmillan, 2018.

Peltier, L. F. *Orthopedics: A History and Iconography*. San Francisco: Norman, 1993.

Rifkin, W. J., J. A. David, N. M. Plana, et al. "Achievements and Challenges in Facial Transplantation." *Annals of Surgery* 268 (2018): 260–270.

Schlich, T. *The Origins of Organ Transplantation: Surgery and Laboratory Science, 1880–1930*. Rochester, NY: University of Rochester Press, 2010.

Shumacker, H. B. *The Evolution of Cardiac Surgery*. Bloomington: Indiana University Press, 1992.

Stark, T. *Knife to the Heart: The Story of Transplant Surgery*. London: Macmillan, 1996.

Thompson, T. *Hearts: Of Surgeons and Transplants, Miracles and Disasters along the Cardiac Frontier*. New York: McCall, 1971.

Tilney, N. L. *Invasion of the Body: Revolutions in Surgery*. Cambridge, MA: Harvard University Press, 2011.

———. *Transplant, from Myth to Reality*. New Haven: Yale University Press, 2003.

PART VI—THE PRESENT AND THE FUTURE

Chapter 19. Changes

Ali, A. M., and C. L. McVay. "Women in Surgery: A History of Adversity, Resilience, and Accomplishment." *Journal of the American College of Surgeons* 223 (2016): 670–673.

Brody, H. J., and W. P. Coleman. "What's in a Name? Are We Dermatologic Surgeons or Surgical Dermatologists?" *Archives of Dermatology* 136 (2000): 1406–1407.

Davis, C. J., and C. J. Filipi. "A History of Endoscopic Surgery." In *Principles of Laparoscopic Surgery*, edited by M. E. Arregui, R. J. Fitzgibbons, N. Katkhouda, et al., 3–20. New York: Springer-Verlag, 1995.

Gaidy, A. D., L. Tremblay, D. Nakayama, et al. "The History of Surgical Staplers: A Combination of Hungarian, Russian, and American Innovation." *American Surgery* 85 (2019): 563–566.

Fingerete, A. L., A. E. Fingerete, and M. A. Hardy. "Mark M. Ravitch: Historian and Innovator." *Journal of Surgical Education* 68 (2011): 155–158.

Harrell, A. G., and B. T. Heniford. "Minimally Invasive Abdominal Surgery: Lux et Veritas Past, Present, and Future." *American Journal of Surgery* 190 (205): 239–243.

Husser, W., and L. Neumayer. "Olga Jonasson, MD, Surgeon, Mentor, Teacher, Friend." *Annals of Surgery* 244 (2006): 839–840.

Kalan, S., S. Chauhan, R. F. Coelho, et al. "History of Robotic Surgery." *Journal of Robotic Surgery* 4 (2010): 141–147.

Kelley, W. E. "The Evolution of Laparoscopy and the Revolution in Surgery in the Decade of the 1990s." *Journal of the Society of Laparoendoscopic Surgeons* 12 (2008): 351–357.

Litynski, G. "Endoscopic Surgery: The History, the Pioneers." *World Journal of Surgery* 23 (1999): 745–753.

Mead, K. C. *A History of Women in Medicine from the Earliest Times to the Beginning of the Nineteenth Century*. Haddam, CT: Haddam Press, 1938.

More, E. S., E. Fee, and M. Parry, eds. *Women Physicians and the Cultures of Medicine*. Baltimore: Johns Hopkins University Press, 2009.

Mueller, C. L., and G. M. Fried. "Emerging Technology in Surgery: Informatics, Robotics, Electronics." In *Sabiston Textbook of Surgery: The Biological Basis of Modern Surgical Practice*, edited by C. M. Townsend, R. D. Beauchamp, B. M. Evers, et al., 393–406. Philadelphia: Elsevier, 2017.

Pastena, J. A. "Women in Surgery: An Ancient Tradition." *Archives of Surgery* 128 (1993): 622–626.

Rishworth, S. "A Short History of Women Surgeons in the College." *Bulletin of the American College of Surgeons* 87 (2002): 34–35.

Rosenberg, L., and T. Schlich. "Surgery: Down for the Count?" *Canadian Medical Association Journal* 184 (2012): 496.

Rutkow, I. M., ed. *Socioeconomics of Surgery*. St. Louis: C.V. Mosby, 1989.

Rutkow, I. M. "'Unnecessary Surgery'; An Update." *Surgery* 84 (1978): 671–678.

———. "Unnecessary Surgery: What Is It?" *Surgical Clinics of North America.* 62 (1982): 613–625.

Schlich, T., and C. Crenner, eds. *Technological Change in Modern Surgery: Historical Perspectives on Innovation*. Rochester, NY: University of Rochester Press, 2017.

Semm, K. "The History of Endoscopy." In *Laparoscopic Surgery: An Atlas for General Surgeons*, edited by G. C. Vitale, J. S. Sanfilippo, and J. Perissat, 3–11. Philadelphia: J. B. Lippincott, 1995.

Surgery in the United States: A Summary Report of the Study on Surgical Services for the United States. 3 vols. Chicago: American College of Surgeons & American Surgical Association, 1976.

Whitfield, N. "A Revolution through the Keyhole: Technology, Innovation, and the Rise of Minimally Invasive Surgery." In *The Palgrave Handbook of the History of Surgery*, edited by T. Schlich, 525–548. London: Palgrave Macmillan, 2018.

Wirtzfeld, D. A. "The History of Women in Surgery." *Canadian Journal of Surgery* 52 (2009): 317–320.

Wyman, A. L. "The Surgeoness: The Female Practitioner of Surgery 1400–1800." *Medical History* 28 (1984): 22–41.

Zetka, J. R. *Surgeons and the Scope*. Ithaca, NY: Cornell University Press, 2003.

PHOTO CREDITS

1. Author's collection
2. Wikimedia Foundation
3. Metropolitan Museum of Art, Harris Brisbane Dick Fund, 1917
4. Author's collection
5. Author's collection
6. Wellcome Collection. Attribution 4.0 International (CC BY 4.0)
7. Wikimedia Commons
8. Structurae/Jacques Mossot
9. Author's collection
10. Wikimedia Commons
11. Wikimedia Commons
12. Library of Congress
13. Author's collection
14. *Frank Leslie's Illustrated Weekly*, July 26, 1856
15. National Library of Medicine
16. United States World War One Centennial Commission
17. Author's collection
18. Wikimedia Commons
19. Wikimedia Commons
20. AP Photo/Charles Tasnadi
21. Author's collection
22. Wikimedia Commons
23. Getty Images/Bettman
24. Wikimedia Commons

INDEX

ABOUT THE AUTHOR

Ira **Rutkow** is a general surgeon and historian of American medicine. He also holds a doctorate of public health from Johns Hopkins University. Among Dr. Rutkow's books are several encyclopedic works on surgical history: *Surgery: An Illustrated History*, named a *New York Times* Notable Book of the Year; *American Surgery: An Illustrated History*; and a two-volume bibliography, *The History of Surgery in the United States, 1775–1900*. He is the author of three other books, *Seeking the Cure*, *James A. Garfield*, and *Bleeding Blue and Gray*. Dr. Rutkow and his wife divide their time between New York City and a farm in the Hudson Valley.